Advances in Trauma and Orthopedic Surgery

Advances in Trauma and Orthopedic Surgery

Editor

Christian von Rüden

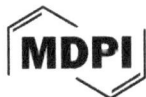

Basel • Beijing • Wuhan • Barcelona • Belgrade • Novi Sad • Cluj • Manchester

Editor
Christian von Rüden
Department of Trauma
Surgery, Orthopaedics and
Hand Surgery
Weiden Medical Center
Weiden
Germany

Editorial Office
MDPI AG
Grosspeteranlage 5
4052 Basel, Switzerland

This is a reprint of articles from the Special Issue published online in the open access journal *Journal of Clinical Medicine* (ISSN 2077-0383) (available at: https://www.mdpi.com/journal/jcm/special_issues/EF6ECZ130F).

For citation purposes, cite each article independently as indicated on the article page online and as indicated below:

Lastname, A.A.; Lastname, B.B. Article Title. *Journal Name* **Year**, *Volume Number*, Page Range.

ISBN 978-3-7258-1579-1 (Hbk)
ISBN 978-3-7258-1580-7 (PDF)
doi.org/10.3390/books978-3-7258-1580-7

© 2024 by the authors. Articles in this book are Open Access and distributed under the Creative Commons Attribution (CC BY) license. The book as a whole is distributed by MDPI under the terms and conditions of the Creative Commons Attribution-NonCommercial-NoDerivs (CC BY-NC-ND) license.

Contents

About the Editor vii

Pietro Regazzoni, Simon Lambert, Jesse B. Jupiter, Norbert Südkamp, Wen-Chih Liu and Alberto A. Fernández Dell'Oca
Homogeneity in Surgical Series: Image Reporting to Improve Evidence
Reprinted from: *J. Clin. Med.* 2023, 12, 1583, doi:10.3390/jcm12041583 1

Stefan Förch, Sabrina Sandriesser, Christian von Rüden, Edgar Mayr and Peter Augat
Cerclage Wiring Improves Biomechanical Stability in Distal Tibia Spiral Fractures Treated by Intramedullary Nailing
Reprinted from: *J. Clin. Med.* 2023, 12, 1770, doi:10.3390/jcm12051770 6

Florian Kellermann, Simon Hackl, Iris Leister, Sven Hungerer, Matthias Militz, Fabian Stuby, et al.
Advances in the Treatment of Implant-Associated Infections of the Pelvis: Eradication Rates, Recurrence of Infection, and Outcome
Reprinted from: *J. Clin. Med.* 2023, 12, 2854, doi:10.3390/jcm12082854 15

Mischa Mühling, Sabrina Sandriesser, Claudio Glowalla, Sven Herrmann, Peter Augat and Sven Hungerer
Risk of Interprosthetic Femur Fracture Is Associated with Implant Spacing—A Biomechanical Study
Reprinted from: *J. Clin. Med.* 2023, 12, 3095, doi:10.3390/jcm12093095 23

Magalie Meinert, Christian Colcuc, Eva Herrmann, Johannes Harbering, Yves Gramlich, Marc Blank, et al.
Septic History Limits the Outcome of Tibiotalocalcaneal Arthrodesis
Reprinted from: *J. Clin. Med.* 2023, 12, 3422, doi:10.3390/jcm12103422 33

Alejandro Lorente, Leire Pelaz, Pablo Palacios, Iker J. Bautista, Gonzalo Mariscal, Carlos Barrios and Rafael Lorente
Arthroscopic vs. Open-Ankle Arthrodesis on Fusion Rate in Ankle Osteoarthritis Patients: A Systematic Review and Meta-Analysis
Reprinted from: *J. Clin. Med.* 2023, 12, 3574, doi:10.3390/jcm12103574 44

Francesca Veronesi, Melania Maglio, Silvia Brogini, Antonio Mazzotti, Elena Artioli and Gianluca Giavaresi
A Systematic Review of the Retrograde Drilling Approach for Osteochondral Lesion of the Talus: Questioning Surgical Approaches, Outcome Evaluation and Gender-Related Differences
Reprinted from: *J. Clin. Med.* 2023, 12, 4523, doi:10.3390/jcm12134523 56

Julie Manon, Vladimir Pletser, Michael Saint-Guillain, Jean Vanderdonckt, Cyril Wain, Jean Jacobs, et al.
An Easy-To-Use External Fixator for All Hostile Environments, from Space to War Medicine: Is It Meant for Everyone's Hands?
Reprinted from: *J. Clin. Med.* 2023, 12, 4764, doi:10.3390/jcm12144764 74

Julia Rehme-Röhrl, Korbinian Sicklinger, Andreas Brand, Julian Fürmetz, Carl Neuerburg, Fabian Stuby and Christian von Rüden
Early Internal Fixation of Concomitant Clavicle Fractures in Severe Thoracic Trauma Prevents Posttraumatic Pneumonia
Reprinted from: *J. Clin. Med.* 2023, 12, 4878, doi:10.3390/jcm12154878 90

Abraham Reyes-Valdés, Mirna Martínez-Ledezma, David Fernández-Quezada, José Guzmán-Esquivel and Martha Irazema Cárdenas-Rojas
Prevalence and Characteristics of Patients Requiring Surgical Reinterventions for Ankle Fractures
Reprinted from: *J. Clin. Med.* **2023**, *12*, 5843, doi:10.3390/jcm12185843 99

Steffen Bernd Rosslenbroich, Chang-Wug Oh, Thomas Kern, John Mukhopadhaya, Michael Johannes Raschke, Ulrich Kneser and Christian Krettek
Current Management of Diaphyseal Long Bone Defects—A Multidisciplinary and International Perspective
Reprinted from: *J. Clin. Med.* **2023**, *12*, 6283, doi:10.3390/jcm12196283 107

Patrick Ziegler, Sven Maier, Fabian Stuby, Tina Histing, Christoph Ihle, Ulrich Stöckle and Markus Gühring
Clinical Outcome of Carbon Fiber Reinforced Polyetheretherketone Plates in Patients with Proximal Humeral Fracture: One-Year Follow-Up
Reprinted from: *J. Clin. Med.* **2023**, *12*, 6881, doi:10.3390/jcm12216881 122

Niklas Grüneweller, Julia Leunig, Ivan Zderic, Boyko Gueorguiev, Dirk Wähnert and Thomas Vordemvenne
Stabilization of Traumatic Iliosacral Instability Using Innovative Implants: A Biomechanical Comparison
Reprinted from: *J. Clin. Med.* **2024**, *13*, 194, doi:10.3390/jcm13010194 131

Artur Kruszewski, Szczepan Piszczatowski, Piotr Piekarczyk, Piotr Cieślik and Krzysztof Kwiatkowski
Weak Points of Double-Plate Stabilization Used in the Treatment of Distal Humerus Fracture through Finite Element Analysis
Reprinted from: *J. Clin. Med.* **2024**, *13*, 1034, doi:10.3390/jcm13041034 143

Simon Hackl, Christian von Rüden, Katharina Trenkwalder, Lena Keppler, Christian Hierholzer and Mario Perl
Long-Term Outcomes Following Single-Stage Reamed Intramedullary Exchange Nailing in Apparently Aseptic Femoral Shaft Nonunion with Unsuspected Proof of Bacteria
Reprinted from: *J. Clin. Med.* **2024**, *13*, 1414, doi:10.3390/jcm13051414 159

Marcin Pelc, Krystian Kazubski, Wiktor Urbański, Paweł Leyko, Joanna Kochańska-Bieri, Łukasz Tomczyk, et al.
Balance and Weight Distribution over the Lower Limbs Following Calcaneal Fracture Treatment with the Ilizarov Method
Reprinted from: *J. Clin. Med.* **2024**, *13*, 1676, doi:10.3390/jcm13061676 175

Jun-Hyuk Lim, Yeong-Seub Ahn, Sungmin Kim and Myung-Sun Kim
Novel Use of a Fibular Strut Allograft with Fibular Head in an Elderly Patient with Proximal Humeral Fracture and Severe Metaphyseal Comminution: An Alternative to Shoulder Arthroplasty
Reprinted from: *J. Clin. Med.* **2024**, *13*, 2200, doi:10.3390/jcm13082200 189

About the Editor

Christian von Rüden

Christian von Rüden, MD MSc, is Chief Physician at the Department for Trauma Surgery, Orthopaedics, and Hand Surgery at the Weiden Medical Center, Bavaria, Germany. He holds an associate professorship at the Paracelsus Medical University Salzburg, Austria, and conducts research at the Institute for Biomechanics at the BG Unfallklinik Murnau, Germany. His specialties include pelvic surgery and nonunion treatment as well as polytrauma management.

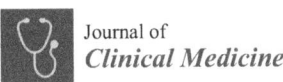

Viewpoint

Homogeneity in Surgical Series: Image Reporting to Improve Evidence

Pietro Regazzoni [1,*,†], Simon Lambert [2], Jesse B. Jupiter [3,†], Norbert Südkamp [4,†], Wen-Chih Liu [3,5] and Alberto A. Fernández Dell'Oca [6,7]

1. Department of Trauma Surgery, University Hospital Basel, 4031 Basel, Switzerland
2. Department of Trauma and Orthopaedics, University College London Hospital, London NW1 2BU, UK
3. Hand and Arm Center, Department of Orthopedics, Massachusetts General Hospital, Boston, MA 02114, USA
4. Department of Orthopedics and Trauma Surgery, Medical Center, Faculty of Medicine, Albert-Ludwigs-University of Freiburg, 79106 Freiburg, Germany
5. Kaohsiung Medical University Hospital, School of Medicine, College of Medicine, Kaohsiung Medical University, Kaohsiung 80756, Taiwan
6. Department of Traumatology, The British Hospital, Montevideo 11600, Uruguay
7. Residency Program in Traumatology and Orthopedics, University of Montevideo, Montevideo 11600, Uruguay
* Correspondence: p_regazzoni@bluewin.ch; Tel.: +41-79-640-02-86
† Pietro Regazzoni, Jesse B. Jupiter, and Norbert Südkamp are professors emeriti.

Abstract: Good clinical practice guidelines are based on randomized controlled trials or clinical series; however, technical performance bias among surgical trials is under-assessed. The heterogeneity of technical performance within different treatment groups diminishes the level of evidence. Surgeon variability with different levels of experience—technical performance levels even after certification—influences surgical outcomes, especially in complex procedures. Technical performance quality correlates with the outcomes and costs and should be measured by image or video-photographic documentation of the surgeon's view field during the procedures. Such consecutive, completely documented, unedited observational data—in the form of intra-operative images and a complete set of eventual radiological images—improve the surgical series' homogeneity. Thereby, they might reflect reality and contribute towards making necessary changes for evidence-based surgery.

Keywords: randomized controlled trials; evidence-based surgery; evidence-based medicine; ICUC; technical performance bias; image-based performance assessments

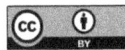

A recent review of the effectiveness of ten orthopedic procedures [1] noted "that most of these procedures recommended by national guidelines and used by surgeons have insufficient readily available high-quality evidence on their clinical effectiveness, which is mainly because of a lack of definitive trials." In the absence of clinically meaningful evidence from high-quality trials, clinicians are obliged to follow the advice of the late David Sackett when discussing options for treatment with patients: "integrating individual clinical expertise with the best external clinical evidence from systematic research" [2], which often relies on consensus statements or advisory guidelines from specific institutions or professional bodies, e.g., NHS England. Evidence-Based Interventions: Guidance for CCGs [3].

A question that follows from the conclusions of this otherwise excellent article concerns whether the essential reasons for this thought-provoking conclusion have been identified, from which reliable solutions can be derived. We offer some points for debate and discussion, with a potential way forward for this challenging problem.

One obvious factor implicated, but rarely measured or assessed, in the variance within operative and non-operative treatment groups is the inter-operator variance in technical performance, whether of operative or non-operative treatment. This inevitably produces a technical performance bias (TPB) as a fundamental problem for surgical trials. The variance occurs not only during surgeons' learning curves but also among certified professionals. The value and expectations of evidence-based medicine are undisputed [1,4–8]; however, for surgical trials, TPB limits the scientific adequacy of a trial and its applicability (generalizability) and acceptance [6,9,10]. Insufficient contemporaneous intraoperative performance documentation confounds a secondary analysis of the technical quality of the reported surgical procedures, as required by Item 5 of the CONSORT guidelines [7]. It is not easy to conceive how this should be achieved without documenting the technical details of the surgical procedure with still images or video clips of the operation field and all intra-operative images [11]. It is interesting that Blom et al. [1] report that total knee replacement, a procedure highly dependent on the proper use of instrumentation, is one of only two procedures of the ten studied for which there is sufficient evidence to support its use in the specific indication of end-stage osteoarthritis of the knee. By removing variability in the surgeons' performance through instrumentation, including augmented or robotic assistance, the variance in the procedure outcome could be reduced, thus making a comparison with non-operative interventions more meaningful, measurable, and relevant (for instance, in cost-analysis comparisons of treatments). It will be interesting to speculate whether navigated ('robotic') knee replacement will take this further [12], making the individual surgeon's performance even less influential for the outcome [13]. The second procedure, for which there is sufficient evidence for efficacy (carpal tunnel decompression, a procedure in which the essence of technical success is soft tissue handling, i.e., surgical competence), comprises fewer 'steps-to-success' to master, and variability may therefore be minimized between surgeons. The quality of the various technical aspects of surgery, such as the expertise demonstrated in soft tissue handling or the number, force, and amplitude of maneuvers needed for fracture reduction—essential for an assessment of performance and procedure outcome—are not documented in most studies and cannot, therefore, be considered. The homogeneity of the technical aspects of different treatment groups in a clinical study is indispensable in a skill-dependent field such as surgery [14,15] but is rarely reported. Current methods for documenting and selectively recording x-rays without unedited contemporaneous, e.g., a video–photographic representation of procedures, do not appear sufficient to guarantee the needed homogeneity. In addition, the complete documentation of all the surgical procedures helps to build up supervised machine-learning models. The latest artificial intelligence (AI) technology assists in the automatic post-production of the key steps of still images and short video clips for a rapid use with a high accuracy. An AI-based surgical platform has played a role in some specific endoscopically assisted procedures [16], and a similar technology may apply to other surgeries in the future.

Currently, the homogeneity of a technical performance within different treatment groups appears so sufficiently poor that the evidence level deteriorates [17]. This has inevitably occurred in frequently cited randomized controlled trials (RCTs) such as the ProFHER study [18,19] regarding the treatment of proximal humerus fractures and the UK heel fracture trial [20] and the UK DRAAFT trial regarding the treatment of distal radius fractures [21]. The conclusions of such studies lead to recommendations that may not be directly relevant to the individual patient and are therefore of limited value in clinical practice [22] Efforts are needed in surgery to produce evidence levels similar to those generated in internal medicine. Justifications for surgical decision-making, such as 'this works in my hands' or 'what my mentor taught me' [23], should be replaced by scientific evidence. Operative procedures, in particular, the experience and preferences of surgeons, which reflect the surgeons' performance, must be stratified. The goal(s) of the treatment must be defined before the intervention, independent of the chosen treatment modality. Subsequently, a surgical outcome is influenced by preoperative expectations [24,25] and surgical performance. The post-procedure assessment of whether the goals were met in the different treatment groups is indispensable: the decrement (including complications caused by suboptimal surgical performance) after the procedure matters as least as much to patients as the increment of functionality gained. The reasons for differences (decrements) between 'work as planned' and 'work as done' must be analyzed. Goals—such as an 'anatomical' reconstruction of a fracture, not an approximation to it—are sometimes only reached by technically highly skilled surgeons, especially for infrequent pathologies. An unrecorded but poor performance from non-specialized surgeons with wildly different experience levels might lead to poorer outcomes and failure to attain the desired goals [26–28]. TPB compounds the problem of 'group inhomogeneity' inherent to many classifications of disease used in such trials: inconclusive results are almost inevitable.

Clinical trials reported without the contemporaneous recording of imaging data, including video–photographic documentation, permitting an independent retrospective evaluation of both group homogeneity (of the classifications used, patients' characteristics, etc.) and the technical performance quality, lose scientific value. The technical performance quality is measurable and correlates with the outcomes and costs [14,29] in cardiac, visceral, and video-assisted surgery studies. It is difficult to imagine that such correlations should not be valid for other fields of surgery if the technical metrics are adapted. The performance–outcome effect might increase with the complexity of the procedure: discussions could then arise about what is technically straightforward and what is not and at what level of expertise a surgeon must be to accomplish a particular procedure. From one surgeon to another, a critical variability exists in soft tissue handling and the sequence of intricate actions to reach articular congruity. This produces an inevitable and undesired inhomogeneity.

The inherent heterogeneity of complex interventions [17] is well known; nevertheless, surgical RCTs seldom consider potentially different quality levels of the technical performance [30]. This is relevant to RCTs in medicine; as a doctor (surgeon), dependent factors are much more critical. Defining necessary and homogeneous performance quality factors can therefore improve the outcomes. The absence of standards of performance assessments for every surgical specialty cannot be a reason not to initiate an effort to establish them. Intra-operative procedural documentation will be needed to determine a 'performance gap': the difference between a high and a low level of performance of a specific technical act. Quality levels can be defined on the basis of complete intra-operative image documentation [14]. This might comprise a rating of a specific procedure step or the entire procedure; surgical time-to-completion does not necessarily reflect either expertise or accuracy but is often used as a surrogate for these performance dimensions. Such performance assessments are still to be clearly defined but all will likely be image-based [31]. To assume that a defined written protocol guarantees that all procedures follow a uniform sequence of actions according to the protocol are illusory. This is particularly true in trauma due to the essential variations from one case to another, which are difficult to depict in a classification.

In one attempt to contribute to this lack of standards, the ICUC working group [32] has developed a concept for complete and detailed image-based reporting, including unedited, contemporaneous, and complete photo-documentation of entire procedures. Such documentation has the potential to overcome the previously mentioned TPB as it allows secondary, retrospective, and independent analysis [32]. The completeness of the record allows significant help for learning by providing images of technical details. It also defines the value of the initiative: all critical or key steps and potential shortcomings are included [6,33]. The evidence-based justification of technical practices based on RCTs in (orthopedic) surgery is a laudable goal but equally challenging to realize. There are relevant reasons for this reality.

First, the standardization of the key steps of any surgical procedure is not only difficult—especially in multi-center trials—but also insufficient if no agreed metrics for secondary analysis and comparison exist. Second, technical performance bias or inhomogeneity (within study groups containing very different elements or classifications applied to such groups) are the basis of imprecise or even incorrect conclusions, which therefore 'permit' a reversion to less evidence-based medicine. Finally, RCT data represent 'work as planned' (according to a research protocol); the attainment of 'work as planned' (the ideal outcome) rather than 'work as done' (the actual outcome) is possibly only realized by a minority of surgeons, and not representative of what most surgeons do in their daily practice. Consecutive, completely documented, unedited observational data might reflect reality more precisely while fulfilling the requirements of the Cochrane Collaboration [11].

Consequences and Conclusions

Transparent (unedited) intraoperative image data, allowing a retrospective analysis, are indispensable to avoid a technical performance bias and assure the homogeneity of treatment groups in surgical trials. Complete, continuous clinical series can represent 'real world data' better than RCTs if they avoid these biases. The incidence of inconclusive results, frequent in surgical RCTs, could diminish. Following the ICUC concept of a complete intra-operative image documentation of surgical procedures, we can obtain data allowing for a retrospective analysis. This would contribute to necessary changes toward evidence-based surgery (EBS).

Author Contributions: Conceptualization, P.R.; writing—original draft preparation, P.R.; writing review and editing, S.L., J.B.J., N.S., W.-C.L. and A.A.F.D. All authors have read and agreed to the published version of the manuscript.

Funding: This research received no external funding.

Institutional Review Board Statement: Not applicable.

Informed Consent Statement: Not applicable.

Data Availability Statement: Not applicable.

Conflicts of Interest: Pietro Regazzoni and Alberto A. Fernández Dell'Oca co-founded ICUC, and Jesse B. Jupiter is the head of upper limb of ICUC.

References

1. Blom, A.W.; Donovan, R.L.; Beswick, A.D.; Whitehouse, M.R.; Kunutsor, S.K. Common elective orthopaedic procedures and their clinical effectiveness: Umbrella review of level 1 evidence. *BMJ* **2021**, *374*, n1511. [CrossRef] [PubMed]
2. Sackett, D.L.; Rosenberg, W.M.; Gray, J.A.; Haynes, R.B.; Richardson, W.S. Evidence based medicine: What it is and what it isn't. *BMJ* **1996**, *312*, 71–72. [CrossRef] [PubMed]
3. England, N. Evidence-Based Interventions: Guidance for CCGs. Available online: https://www.engage.england.nhs.uk/consultation/evidence-based-interventions/user_uploads/evidence-based-interventions-consultation-document-1.pdf (accessed on 25 November 2022).
4. Berlin, J.A.; Golub, R.M. Meta-analysis as evidence: Building a better pyramid. *JAMA* **2014**, *312*, 603–605. [CrossRef] [PubMed]
5. Ebell, M.H.; Sokol, R.; Lee, A.; Simons, C.; Early, J. How good is the evidence to support primary care practice? *Evid. Based Med.* **2017**, *22*, 88–92. [CrossRef] [PubMed]
6. Greenhalgh, T.; Howick, J.; Maskrey, N.; Evidence Based Medicine Renaissance Group. Evidence based medicine: A movement in crisis? *BMJ* **2014**, *348*, g3725. [CrossRef]
7. Saitz, R. Evidence-Based Medicine these 7 years: Time for the editor to go on permanent sabbatical. *Evid. Based Med.* **2017**, *22*, 79–80. [CrossRef]
8. Ubel, P.A. Medical Facts versus Value Judgments—Toward Preference-Sensitive Guidelines. *N. Engl. J. Med.* **2015**, *372*, 2475–2477. [CrossRef]
9. McCulloch, P.; Taylor, I.; Sasako, M.; Lovett, B.; Griffin, D. Randomised trials in surgery. Problems and possible solutions. *BMJ* **2002**, *324*, 1448–1451. [CrossRef]
10. Paradis, C. Bias in surgical research. *Ann. Surg.* **2008**, *248*, 180–188. [CrossRef]
11. Gøtzsche, P.C. We need access to all data from all clinical trials. *Cochrane Database Syst. Rev.* **2011**, *12*, ED000035. [CrossRef]
12. Choi, B.S.; Kim, S.E.; Yang, M.; Ro, D.H.; Han, H.S. Functional alignment with roboticarm assisted total knee arthroplasty demonstrated better patient-reported outcomes than mechanical alignment with manual total knee arthroplasty. *Knee Surg. Sport. Traumatol. Arthrosc. Off. J. ESSKA* **2022**. Online ahead of print. [CrossRef]
13. Sinclair, S.T.; Klika, A.K.; Jin, Y.; Higuera, C.A.; Piuzzi, N.S.; Cleveland Clinic OME Arthroplasty Group. The Impact of Surgeon Variability on Patient-Reported Outcome Measures, Length of Stay, Discharge Disposition, and 90-Day Readmission in TKA. *J. Bone Jt. Surgery. Am. Vol.* **2022**, *104*, 2016–2025. [CrossRef]
14. Birkmeyer, J.D.; Finks, J.F.; O'Reilly, A.; Oerline, M.; Carlin, A.M.; Nunn, A.R.; Dimick, J.; Banerjee, M.; Birkmeyer, N.J.; Michigan Bariatric Surgery, C. Surgical skill and complication rates after bariatric surgery. *N. Engl. J. Med.* **2013**, *369*, 1434–1442. [CrossRef] [PubMed]
15. Hawe, P.; Shiell, A.; Riley, T. Complex interventions: How "out of control" can a randomised controlled trial be? *BMJ* **2004**, *328*, 1561–1563. [CrossRef] [PubMed]

16. Bar, O.; Neimark, D.; Zohar, M.; Hager, G.D.; Girshick, R.; Fried, G.M.; Wolf, T.; Asselmann, D. Impact of data on generalization of AI for surgical intelligence applications. *Sci. Rep.* **2020**, *10*, 22208. [CrossRef] [PubMed]
17. Murad, M.H.; Asi, N.; Alsawas, M.; Alahdab, F. New evidence pyramid. *Evid. Based Med.* **2016**, *21*, 125–127. [CrossRef]
18. Launonen, A.P.; Lepola, V.; Flinkkila, T.; Laitinen, M.; Paavola, M.; Malmivaara, A. Treatment of proximal humerus fractures in the elderly: A systemic review of 409 patients. *Acta Orthop.* **2015**, *86*, 280–285. [CrossRef]
19. Rangan, A.; Handoll, H.; Brealey, S.; Jefferson, L.; Keding, A.; Martin, B.C.; Goodchild, L.; Chuang, L.H.; Hewitt, C.; Torgerson, D.; et al. Surgical vs nonsurgical treatment of adults with displaced fractures of the proximal humerus: The PROFHER randomized clinical trial. *JAMA* **2015**, *313*, 1037–1047. [CrossRef]
20. Griffin, D.; Parsons, N.; Shaw, E.; Kulikov, Y.; Hutchinson, C.; Thorogood, M.; Lamb, S.E.; Investigators, U.K.H.F.T. Operative versus non-operative treatment for closed, displaced, intra-articular fractures of the calcaneus: Randomised controlled trial. *BMJ* **2014**, *349*, g4483. [CrossRef]
21. Costa, M.L.; Achten, J.; Plant, C.; Parsons, N.R.; Rangan, A.; Tubeuf, S.; Yu, G.; Lamb, S.E. UK DRAFFT: A randomised controlled trial of percutaneous fixation with Kirschner wires versus volar locking-plate fixation in the treatment of adult patients with a dorsally displaced fracture of the distal radius. *Health Technol. Assess* **2015**, *19*, 1–124. [CrossRef]
22. Kerr, S.; Warwick, D.; Haddad, F.S. Cost-effectiveness studies: Who is the key stakeholder? *Bone Jt. J* **2019**, *101*, 1321–1324. [CrossRef] [PubMed]
23. Hageman, M.G.; Guitton, T.G.; Ring, D.; Science of Variation, G. How surgeons make decisions when the evidence is inconclusive. *J. Hand Surg.* **2013**, *38*, 1202–1208. [CrossRef] [PubMed]
24. Chahla, J.; Beck, E.C.; Nwachukwu, B.U.; Alter, T.; Harris, J.D.; Nho, S.J. Is There an Association Between Preoperative Expectations and Patient-Reported Outcome After Hip Arthroscopy for Femoroacetabular Impingement Syndrome? *Arthroscopy* **2019**, *35*, 3250–3258 e3251. [CrossRef] [PubMed]
25. Factor, S.; Neuman, Y.; Vidra, M.; Shalom, M.; Lichtenstein, A.; Amar, E.; Rath, E. Violation of expectations is correlated with satisfaction following hip arthroscopy. *Knee Surg. Sport. Traumatol. Arthrosc. Off. J. ESSKA* **2022**. Online ahead of print. [CrossRef] [PubMed]
26. Berkes, M.B.; Little, M.T.; Lorich, D.G. Open reduction internal fixation of proximal humerus fractures. *Curr. Rev. Musculoskelet. Med.* **2013**, *6*, 47–56. [CrossRef] [PubMed]
27. Olerud, P.; Ahrengart, L.; Ponzer, S.; Saving, J.; Tidermark, J. Hemiarthroplasty versus nonoperative treatment of displaced 4-part proximal humeral fractures in elderly patients: A randomized controlled trial. *J. Shoulder Elb. Surg.* **2011**, *20*, 1025–1033. [CrossRef] [PubMed]
28. Olerud, P.; Ahrengart, L.; Ponzer, S.; Saving, J.; Tidermark, J. Internal fixation versus nonoperative treatment of displaced 3-part proximal humeral fractures in elderly patients: A randomized controlled trial. *J. Shoulder Elb. Surg.* **2011**, *20*, 747–755. [CrossRef]
29. Trehan, A.; Barnett-Vanes, A.; Carty, M.J.; McCulloch, P.; Maruthappu, M. The impact of feedback of intraoperative technical performance in surgery: A systematic review. *BMJ Open* **2015**, *5*, e006759. [CrossRef]
30. McArdle, C.S.; Hole, D. Impact of variability among surgeons on postoperative morbidity and mortality and ultimate survival. *BMJ* **1991**, *302*, 1501–1505. [CrossRef]
31. Regazzoni, P.; Fernandez, A.; Perren, S.M. Balancing Success and Risk in Orthopedic Trauma Surgery: The Ridge-Walking between Sound Accepting "Good" and Risky Striving for "Better". *Acta Chir. Orthop. Traumatol. Cechoslov.* **2016**, *83*, 9–15.
32. Regazzoni, P.; Giannoudis, P.V.; Lambert, S.; Fernandez, A.; Perren, S.M. The ICUC((R)) app: Can it pave the way for quality control and transparency in medicine? *Injury* **2017**, *48*, 1101–1103. [CrossRef] [PubMed]
33. Sherman, R.E.; Anderson, S.A.; Dal Pan, G.J.; Gray, G.W.; Gross, T.; Hunter, N.L.; LaVange, L.; Marinac-Dabic, D.; Marks, P.W.; Robb, M.A.; et al. Real-World Evidence—What Is It and What Can It Tell Us? *N. Engl. J. Med.* **2016**, *375*, 2293–2297. [CrossRef] [PubMed]

Disclaimer/Publisher's Note: The statements, opinions and data contained in all publications are solely those of the individual author(s) and contributor(s) and not of MDPI and/or the editor(s). MDPI and/or the editor(s) disclaim responsibility for any injury to people or property resulting from any ideas, methods, instructions or products referred to in the content.

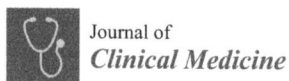

Article

Cerclage Wiring Improves Biomechanical Stability in Distal Tibia Spiral Fractures Treated by Intramedullary Nailing

Stefan Förch [1,†], Sabrina Sandriesser [2,3,*,†], Christian von Rüden [2,3,4], Edgar Mayr [1] and Peter Augat [2,3]

1 Department of Trauma, Orthopaedic, Plastic and Hand Surgery, University Hospital of Augsburg, Stenglinstrasse 2, 86156 Augsburg, Germany
2 Institute for Biomechanics, BG Unfallklinik Murnau, Prof. Küntscher Str. 8, 82418 Murnau, Germany
3 Institute for Biomechanics, Paracelsus Medical University, Strubergasse 21, 5020 Salzburg, Austria
4 Department of Trauma Surgery, BG Unfallklinik Murnau, Prof. Küntscher Str. 8, 82418 Murnau, Germany
* Correspondence: sabrina.sandriesser@bgu-murnau.de
† These authors contributed equally to this work.

Abstract: Background: Partial weight-bearing after operatively treated fractures has been the standard of care over the past decades. Recent studies report on better rehabilitation and faster return to daily life in case of immediate weight-bearing as tolerated. To allow early weight-bearing, osteosynthesis needs to provide sufficient mechanical stability. The purpose of this study was to investigate the stabilizing benefits of additive cerclage wiring in combination with intramedullary nailing of distal tibia fractures. Methods: In 14 synthetic tibiae, a reproducible distal spiral fracture was treated by intramedullary nailing. In half of the samples, the fracture was further stabilized by additional cerclage wiring. Under clinically relevant partial and full weight-bearing loads the samples were biomechanically tested and axial construct stiffness as well as interfragmentary movements were assessed. Subsequently, a 5 mm fracture gap was created to simulate insufficient reduction, and tests were repeated. Results: Intramedullary nails offer already high axial stability. Thus, axial construct stiffness cannot be significantly enhanced by an additive cerclage (2858 ± 958 N/mm NailOnly vs. 3727 ± 793 N/mm Nail + Cable; $p = 0.089$). Under full weight-bearing loads, additive cerclage wiring in well-reduced fractures significantly reduced shear ($p = 0.002$) and torsional movements ($p = 0.013$) and showed similar low movements as under partial weight-bearing (shear 0.3 mm, $p = 0.073$; torsion 1.1°, $p = 0.085$). In contrast, additional cerclage had no stabilizing effect in large fracture gaps. Conclusions: In well-reduced spiral fractures of the distal tibia, the construct stability of intramedullary nailing can be further increased by additional cerclage wiring. From a biomechanical point of view, augmentation of the primary implant reduced shear movement sufficiently to allow immediate weight-bearing as tolerated. Especially, elderly patients would benefit from early post-operative mobilization, which allows for accelerated rehabilitation and a faster return to daily activities.

Keywords: cable; cerclage; tibia shaft; comminuted fracture; intramedullary nailing; biomechanics

Citation: Förch, S.; Sandriesser, S.; von Rüden, C.; Mayr, E.; Augat, P. Cerclage Wiring Improves Biomechanical Stability in Distal Tibia Spiral Fractures Treated by Intramedullary Nailing. J. Clin. Med. 2023, 12, 1770. https://doi.org/10.3390/jcm12051770

Academic Editors: Yuichi Hoshino and Andreas Neff

Received: 12 January 2023
Revised: 16 February 2023
Accepted: 21 February 2023
Published: 22 February 2023

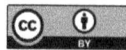

Copyright: © 2023 by the authors. Licensee MDPI, Basel, Switzerland. This article is an open access article distributed under the terms and conditions of the Creative Commons Attribution (CC BY) license (https://creativecommons.org/licenses/by/4.0/).

1. Introduction

Fractures of the tibial shaft represent the most common long bone fractures [1]. After operative fracture fixation, partial weight-bearing is still considered the post-operative treatment of choice according to the AO surgery reference [2]. However, the recent literature supports the need for a shift in the post-operative weight-bearing regimen toward early mobilization [3,4]. Especially in the geriatric patient population, immediate weight-bearing as tolerated is becoming more prevalent and is treated as one of the key elements for successful rehabilitation [5]. Thus, immediate loading of the treated limb implies the need for increased implant stability.

In combination with a distal tibia locking plate, additive cable cerclage wiring has already been proven from a biomechanical aspect, to increase construct stability and allow for immediate post-operative weight-bearing [6,7]. Promising first clinical results emphasize the beneficial stabilizing effect of supplemental cerclage wiring in distal tibia spiral fractures [8]. A minimally invasive technique guarantees a careful and safe cerclage insertion with only 3% of cerclages inducing local tissue irritation [8]. Moreover, a recent literature review could not find any direct link between cerclage wiring on the periosteal blood supply and delayed or inhibited fracture healing [9].

In extra-articular tibia fractures, intramedullary nailing offers a suitable alternative that ensures satisfactory clinical outcomes [10]. Nailing seems slightly superior in terms of post-operative complications and infection rates [11], but appears to be associated with higher malunion rates [10]. To achieve sufficient fracture reduction and to stabilize a torsional fracture of the tibia, the use of cerclage wires has already been suggested [8,12,13]. Nonetheless, the stabilizing effect of cerclage wiring in combination with a tibia nail in a realistic fracture model has not yet been investigated in biomechanical studies.

Thus, the aim of this biomechanical study was to investigate additional cerclage wiring in combination with intramedullary nailing for the fixation of distal tibia spiral fractures. We hypothesized that in a well-reduced fracture, an additional cable cerclage will reduce interfragmentary movements under full weight-bearing conditions. Furthermore, we assumed that additional cerclage wiring has a limited stabilizing effect at a larger fracture gap or comminuted fracture zone.

2. Materials and Methods

For this biomechanical study, a spiral shaft fracture (AO/OTA 42-A1.1c) was cut with the help of a custom-made sawing template at the distal third of synthetic composite tibiae (large left, fourth generation, Sawbones Europe AB, Malmoe, Sweden). A total number of fourteen samples were reproducibly fractured and instrumented with a standard tibia nail (T2 tibia nail standard, ø 11 × 390 mm, Stryker GmbH & Co. KG, Duisburg, Germany) by using another template for fragment reposition. Implantation was conducted by an experienced trauma surgeon and led to a complete reduction of the fracture gap in all samples. Distally, the nail was locked freehand by placing all three screw options. At the proximal tibia, two screws were placed via the targeting device, and the most proximal screw was omitted.

Half of the samples were tested as solitary nail fixation ($n = 7$ NailOnly) and in the other half the fracture was further stabilized by a supplemental steel cable cerclage ($n = 7$ Nail + Cable) (ø 1.7 mm, DePuy Synthes Companies, Oberdorf, Switzerland) looped around the fracture zone (Figure 1a). According to the manufacturer's recommendation, the cerclage was tightened under a tension of 50 kg and closed by a crimp mechanism.

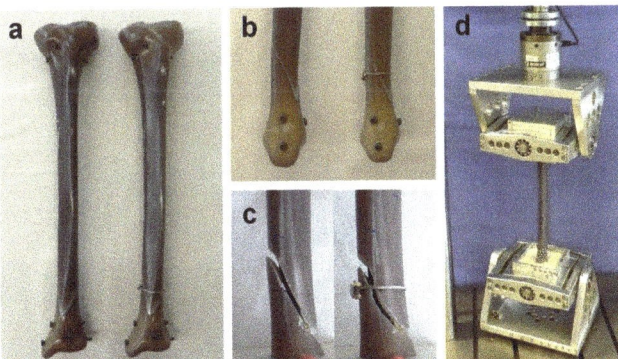

Figure 1. Synthetic tibia sample and test setup: (**a**) frontal view on the instrumented tibia with the solitary nail and with supplemental cable cerclage wiring around the fracture zone; (**b**) medial view on the distal tibia with a reduced fracture gap; (**c**) 5 mm fracture gap; (**d**) test setup with two cardan joints to avoid constraining forces.

Prior to mechanical testing the tibiae were aligned vertically and were embedded in polyurethane (RenCast FC 53 A/B + filler DT 082, Huntsman, The Woodlands, TX, USA) at both ends to achieve a resulting working length of 295 mm. To avoid embedding the implant, the nail entry point as well as the screw heads and the slightly protruding screw tips were covered with modeling clay.

Mechanical testing was performed on a servo-hydraulic testing machine (Instron 8874, Dynacell, measuring range ± 10 kN, accuracy ± 2% and ±100 Nm, accuracy ±1%, Instron Structural Testing GmbH, High Wycombe, UK) with cardan joints to avoid constraining forces (Figure 1d). The load protocol covered clinically relevant partial (20 kg) as well as full (75 kg) weight-bearing loads and was adopted from previous studies [6,7]. To settle each construct, an axial sinusoidal load of 10–200 N at a frequency of 1 Hz was applied for a total of 100 cycles, followed by a pure axial ramp up to 200 N at a velocity of 0.1 mm/s to determine initial axial construct stiffness by analyzing the linear portion of the force–displacement curve.

The first part of the load protocol consisted of quasi-static testing under combined axial and torsional loads of approximately 20 kg partial (200 N and 2 Nm) and 75 kg full weight-bearing loads (750 N and 7 Nm). In this specific test setup, the applied torsion mimicked internal rotation.

After quasi-static testing, each sample underwent a dynamic load protocol to simulate clinically relevant post-operative loading. Torsional loading was applied at a frequency of 0.5 Hz, alternating between ±4 Nm. Axial sinusoidal loading was applied at 1 Hz, starting between 50 N (valley) and 200 N (peak), and peak load increased by 50 N after every 1000 cycles. Tests were terminated when reaching a load maximum of 2000 N.

Finally, to mimic a more complex, comminuted, or incompletely reduced fracture condition, an interfragmentary gap of 5 mm was created in each construct by manually grinding material along the fracture line (Figure 1c). To investigate imperfect cerclage tension, the cable cerclage was kept in place and has not been replaced. The same quasi-static tests under partial and full weight-bearing loads were conducted and the results were compared to the well-reduced samples.

To determine interfragmentary movements, small adhesive marker points were attached along the fracture line on the proximal and distal fragments and these points were tracked by an optical 3D motion tracking system (ARAMIS Professional 5 M, GOM GmbH, Braunschweig, Germany). For quasi-static testing pictures were taken at each unloaded and loaded state and for dynamic testing movements at the maximum load of 2000 N were analyzed. Translational and rotational movements in the fracture gap were evaluated. The coordinate system was aligned in a way that the vertical axis was oriented along the tibial shaft axis and defined axial movement. Sagittal and frontal axes were defined according to the respective anatomical orientations. Shear movements were defined as movement in the transverse plane. Rotational movements were calculated as rotation around the tibial shaft axis and sagittal axis. To guarantee reproducible data processing, the origin of the coordinate system was placed at the same position for all specimens.

Axial construct stiffness was calculated by dividing the force by the deformation along the vertical shaft axis. Axial, shear, and rotational movements were assessed at partial (200 N), full (750 N), and maximum (2000 N) loading. For statistical analysis, data were tested for normal distribution using Shapiro–Wilk tests. Axial stiffness was statistically compared using unpaired t-tests. For quasi-static loading, the reduced condition was compared to the gap condition using Wilcoxon tests for paired samples, and Mann–Whitney tests for unpaired comparisons with and without additive cerclage. For dynamic loading, the NailOnly group was compared to the Nail + Cable group using unpaired *t*-tests (SPSS Statistics, Version 26, IBM, Armonk, NY, USA). Values are given as mean and standard deviation.

3. Results

Solitary nail fixation already achieved high axial construct stiffness and could not be significantly increased by a supplemental cable cerclage (2858 ± 958 N/mm NailOnly vs. 3727 ± 793 N/mm Nail + Cable; $p = 0.089$). The 5 mm gap condition reduced axial stiffness for NailOnly (1283 ± 538 N/mm; $p = 0.003$) as well as for Nail + Cable (1028 ± 271 N/mm; $p < 0.001$).

Under quasi-static loading, well-reduced constructs showed significantly less interfragmentary movement ($p \leq 0.018$) compared to constructs with remaining gap condition for all loading scenarios, except for axial movement under partial weight-bearing showing no movement at all ($p = 0.684$) (Figure 2).

Under full weight-bearing, axial movement remained below 0.2 mm and 0.5 mm for reduced condition and gap condition, respectively. Both cases showed little axial movements with no further stabilization by additional cerclage wiring.

In the well-reduced fracture condition, shear movement amounted to 0.7 ± 0.1 mm under full weight-bearing. Additional cerclage wiring significantly reduced shear movement to 0.3 ± 0.1 mm ($p = 0.002$), which was comparable to the shear movement under partial weight-bearing without cable (0.2 ± 0.1 mm; $p = 0.073$). For the gap condition, shear movement increased to 1.3 ± 0.3 mm and could not be reduced by an additive cable cerclage (1.0 ± 0.3 mm; $p = 0.073$).

The highest rotation around the shaft axis was observed for the NailOnly group under full weight-bearing, with 2.5 ± 0.5° for the reduced condition and up to 230% higher rotations for the gap condition (5.9 ± 0.9°). In the reduced condition, the addition of a cable cerclage significantly restricted rotations to 1.1 ± 0.8° ($p = 0.013$), which was comparable to partial weight-bearing ($p = 0.085$). In the gap condition, no further reduction was achieved by additional cerclage wiring.

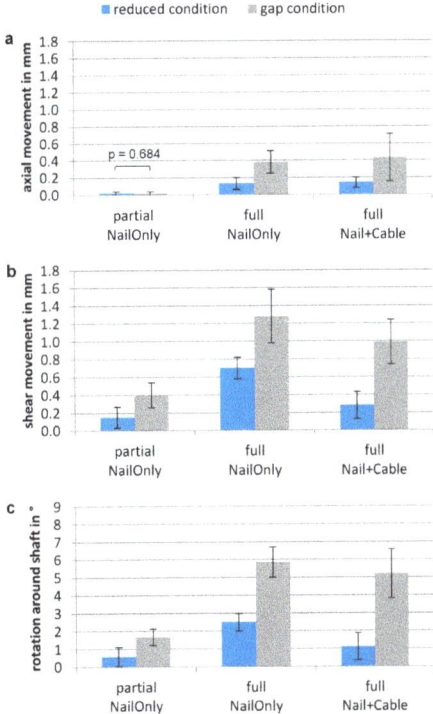

Figure 2. Interfragmentary motion under quasi-static partial and full weight-bearing loads for a well-reduced fracture condition and for a gap condition. Differences between NailOnly group and

Nail + Cable group are shown for (**a**) axial movement in mm; (**b**) shear movement in mm and (**c**) rotation around the shaft axis in °. Values are given as mean ± standard deviation. Movements in the gap condition were significantly larger ($p \leq 0.018$) compared to the reduced condition, if not otherwise indicated.

All samples survived dynamic loading up to 2000 N without any construct failure. The cerclage wiring significantly reduced translational movements by 63% for axial ($p = 0.032$) and by 62% for shear movements ($p = 0.006$) (Figure 3). Rotational movements were generally at a low level of less than 0.5°. With an additional cable cerclage, rotations were reduced by 36% around the shaft axis ($p = 0.315$) and by 50% around the sagittal axis ($p = 0.086$), but without statistical significance.

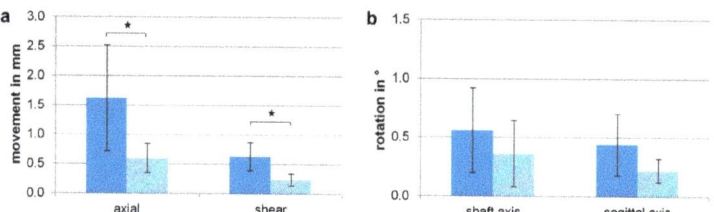

Figure 3. Resulting motion for the reduced fracture condition at maximum applied load of 2000 N and 4 Nm after dynamic loading of the NailOnly (solid bar) and the Nail + Cable (dashed bar) groups for (**a**) axial and shear movements and (**b**) rotational movements around the shaft axis and the sagittal axis. Values are given as mean ± standard deviation and significant differences are marked by the asterisk symbol (* $p < 0.05$).

4. Discussion

Distal tibia shaft fractures can be reliably stabilized by intramedullary nailing. In this study, it has been demonstrated that for well-reduced spiral fractures, the stabilization can be further increased by applying cerclage wiring around the fracture zone. The additional stabilization especially reduced shear movements at the fracture site, which is considered of particular importance for an undisturbed fracture healing process. The extent of added construct stiffness and movement reduction suggests that spiral fractures of the distal tibia are to be allowed for immediate weight-bearing as tolerated without the risk of construct failure, and loss of reduction of malalignment.

As interfragmentary movements play a crucial role in callus formation and fracture healing, a supplemental cerclage serves not only as a temporary reduction tool during nail insertion but improves the overall stability of the fracture fixation [14,15]. The results of the present study show that only in well-reduced fractures the cerclage provides increased construct stability. Larger fracture gaps of 5 mm simulating a comminuted fracture zone, resulted in significantly higher movements, which could not be reduced by the addition of a cable cerclage. The reported results underline the importance of a good reduction for the stability of osteosynthesis. In clinical practice, the insertion of a cerclage for spiral fractures often allows anatomical reduction.

Depending on the localization and type of fracture, a cerclage has no stabilizing effect in comminuted or transverse fracture patterns but develops its potential in spiral and oblique fractures [16]. In other orthopedic and trauma surgeries, e.g., the femoral shaft, additional cerclage wires experience broad approval and contribute to the overall stability of the osteosynthesis [17–20].

Only a few studies support the use of additional cerclage wiring in combination with intramedullary nailing for the stabilization of spiral fractures of the distal tibia. A recent study was published promising clinical results on 96 tibia shaft spiral fractures treated with additive cerclages to increase the stability of the osteosynthesis [8]. Huang et al. reported on effective and simplified fracture reduction in oblique and spiral fractures and improved fixation stability due to additional cerclage wiring [13]. Habernek published 37 cases of torsional tibia fractures treated by intramedullary nailing and percutaneous cerclage wiring, already more than 30 years ago [12]. In addition to the advantages in fracture reduction, he reported on early full weight-bearing and benefits in fracture healing. However, the concept of early weight-bearing did not gain acceptance and the recommendation of partial weight-bearing prevailed.

In recent years, more and more literature emerged, questioning the restrictions in postoperative weight-bearing and initiating a discussion towards early loading as tolerated [3,5]. It was found that, especially in elderly patients, immediate mobilization reduced postoperative complications, led to successful rehabilitation, and improved the overall outcome after hip fractures [3,5,21,22] as well as after fractures of the distal femur [4,23]. A randomized controlled trial investigating 115 patients after surgically treating ankle fractures revealed that immediate mobilization and weight-bearing as tolerated led to faster return to work and improved functional outcomes [24]. According to Gross et al. immediate weight-bearing after intramedullary nailing of isolated distal tibia shaft fractures (AO/OTA type 42-A and 42-B) is not related to complications or adverse events [25]. To our knowledge, this randomized controlled trial is the only study investigating a comparable fracture type to the present study (AO/OTA 42-A1.1c) and supporting the concept of early loading. However, all these mentioned studies examine the effect of immediate weight-bearing from a clinical perspective. Our present study investigates for the first time the biomechanical performance, including construct stiffness and interfragmentary motion, of distal tibia fractures treated by intramedullary nailing and supplemental cerclage wiring.

Depending on fracture height and involvement of the ankle joint, fractures at the distal tibia can also be treated by plate osteosynthesis. A previous study showed that in combination with a distal tibia locking plate, an additive cerclage has been proven to increase overall construct stability to allow for immediate weight-bearing, from a biomechanical point of view [6]. Investigating the same fracture model, the current findings reveal increased axial construct stiffness, irrespective of the use of an additive cerclage. Due to the principle of load transfer, intramedullary implants show higher axial stiffness compared to extramedullary locking plates [26]. In our study, axial stiffness ranges between 2800 and 3700 N/mm, which is within the favorable range above 2500 N/mm for fracture gaps smaller than 3 mm [27].

Accordingly, for fracture gaps smaller than 3 mm, interfragmentary movements of 0.2 to 1.0 mm offer perfect conditions for bone healing [28]. Thus, micromotions in the fracture gap seem favorable for callus formation and fracture healing [28]. In a study by Epari et al., a clear relationship was found between the stability of osteosynthesis and the mechanical strength of the healing bone [29]. It is therefore concluded that moderate degrees of axial stability are related to a higher callus strength [29]. These findings are true for axial stability. However, sufficient reduction of shear movements is equally important for bone healing [14]. From a clinical point of view, increasing the stability of the fracture fixation allows for an earlier and less restricted mobilization of the patient as compared to fractures with insufficient reduction or imperfect alignment. Alignment, reduction, and stabilization result in load sharing between osteosynthesis implant and bone and have been shown to result in a more favorable healing outcome [30,31].

Relating to clinical aspects, nailing and plating of extra-articular distal tibia fractures show both satisfactory results [10]. Nailing seems slightly superior in terms of postoperative complications, infection rates, and reduced surgery time, but poses the risk of higher malunion rates [11,32–35]. To reduce the risk of malunion, proper alignment, and sufficient fracture reduction can be achieved by an additional cerclage looped around the fracture zone. Our study demonstrates that an additive cerclage cannot increase axial construct stiffness, but significantly lowers shear movements in the fracture gap. The current literature agrees on the fact that satisfactory surgical treatment of tibia shaft fractures is challenging to achieve and implant selection should be carefully made for each individual patient [10].

Implant flexibility and as a consequence the amount of interfragmentary movement, especially shear movement in the transverse plane, strongly depends on the diameter of the intramedullary nail [36]. It is therefore recommended to use thicker nail diameters in order to achieve adequate implant stability. Sufficient reduction of shear movements is also essential to trigger the onset of callus formation and to achieve adequate fracture healing [14,29]. Another study confirmed that good reduction of the fragments with small fracture gaps promotes healing and induces good revascularization [37]. Nonetheless, the blood supply and tissue irritation at distal tibia fractures still remain the subject of controversial discussion, especially when using additive cerclage wires. Even though there is only little soft tissue covering the lower third of the tibia, no correlation between impaired healing and cerclage wiring directly on the periosteum was found in a clinical study reporting on the first promising results [8]. The radially oriented blood vessels are not disrupted by cerclage wiring when following a minimally invasive approach and tissue-preserving implantation [16]. A careful cerclage insertion is of particular importance in elderly patients with reduced bone quality.

Limitations of this study include the inherent weakness of biomechanical in vitro studies to not represent in vivo situations and healing processes. Instead of human specimens, synthetic bone models have been used to exclude inter-specimen variability and to focus on implant fixation and the stabilizing effect of additive cerclage wiring [38]. Cut-through or failure of the cerclage could not be induced in these synthetic bones and was not the subject of this study. The cerclage was not replaced after dynamic loading to maintain imperfect cerclage tension and incomplete fracture reduction. According to the surgical guidelines final reaming should be 1.0 to 1.5 mm larger than the nail diameter to be used. Due to compressed and dense foam mimicking cancellous bone in the synthetic model, the intramedullary canal was reamed to 13 mm for the use of tibia nails with 11 mm diameter. The absence of muscles and soft tissue has been partly compensated for by applying a physiologic and clinically relevant load scenario of combined axial and torsional loads. Post-operative loading was simulated under moderate as well as full weight-bearing conditions to identify the stabilizing effect of additional cerclage wiring. The decision to investigate only steel cable cerclages is based on findings from the previous literature. Different cerclage materials have been tested in a biomechanical setup, revealing that steel cable cerclages show the largest reduction in interfragmentary motion [6,7].

5. Conclusions

In conclusion, from a biomechanical point of view, a well-reduced spiral fracture of the distal tibia is adequately stabilized by intramedullary nailing. Applying an additional cable cerclage increases shear stability, allowing the patient to bear full weight. In case of a larger fracture gap, additional cerclage wiring cannot adequately reduce interfragmentary movements. Therefore, post-operative rehabilitation should be in accordance with the type of fracture and the stability of the fixation. To further investigate the effect of additional cerclage wiring in distal tibia spiral fractures, further clinical trials are needed.

Author Contributions: Conceptualization, S.F. and E.M.; methodology, all authors; preparation and implantation, S.S. and S.F.; investigation, S.S.; data collection, S.F., S.S. and P.A.; formal analysis and discussion, all authors; writing—original draft preparation, S.S.; writing—review and editing, S.F., C.v.R., E.M. and P.A.; supervision, P.A. and E.M. All authors have read and agreed to the published version of the manuscript.

Funding: This research received no external funding.

Institutional Review Board Statement: Ethical approval is not required for studies not involving human or animal tissue.

Informed Consent Statement: Not applicable for studies not involving humans.

Data Availability Statement: Data relating to this study are available from the corresponding author upon reasonable request.

Acknowledgments: The steel cable cerclages were provided free of charge by DePuy Synthes.

Conflicts of Interest: The authors declare no conflict of interest.

References

1. Larsen, P.; Elsoe, R.; Hansen, S.H.; Graven-Nielsen, T.; Laessoe, U.; Rasmussen, S. Incidence and epidemiology of tibial shaft fractures. *Injury* **2015**, *46*, 746–750. [CrossRef] [PubMed]
2. White, R.; Camuso, M. AO Surgery Reference-Intramedullary Nailing. Available online: https://surgeryreference.aofoundation.org/orthopedic-trauma/adult-trauma/tibial-shaft/simple-fracture-spiral/intramedullary-nailing#aftercare (accessed on 6 February 2023).
3. Baer, M.; Neuhaus, V.; Pape, H.C.; Ciritsis, B. Influence of mobilization and weight bearing on in-hospital outcome in geriatric patients with hip fractures. *SICOT J.* **2019**, *5*, 4. [CrossRef] [PubMed]
4. Consigliere, P.; Iliopoulos, E.; Ads, T.; Trompeter, A. Early versus delayed weight bearing after surgical fixation of distal femur fractures: A non-randomized comparative study. *Eur. J. Orthop. Surg. Traumatol.* **2019**, *29*, 1789–1794. [CrossRef] [PubMed]
5. Kammerlander, C.; Pfeufer, D.; Lisitano, L.A.; Mehaffey, S.; Bocker, W.; Neuerburg, C. Inability of Older Adult Patients with Hip Fracture to Maintain Postoperative Weight-Bearing Restrictions. *J. Bone Joint Surg. Am.* **2018**, *100*, 936–941. [CrossRef]
6. Sandriesser, S.; Förch, S.; Mayr, E.; Schrödl, F.; von Rüden, C.; Augat, P. Supplemental cerclage wiring in angle stable plate fixation of distal tibial spiral fractures enables immediate post-operative full weight-bearing: A biomechanical analysis. *Eur. J. Trauma Emerg. Surg.* **2020**, *48*, 621–628. [CrossRef]
7. Förch, S.; Sandriesser, S.; Mayr, E.; Schrödl, F.; von Rüden, C.; Augat, P. Biomechanical comparison of different cerclage types in addition to an angle stable plate osteosynthesis of distal tibial fractures. *Injury* **2021**, *52*, 2126–2130. [CrossRef]
8. Förch, S.; Reuter, J.; von der Helm, F.; Lisitano, L.; Hartwig, C.; Sandriesser, S.; Nuber, S.; Mayr, E. A minimally invasive cerclage of the tibia in a modified Goetze technique: Operative technique and first clinical results. *Eur. J. Trauma Emerg. Surg.* **2021**, *48*, 3115–3122. [CrossRef]
9. Förch, S.; Sandriesser, S.; Fenwick, A.; Mayr, E. Impairment of the blood supply by cerclages: Myth or reality? An overview of the experimental study situation. *Unfallchirurg* **2020**, *124*, 231–240. [CrossRef]
10. Bleeker, N.J.; van de Wall, B.J.M.; FFA, I.J.; Doornberg, J.N.; Kerkhoffs, G.; Jaarsma, R.L.; Knobe, M.; Link, B.C.; Babst, R.; Beeres, F.J.P. Plate vs. nail for extra-articular distal tibia fractures: How should we personalize surgical treatment? A meta-analysis of 1332 patients. *Injury* **2021**, *52*, 345–357. [CrossRef]
11. Ekman, E.; Lehtimäki, K.; Syvänen, J.; Saltychev, M. Comparison Between Nailing and Plating in the Treatment of Distal Tibial Fractures: A Meta-Analysis. *Scand. J. Surg.* **2021**, *110*, 115–122. [CrossRef]
12. Habernek, H. Percutaneous cerclage wiring and interlocking nailing for treatment of torsional fractures of the tibia. *Clin. Orthop. Relat. Res.* **1991**, *267*, 164–168. [CrossRef]
13. Huang, M.T.; Lin, C.J. Percutaneous cerclage wiring-assisted interlocking nailing for torsional tibia fractures: A modification with improved safety and simplicity. *J. Trauma* **2011**, *71*, 1054–1058. [CrossRef]
14. Augat, P.; Burger, J.; Schorlemmer, S.; Henke, T.; Peraus, M.; Claes, L. Shear movement at the fracture site delays healing in a diaphyseal fracture model. *J. Orthop. Res.* **2003**, *21*, 1011–1017. [CrossRef]
15. Bliemel, C.; Anrich, B.; Knauf, T.; Oberkircher, L.; Eschbach, D.; Klasan, A.; Debus, F.; Ruchholtz, S.; Baumlein, M. More than a reposition tool: Additional wire cerclage leads to increased load to failure in plate osteosynthesis for supracondylar femoral shaft fractures. *Arch. Orthop. Trauma Surg.* **2020**, *141*, 1197–1205. [CrossRef]
16. Perren, S.M.; Fernandez Dell'oca, A.; Regazzoni, P. Fracture Fixation Using Cerclage, Research Applied to Surgery. *Acta Chir. Orthop. Traumatol. Cech.* **2015**, *82*, 389–397.
17. Gordon, K.; Winkler, M.; Hofstadter, T.; Dorn, U.; Augat, P. Managing Vancouver B1 fractures by cerclage system compared to locking plate fixation-a biomechanical study. *Injury* **2016**, *47* (Suppl. S2), S51–S57. [CrossRef]
18. Apivatthakakul, T.; Siripipattanamongkol, P.; Oh, C.W.; Sananpanich, K.; Phornphutkul, C. Safe zones and a technical guide for cerclage wiring of the femur: A computed topographic angiogram (CTA) study. *Arch. Orthop. Trauma Surg.* **2018**, *138*, 43–50. [CrossRef]
19. Codesido, P.; Mejia, A.; Riego, J.; Ojeda-Thies, C. Subtrochanteric fractures in elderly people treated with intramedullary fixation: Quality of life and complications following open reduction and cerclage wiring versus closed reduction. *Arch. Orthop. Trauma Surg.* **2017**, *137*, 1077–1085. [CrossRef]
20. Hoskins, W.; Bingham, R.; Joseph, S.; Liew, D.; Love, D.; Bucknill, A.; Oppy, A.; Griffin, X. Subtrochanteric fracture: The effect of cerclage wire on fracture reduction and outcome. *Injury* **2015**, *46*, 1992–1995. [CrossRef]
21. Ottesen, T.D.; McLynn, R.P.; Galivanche, A.R.; Bagi, P.S.; Zogg, C.K.; Rubin, L.E.; Grauer, J.N. Increased complications in geriatric patients with a fracture of the hip whose postoperative weight-bearing is restricted: An analysis of 4918 patients. *Bone Joint J.* **2018**, *100-B*, 1377–1384. [CrossRef]
22. Pfeufer, D.; Zeller, A.; Mehaffey, S.; Bocker, W.; Kammerlander, C.; Neuerburg, C. Weight-bearing restrictions reduce postoperative mobility in elderly hip fracture patients. *Arch. Orthop. Trauma Surg.* **2019**, *139*, 1253–1259. [CrossRef] [PubMed]

23. Paulsson, M.; Ekholm, C.; Jonsson, E.; Geijer, M.; Rolfson, O. Immediate Full Weight-Bearing Versus Partial Weight-Bearing After Plate Fixation of Distal Femur Fractures in Elderly Patients. A Randomized Controlled Trial. *Geriatr. Orthop. Surg. Rehabil.* **2021**, *12*, 21514593211055889. [CrossRef] [PubMed]
24. Smeeing, D.P.J.; Houwert, R.M.; Briet, J.P.; Groenwold, R.H.H.; Lansink, K.W.W.; Leenen, L.P.H.; van der Zwaal, P.; Hoogendoorn, J.M.; van Heijl, M.; Verleisdonk, E.J.; et al. Weight-bearing or non-weight-bearing after surgical treatment of ankle fractures: A multicenter randomized controlled trial. *Eur. J. Trauma Emerg. Surg.* **2020**, *46*, 121–130. [CrossRef] [PubMed]
25. Gross, S.C.; Galos, D.K.; Taormina, D.P.; Crespo, A.; Egol, K.A.; Tejwani, N.C. Can Tibial Shaft Fractures Bear Weight After Intramedullary Nailing? A Randomized Controlled Trial. *J. Orthop. Trauma* **2016**, *30*, 370–375. [CrossRef] [PubMed]
26. Hoegel, F.W.; Hoffmann, S.; Weninger, P.; Bühren, V.; Augat, P. Biomechanical comparison of locked plate osteosynthesis, reamed and unreamed nailing in conventional interlocking technique, and unreamed angle stable nailing in distal tibia fractures. *J. Trauma Acute Care Surg.* **2012**, *73*, 933–938. [CrossRef]
27. Claes, L. Mechanobiology of fracture healing part 2:Relevance for internal fixation of fractures. *Unfallchirurg* **2017**, *120*, 23–31. [CrossRef]
28. Claes, L. Mechanobiology of fracture healing part 1:Principles. *Unfallchirurg* **2017**, *120*, 14–22. [CrossRef]
29. Epari, D.R.; Kassi, J.P.; Schell, H.; Duda, G.N. Timely fracture-healing requires optimization of axial fixation stability. *J. Bone Joint Surg. Am.* **2007**, *89*, 1575–1585. [CrossRef]
30. Högel, F.; Gerber, C.; Bühren, V.; Augat, P. Reamed intramedullary nailing of diaphyseal tibial fractures: Comparison of compression and non-compression nailing. *Eur. J. Trauma Emerg. Surg.* **2013**, *39*, 73–77. [CrossRef]
31. Gonschorek, O.; Hofmann, G.O.; Bühren, V. Interlocking compression nailing: A report on 402 applications. *Arch. Orthop. Trauma Surg.* **1998**, *117*, 430–437. [CrossRef]
32. Bisaccia, M.; Cappiello, A.; Meccariello, L.; Rinonapoli, G.; Falzarano, G.; Medici, A.; Vicente, C.I.; Piscitelli, L.; Stano, V.; Bisaccia, O.; et al. Nail or plate in the management of distal extra-articular tibial fracture, what is better? Valutation of outcomes. *SICOT J.* **2018**, *4*, 2. [CrossRef]
33. Hu, L.; Xiong, Y.; Mi, B.; Panayi, A.C.; Zhou, W.; Liu, Y.; Liu, J.; Xue, H.; Yan, C.; Abududilibaier, A.; et al. Comparison of intramedullary nailing and plate fixation in distal tibial fractures with metaphyseal damage: A meta-analysis of randomized controlled trials. *J. Orthop. Surg. Res.* **2019**, *14*, 30. [CrossRef]
34. Casstevens, C.; Le, T.; Archdeacon, M.T.; Wyrick, J.D. Management of extra-articular fractures of the distal tibia: Intramedullary nailing versus plate fixation. *J. Am. Acad. Orthop. Surg.* **2012**, *20*, 675–683. [CrossRef]
35. Mao, Z.; Wang, G.; Zhang, L.; Zhang, L.; Chen, S.; Du, H.; Zhao, Y.; Tang, P. Intramedullary nailing versus plating for distal tibia fractures without articular involvement: A meta-analysis. *J. Orthop. Surg. Res.* **2015**, *10*, 95. [CrossRef]
36. Augat, P.; Penzkofer, R.; Nolte, A.; Maier, M.; Panzer, S.; v Oldenburg, G.; Pueschl, K.; Simon, U.; Buhren, V. Interfragmentary movement in diaphyseal tibia fractures fixed with locked intramedullary nails. *J. Orthop. Trauma* **2008**, *22*, 30–36. [CrossRef]
37. Claes, L.; Eckert-Hubner, K.; Augat, P. The fracture gap size influences the local vascularization and tissue differentiation in callus healing. *Langenbecks Arch. Surg.* **2003**, *388*, 316–322. [CrossRef]
38. Gardner, M.J.; Silva, M.J.; Krieg, J.C. Biomechanical testing of fracture fixation constructs: Variability, validity, and clinical applicability. *J. Am. Acad. Orthop. Surg.* **2012**, *20*, 86–93. [CrossRef]

Disclaimer/Publisher's Note: The statements, opinions and data contained in all publications are solely those of the individual author(s) and contributor(s) and not of MDPI and/or the editor(s). MDPI and/or the editor(s) disclaim responsibility for any injury to people or property resulting from any ideas, methods, instructions or products referred to in the content.

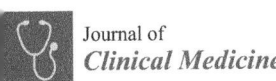

Article

Advances in the Treatment of Implant-Associated Infections of the Pelvis: Eradication Rates, Recurrence of Infection, and Outcome

Florian Kellermann [1,2], Simon Hackl [1], Iris Leister [1], Sven Hungerer [1], Matthias Militz [1], Fabian Stuby [1], Bernhard Holzmann [2] and Jan Friederichs [1,*]

1 Trauma Center Murnau, Prof.-Küntscher-Str. 8, 82418 Murnau, Germany
2 Department of Surgery, Klinikum Rechts der Isar München, 81675 Munich, Germany
* Correspondence: jan.friederichs@bgu-murnau.de; Tel.: +49-8841-484731; Fax: +49-8841-484678

Abstract: Introduction: Surgical site infections after operative stabilization of pelvic and acetabular fractures are rare but serious complications. The treatment of these infections involves additional surgical procedures, high health care costs, a prolonged stay, and often a worse outcome. In this study, we focused on the impact of the different causing bacteria, negative microbiological results with wound closure, and recurrence rates of patients with implant-associated infections after pelvic surgery. Material and Methods: We retrospectively analyzed a study group of 43 patients with microbiologically proven surgical site infections (SSI) after surgery of the pelvic ring or the acetabulum treated in our clinic between 2009 and 2019. Epidemiological data, injury pattern, surgical approach, and microbiological data were analyzed and correlated with long-term follow-up and recurrence of infection. Results: Almost two thirds of the patients presented with polymicrobial infections, with staphylococci being the most common causing agents. An average of 5.7 (±5.4) surgical procedures were performed until definitive wound closure. Negative microbiological swabs at time of wound closure were only achieved in 9 patients (21%). Long-term follow-up revealed a recurrence of infection in only seven patients (16%) with an average interval between revision surgery and recurrence of 4.7 months. There was no significant difference of recurrence rate for the groups of patients with positive/negative microbiology in the last operative revision (71% vs. 78%). A positive trend for a correlation with recurrent infection was only found for patients with a Morel–Lavallée lesion due to run-over injuries (30% vs. 5%). Identified causing bacteria did not influence the outcome and rate of recurrence. Conclusion: Recurrence rates after surgical revision of implant-associated infections of the pelvis and the acetabulum are low and neither the type of causing agent nor the microbiological status at the timepoint of wound closure has a significant impact on the recurrence rate.

Keywords: osteosynthesis; pelvic fractures; infection; eradication; recurrence

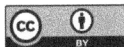

1. Introduction

Unstable pelvic fractures usually result from a high-energy mechanism. Nonoperative treatment of such fractures often leads to significant disabilities. Therefore, various techniques for operative stabilization of both the anterior and posterior pelvic ring have been described [1–3]. However, due to extensive surgical approaches, the long duration of operative procedures, and concomitant soft-tissue damage and postoperative infection rates were reported to be as high as 18–27% in early series for posterior approaches of type C pelvic fractures [4] and have improved to rates below 5% in more recent studies [1]. Similar rates of infection have been reported after the osteosynthetic stabilization of the anterior pelvic ring and operative reconstruction of acetabular fractures [5,6]. Infection rates can be even higher, up to 50%, for open pelvic fractures or complex fractures with concomitant injuries of the rectum or bladder, resulting in worse overall outcomes [7,8].

A recent study by Karakaris et al. analyzed patients with deep infections following operative reconstruction of pelvic fractures and concluded that surgical site infections (SSI) are a rare but serious complication of pelvic surgery, occurring in 2.1% of cases. Injury- and surgery-related risk factors were identified, such as fracture type, high Injury Severity Score (ISS), long duration of surgery, and a posterior sacral approach. Significant patient factors included obesity, diabetes, and alcohol consumption [9]. Interestingly, no significant correlation was observed between surgical site infection and pelvic packing, pelvic arterial embolization (PAE), or Morel–Lavallee lesion, contrary to previous reports [10–12].

A surgical site infection of the pelvis can have serious consequences, such as prolonged hospital stay, increased healthcare costs, possible readmissions, and worse physical, social, and psychological outcomes [9,10]. Conservative treatment is not possible, and a long regimen of operations is required to eradicate the infection without compromising stability and function. Karakaris et al. found that up to 16 operations were necessary to achieve this aim, with a median number of 3 operations. However, complete eradication was achieved in 93% of patients [9].

While the prevention of surgical site infections has improved over the last decades due to advanced surgical techniques, identification of risk factors, and post-operative measures, only a few studies focus on the management and outcome of surgical site infections after pelvic surgery and little is known about treatment algorithms, effectiveness of different measures such as vacuum assistant closure (VAC), causative bacteria, negative microbiological results with wound closure, and long-term results after eradication [9]. There are several case reports and small series, for example, the recent study of Vaidya, where a series of 10 infections after anterior subcutaneous internal fixation of the pelvis were analyzed [13]. The predominant causative agent was *Staphylococcus aureus*; surgical irrigation and debridement, implant removal, and culture-specific antibiotics led to a favorable outcome in all ten patients. This goes in accordance to clinical practice, several case reports, and postoperative deep wound infections of other locations [10–12]. However, to our knowledge, there is no study that focuses on long-term recurrence rates of patients with posttraumatic infections of the pelvis.

Therefore, the aim of our study is to focus on the long-term results of patients with microbiologically proven surgical site infections after pelvic surgery. This rare subgroup of patients has not been previously studied, and no data exist regarding the impact of different causative bacteria, negative microbiological results with wound closure, and recurrence rates.

2. Material and Methods

The retrospective cohort single center study was conducted at our Level One Trauma Center. All patients with microbiologically proven surgical site infections (SSI) after surgery of the pelvic ring or the acetabulum treated in our clinic between 2009 and 2019 were included. The study adhered to ethical standards set by the institutional and national research committee and was approved by the local ethics committee in compliance with the 1964 Helsinki Declaration and its subsequent amendments. Patients provided written informed consent before receiving treatment. Exclusion criteria were patients aged <18 years, and patients with only soft-tissue infections or decubiti as well as infections after endoprosthetic surgery. The study recorded patient data such as sex, age, trauma mechanism, primary fracture classification according to the AO and Letournel systems, primary operative access, procedure, time to infection, number of operations, and length of hospital stay. It also documented the initial microbiological result, changes in detected causative bacteria, and microbiological result at the time of wound closure. Table 1 summarizes the patient data.

Table 1. Clinical characteristics of 43 patients with implant-associated infections of the pelvis and the acetabulum.

Age (years)	45.4 (±15.4)
Male	32 (74.4%)
Female	11 (25.6%)
Early infection (<6 weeks)	24 (56%)
Late infection >6 weeks)	19 (44%)
Days in hospital (median)	45 (7–330)
Number of operations (average)	5.7 (±5.4)
Follow-up (median, months)	98.2 (24–226)

2.1. Surgical Procedure

All patients were treated in our Department of Septic Surgery following a standardized pre-, intra-, and post-operative management protocol. Preoperative management included a thorough clinical examination by the treating surgeon, a CT scan, an evaluation of comorbidities, a detailed analysis of the previous operative procedure, and a standardized blood analysis including all parameters of infection. The standardized intraoperative protocol of the index operation put the focus on the proof of the surgical site infection and the identification of the causing bacteria and thus was strictly followed by the operating surgeon. Surgery was performed under general anesthesia using pre-existent access if possible. Perioperative antibiotic treatment was initiated only after taking at least two swabs, and two pieces of tissue for microbiological and histological examination were taken from representative areas of the affected region. According to the protocol, the empirical antimicrobial regimen was continued until a modification according to the culture results was possible. In the index operation, hardware was removed only when an infection was macroscopically without doubt or had been proven before. If necessary, mechanical stability was restored by external fixation. The removal of the metalwork was followed by a radical debridement with resection of all fibrotic and macroscopically infected tissue of the interphase. After the administration of local antiseptic solution (Octenidin, Polyhexamide), vacuum-assisted closure (VAC) of the surgical site was achieved and a standardized multi-stage surgical revision protocol was started with operative debridement every 5–7 days based on clinical and biochemical parameters, the soft-tissue status, the extent of the infection, and on the virulence of the microorganism. This revision protocol was repeated until short-term cultures were negative, a macroscopically clean soft-tissue status was achieved and clinical and biochemical parameters had improved accordingly. The wound was then finally closed, and test-specific antimicrobial medication was continued for at least 6 weeks after the last surgical intervention.

2.2. Microbiological Examination

To conduct microbiological analysis, at least three dry swabs (MASTASWAB TM, Mast Group Ltd., Bootle, UK) were taken directly from the removed implant, the interface, and from macroscopically suspicious areas of the wound. The swabs were streaked out on Columbia agar with 5% sheep blood, chocolate agar, MacConkey agar, and thioglycolate broth (bioMerieux, Hazelwood, MO, USA). Samples were then incubated at 37 °C in 5% CO_2 or anaerobic conditions for 48 h for short-term culturing; morphologically distinct colonies were identified and antibiotic susceptibility to 28 antibiotics was determined using the Vitek2-machine (bioMerieux, Hazelwood, MO, USA) with standardized definition of minimum inhibitory concentration (MIC) and multi-drug resistance [14]. At least two tissue samples from the interface, non-union, or macroscopically suspicious areas were directly inserted into a sterile containment prefilled with 9 ml of thioglycolate broth (bioMerieux, Hazelwood, MO, USA). After incubation at 37 °C in 5% CO_2 or under anaerobic conditions for at least 14 days (long-term culturing), the suspension was additionally streaked out and proceeded as described above.

2.3. Follow-Up

Patients were followed up in our outpatient department at regular intervals after 6 weeks, 3 months, and 6 months. Follow-up included a clinical examination, systemic inflammatory parameters, and a radiological follow-up. Revision surgery and/or antibiotic treatment due to soft-tissue inflammation was documented. For long-term follow-up, patients were contacted via a short survey or by telephone focusing on recurrence of infection and conservative treatment or revision surgery due to recurrent infection. Loss of follow-up was documented if no contact with the patient was achieved.

2.4. Statistical Analysis

Statistical analysis was performed using IBM SPSS®Statistics for Windows 19.0 (IBM Corp., Armonk, NY, USA). Results of this study are presented as mean values ± standard error of the mean (SEM) or median. Significance was statistically calculated based on the Mann–Whitney U-test or Fisher's exact test. Results were considered to be statistically significant with p values < 0.05.

3. Results

3.1. Epidemiology and Initial Surgical Approach

The study included 43 patients who had confirmed surgical site infections (SSI) following surgery of the pelvic ring or the acetabulum. The epidemiological information of the study participants is outlined in Table 1. Of the 43 patients, 27 (63%) received surgical stabilization of instable pelvic fractures (Type B (n = 11 (26%)) and C (n = 16 (37%))), 5 patients (12%) were treated for surgical site infections after isolated acetabular fractures, and, in 7 patients (16%), surgical intervention addressed the combination of unstable pelvic fracture and acetabular fracture. The remaining four patients comprised of two hemipelvectomies and two unclassified injuries. The injury patterns described above led to a total of 88 initial operative approaches involving the anterior (n = 37), the posterior (n = 43) pelvic ring, the acetabulum (n = 5), and others (n = 3), as shown in Figure 1.

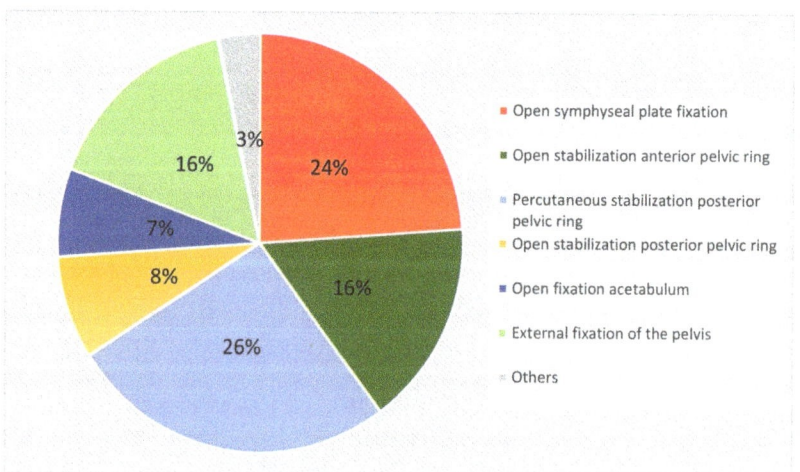

Figure 1. Initial surgical approaches of 43 patients with subsequent implant-associated infections after surgical treatment of fractures of the pelvis and the acetabulum (n = 88).

3.2. Microbiology

The index operation aimed at the removal of all hardware, the identification of the causing agent, and a radical debridement of infected tissue. The identification of the causing pathogen was achieved in all 43 patients revealing a total of 36 different bacteria and fungi (Table S1). Over the course of revision surgery, *Staphylococcus epidermidis* was detected in 26 patients (60.5%) and *Staphylococcus aureus* in 16 patients (37.2%). The eight most frequent species are listed in Figure 2. Almost two thirds of the patients presented with polymicrobial infections (2–8 different bacteria and fungi); monomicrobial infections were observed in 14 patients (32.6%), half of them caused by *Staphylococcus epidermidis* (7 patients), four infections caused by *Staphylococcus aureus*, two by enterococci, and one by clostridium difficile. During the revision surgery, in 21 of 43 patients (48.8%), a change of the bacterial species was observed, while the intraoperative swabs showed a persistent colonization pattern throughout the surgical treatment in 22 patients (51.2%).

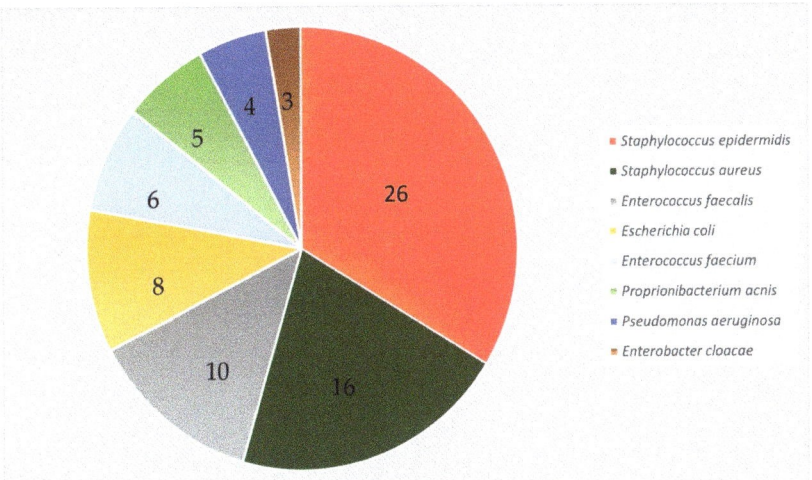

Figure 2. Microbiological results of 43 patients with implant-associated infections after surgical treatment of fractures of the pelvis and the acetabulum. Two thirds of infections were polymicrobial; 36 different bacteria and fungi were detected. The eight most frequent bacteria are listed.

3.3. Eradication Rate and Recurrence of Infection

Revision surgery aimed at the eradication of the infection. However, an eradication with negative swabs at the time point of wound closure was only achieved for 9 patients (21%). A total of 34 wounds still had positive microbiological results in the long-term culture of the last operation (79%).

However, in the long-term follow-up, only seven patients (16%) suffered of a recurrent infection with an average time interval of 4.7 months between revision surgery and recurrence. Nine patients (21%) were lost to follow-up, while twenty-seven patients (63%) showed no signs of infection during a follow-up period ranging from 24 to 226 months. There was no significant correlation between recurrence rate and age, sex, surgical approach, fracture classification, type of osteosynthesis, number of surgical revisions, or early/late surgical site infection. Interestingly, there was no significant difference of recurrence rate for the groups of patients with positive/negative microbiology in the last operative revision (71% vs. 78%). A positive trend for a correlation with recurrent infection was only found for patients with a Morel–Lavallée lesion due to run-over injuries (30% vs. 5%). The identified bacteria did not influence outcome and rate of recurrence, the distribution of the most frequent germs was almost identical in both groups as shown in Table 2.

Table 2. Most frequent causing bacteria of implant-associated infections after pelvic surgery related to recurrence of infection in long-term follow-up. Note that polymicrobial infections were found in almost two thirds of the patients.

Recurrent Infection	Non-Recurrent Infection
n = 7 (16%)	27 (63%)
Staphylococcus epidermidis (57%)	*Staphylococcus epidermidis* (67%)
Enterococcus faecalis (43%)	*Staphylococcus aureus* (39%)
Staphylococcus aureus (29%)	*Enterococcus faecalis* (19%)
	Escherichia coli (19%)
	Enterococcus faecium (17%)
	Pseudomonas aeruginosa (8%)

In summary, the likelihood of implant-associated infection recurrence in the pelvis and acetabulum following surgical revision is relatively low. The recurrence rate is not significantly affected by either the type of causative agent or the microbiological status at the time of wound closure.

4. Discussion

Surgical site infections following pelvic surgery are a rare yet severe complication that often require extended hospitalization, multiple revision surgeries, and prolonged antibiotic therapy. Proper management of soft tissues is crucial, but treating surgeons have noted a high rate of persistent infection and recurrence after revision surgery. Our study, which involved a large group of 43 patients, is the first to show that even after a long-term follow-up of two to nine years, the recurrence rate is relatively low at 16%, indicating a positive prognosis for revision surgery.

In most cases, revision surgery did not manage to completely eradicate the causing bacteria. Only in 9 patients (21%) negative microbiological results were achieved until secondary wound closure. However, the recurrence rate did not significantly differ between patients with a microbiologically eradicated site at the time of wound closure and those with persisting positive swabs. This finding is unexpected and could change the paradigm of postoperative infection treatment after pelvic surgery. Corresponding to our protocol, the eradication procedures of surgical site infections of the pelvis often involve multiple operations over a long period of time, putting a high burden on the patient. Advancements in surgical treatment with a more radical initial debridement in combination with the knowledge gained in our study could lead to fewer operations, shorter hospital stays, lower treatment costs, and less stress for the patient.

One of the largest studies on early reoperation of acetabular fractures due to surgical site infections was published by Ding and coworkers in 2018 [6]. Due to the large study collective, they were able to analyze 56 patients reoperated due to implant-associated infections after operative stabilization of acetabular fractures and reported an infection rate of 7% which is comparable to other reported infection rates after acetabular surgery [15–17]. The median time for postoperative infection occurred at 2.4 weeks after the index operation, with a range of up to 102 weeks. Presumably, the rate of early and late infections is comparable to our study collective where 56% of infections were early infections (<6 weeks). In contrast to our study, microbiological examination proved polymicrobial infections in only approximately one third of the patients while we were able to identify more than one causing agent (up to eight) in two thirds of the patients. Nevertheless, the genus distribution was comparable to our study and other reported results with *Staphylococcus aureus*, *Staphylococcus epidermidis*, and *Enterococcus faecalis* being the most common bacteria [16,17]. In contrast, Torbert et al. detected a higher percentage of gram-negative bacteria with up to 63% of all infections [18]. Although many of the prevailing studies describe the standard surgical procedure for the treatment of deep surgical site infections of the pelvis, there is little information about the success of these operations. In their study, Suzuki and coworkers describe a mean of 3.3 surgical revisions for a deep infection with a range of 1–13 operations [17]. Only 40% of the cases necessitated implant removal, and culture specific local and systemic antibiotic therapy was administered according to international standards. However, no information regarding long-term success and recurrence rates is provided.

The Morel–Lavallée lesion is described as an internal degloving injury caused by shear forces on the soft tissue of the pelvis, a frequent concomitant injury of severe pelvic fractures. Due to the severity of the fracture and of other concomitant injuries, the Morel–Lavallée lesion is often underestimated and undertreated. Several studies have proven that the risk of soft-tissue infection of this lesion is high [17,19,20] and the risk of a surgical sight infection even on other locations of the pelvis is increased [17,21]. Our study adds the important results, that the recurrence rate after revision surgery of implant-associated infections of the pelvis is higher in patients with an initial Morel–Lavallée lesion. This finding is significant and should be considered when determining the appropriate surgical treatment for infections in the pelvis.

There are certain limitations of this retrospective single center cohort study. The surgical treatment in a single center might lead to a selection bias; the heterogeneous operative approaches might also act as confounding factors. However, the series of 43 patients operatively revised for implant-associated infections of the pelvis is the largest series found in the literature.

5. Conclusions

In summary, our study's findings may contribute to advancements in surgical treatments for implant-associated infections following pelvic surgery. Contrary to the belief that these infections are difficult to treat and have a poor prognosis with a high recurrence rate, our long-term follow-up showed a recurrence in only 16% of patients. Furthermore, our data suggests that performing one or more negative swabs prior to wound closure may not be necessary for successful therapy, as recurrence rates were similar for both negative and positive wound closures. This implies that fewer operations may be required to achieve treatment success. Nevertheless, we recommend thorough soft-tissue management and potentially more aggressive surgical debridement for patients with previous soft-tissue problems such as the Morel–Lavallée lesion.

Supplementary Materials: The following supporting information can be downloaded at: https://www.mdpi.com/article/10.3390/jcm12082854/s1, Table S1. All detected bacteria and fungi, the first eight bacterial were detected in twice, all other bacteria and fungi were only detected once.

Author Contributions: Conceptualization, S.H. (Sven Hungerer), M.M., B.H. and J.F.; methodology, J.F.; formal analysis, F.K., S.H. (Simon Hackl), I.L. and S.H. (Sven Hungerer); investigation, F.K. and J.F.; resources, F.K.; data curation, J.F.; writing—original draft, F.K. and J.F.; writing—review and editing, S.H. (Simon Hackl) and J.F.; supervision, F.S. and B.H. All authors have read and agreed to the published version of the manuscript.

Funding: This research received no external funding.

Institutional Review Board Statement: The study was conducted in accordance with the Declaration of Helsinki and approved by the Institutional Review Board (or Ethics Committee) of the BLAEK (Bayerische Landesärztekammer, No. 2023-1039).

Informed Consent Statement: Patients provided written informed consent.

Data Availability Statement: Data are not available due to privacy and ethical restrictions.

Conflicts of Interest: The authors declare no conflict of interest.

References

1. Stover, M.D.; Sims, S.; Matta, J. What is the infection rate of the posterior approach to type C pelvic injuries? *Clin. Orthop. Relat. Res.* **2012**, *470*, 2142–2147. [CrossRef] [PubMed]
2. Kellam, J.F.; McMurtry, R.Y.; Paley, D.; Tile, M. The unstable pelvic fracture. *Operative treatment. Orthop. Clin. North Am.* **1987**, *18*, 25–41. [PubMed]
3. Vaidya, R.; Kubiak, I.N.; Bergin, P.F.; Dombroski, D.G.; Critchlow, R.J.; Sethi, A.; Starr, A.J. Complications of anterior subcutaneous internal fixation for unstable pelvis fractures: A multicenter study. *Clin. Orthop. Relat. Res.* **2012**, *470*, 2124–2131. [CrossRef] [PubMed]
4. Goldstein, A.; Phillips, T.; Sclafani, S.J.; Scalea, T.; Duncan, A.; Goldstein, J.; Panetta, T.; Shaftan, G. Early open reduction and internal fixation of the disrupted pelvic ring. *J. Trauma. Inj. Infect. Crit. Care.* **1986**, *26*, 325–333. [CrossRef] [PubMed]
5. Morris, S.A.C.; Loveridge, J.; Smart, D.K.A.; Ward, A.J.; Chesser, T.J.S. Is fixation failure after plate fixation of the symphysis pubis clinically important? *Clin. Orthop. Relat. Res.* **2012**, *470*, 2154–2160. [CrossRef] [PubMed]
6. Ding, A.; O'Toole, R.V.; Castillo, R.; Reahl, B.; Montalvo, R.; Nascone, J.W.; Sciadini, M.F.; Carlini, A.R.; Manson, T.T. Risk Factors for early reoperation after operative treatment of Acetabular Fractures. *J. Orthop. Trauma* **2018**, *32*, 251–257. [CrossRef] [PubMed]
7. Song, W.; Zhou, D.; Xu, W.; Zhang, G.; Wang, C.; Qiu, D.; Dong, J. Factors of pelvic infection and death in patients with open pelvic fractures and rectal injuries. *Surg. Infect.* **2017**, *18*, 711–715. [CrossRef] [PubMed]
8. Yao, H.H.; Esser, M.; Grummet, J.; Atkins, C.; Royce, P.; Hanegbi, U. Lower risk of pelvic metalware infection with operative repair of concurrent bladder rupture. *ANZ J. Surg.* **2018**, *88*, 560–564.
9. Kanakaris, N.K.; Ciriello, V.; Stavrou, P.Z.; West, R.M.; Giannoudis, P.V. Deep infection following reconstruction of pelvic fractures: Prevalence, characteristics and predisposing risk factors. *Eur. J. Trauma Emerg. Surg.* **2021**, *48*, 3701–3709. [CrossRef] [PubMed]
10. Whitehouse, J.D.; Friedman, N.D.; Kirkland, K.B.; Richardson, W.J.; Sexton, D.J. The impact of surgical-site infections following orthopedic surgery at a community hospital and a university hospital: Adverse quality of life, excess length of stay and extra cost. *Infect Control Hosp. Epidemiol.* **2002**, *23*, 183–189. [CrossRef] [PubMed]
11. Manson, T.T.; Perdue, P.W.; Pollack, A.N.; O'Toole, R.V. Embolization of pelvic arterial injury is a risk factor for deep infection after acetabular fracture surgery. *J. Orthop. Trauma* **2012**, *27*, 11–15. [CrossRef] [PubMed]
12. Papakostidis, C.; Giannoudis, P.V. Pelvic ring injuries with haemodynamic instability: Efficacy of pelvic packing, a systematic review. *Injury* **2009**, *40*, 53–61. [CrossRef] [PubMed]
13. Vaidya, R.; Amar, K.; Woodburry, D.; Washington, A. Infection after the use of INFIX in pelvic ring injuries. *SICOT J.* **2021**, *7*, 1–6. [CrossRef] [PubMed]
14. Brown, D.F.; Wootton, M.; Howe, R.A. Antimicrobial susceptibility testing break-points and methods from BSAC to EUCAST. *J. Antimicrob. Chemother.* **2016**, *71*, 3–5. [CrossRef] [PubMed]
15. Sagi, C.H.; Dziadosz, D.; Mir, H.; Virani, N.; Olson, C. Obesity, Leukocytosis, Embolization, and Injury Severity increase the risk for deep postoperative Wound Infection after Pelvic and Acetabular Surgery. *J. Orthop. Trauma* **2013**, *27*, 6–10. [CrossRef] [PubMed]
16. Iqbal, F.; Younus, S.; Asmatullah; Bin Zia, O.; Khan, N. Surgical Site Infection following fixation of acetabular fractures. *Hip. Pelvis.* **2017**, *29*, 176–181. [CrossRef] [PubMed]
17. Suzuki, T.; Morgan, S.J.; Smith, W.R.; Stahel, P.F.; Gillani, S.A.; Hak, D.J. Postoperative surgical site infection following acetabular fracture fixation. *Injury* **2010**, *41*, 396–399. [CrossRef] [PubMed]
18. Torbert, J.T.; Joshi, M.; Moraff, A.; Matuszewski, P.E.; Holmes, A.; Pollak, A.M.; O'Toole, O.V. Current bacterial speciation and antibiotic resistance in deep infection after operative fixation of fractures. *J. Orthop. Trauma* **2015**, *29*, 7–17. [CrossRef] [PubMed]
19. Letournel, E.; Judet, R. *Fractures of the Acetabulum*; Springer: Berlin, Germany, 1993.
20. Hak, D.J.; Olson, S.A.; Matta, J.M. Diagnosis and management of closed internal degloving injuries associated with pelvic and acetabular fractures: The Morel-Lavallée lesion. *J. Trauma* **1997**, *42*, 1046–1051. [CrossRef] [PubMed]
21. Tseng, S.; Tornetta, P., 3rd. Percutaneous management of Morel-Lavallée lesions. *J. Bone Joint Surg. Am.* **2006**, *88*, 92–96. [PubMed]

Disclaimer/Publisher's Note: The statements, opinions and data contained in all publications are solely those of the individual author(s) and contributor(s) and not of MDPI and/or the editor(s). MDPI and/or the editor(s) disclaim responsibility for any injury to people or property resulting from any ideas, methods, instructions or products referred to in the content.

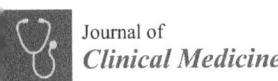

Article

Risk of Interprosthetic Femur Fracture Is Associated with Implant Spacing—A Biomechanical Study

Mischa Mühling [1,2,†], Sabrina Sandriesser [1,2,†], Claudio Glowalla [3], Sven Herrmann [1,2], Peter Augat [1,2] and Sven Hungerer [1,2,3,*]

[1] Institute for Biomechanics, BG Unfallklinik Murnau, Prof. Küntscher Str. 8, 82418 Murnau, Germany; mischa.muehling@bgu-murnau.de (M.M.)
[2] Institute for Biomechanics, Paracelsus Medical University, Strubergasse 21, 5020 Salzburg, Austria
[3] Department of Arthroplasty, BG Unfallklinik Murnau, Prof. Küntscher Str. 8, 82418 Murnau, Germany
* Correspondence: sven.hungerer@bgu-murnau.de
† These authors contributed equally to this work.

Abstract: Background: Ipsilateral revision surgeries of total hip or knee arthroplasties due to periprosthetic fractures or implant loosening are becoming more frequent in aging populations. Implants in revision arthroplasty usually require long anchoring stems. Depending on the residual distance between two adjacent knee and hip implants, we assume that the risk of interprosthetic fractures increases with a reduction in the interprosthetic distance. The aim of the current study was to investigate the maximum strain within the femoral shaft between two ipsilateral implants tips. Methods: A simplified physical model consisting of synthetic bone tubes and metallic implant cylinders was constructed and the surface strains were measured using digital image correlation. The strain distribution on the femoral shaft was analyzed in 3-point- and 4-point-bending scenarios. The physical model was transferred to a finite element model to parametrically investigate the effects of the interprosthetic distance and the cortical thickness on maximum strain. Strain patterns for all parametric combinations were compared to the reference strain pattern of the bone without implants. Results: The presence of an implant reduced principal strain values but resulted in distinct strain peaks at the locations of the implant tips. A reduced interprosthetic distance and thinner cortices resulted in strain peaks of up to 180% compared to the reference. At low cortical thicknesses, the strain peaks increased exponentially with a decrease in the interprosthetic distance. An increasing cortical thickness reduced the peak strains at the implant tips. Conclusions: A minimum interprosthetic distance of 10 mm seems to be crucial to avoid the accumulation of strain peaks caused by ipsilateral implant tips. Interprosthetic fracture management is more important in patients with reduced bone quality.

Keywords: interprosthetic fracture; kissing implants; total hip arthroplasty; total knee arthroplasty

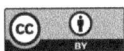

1. Introduction

The number of total hip arthroplasties (THA) and total knee arthroplasties (TKA) is increasing worldwide in industrial countries with an ageing population as there is a positive correlation of osteoarthritis with age [1,2]. As a result, the frequency of revision surgeries after THA or TKA is also increasing. The most common reasons for revision surgery are infection, implant loosening or periprosthetic fractures [3–5]. Revision surgery of hip and knee arthroplasty is often associated with longer anchoring stems and requires significant surgical expertise [6,7]. Problems arise in patients with ipsilateral adjacent hip and knee implants with only a short residual length between implants. The risk of interprosthetic fractures is high because of the reduced bone quality in elderly patients and is further elevated by implant rigidity [8]. Megaprostheses, such as total femur replacement, as alternative treatment options are associated with high rates of intraoperative morbidity, postoperative infection and dislocation [9,10]. Therefore, the preferred surgical strategy is to preserve the native bone and minimize the risk of interprosthetic fractures.

At least four factors contribute to the strength of the femoral bone in between two ipsilateral adjacent femoral implants: the distance between the two implants, the cortical thickness, the bone quality and the anchoring technique [11–13]. Tight interprosthetic distances are thought to lead to excessive strain on the bone between the two implant tips, increasing the risk of an interprosthetic fracture. Soenen et al. showed in a finite element study that the risk of fracture increased for interprosthetic distances smaller than 110 mm, but did not investigate implant distances less than 50 mm [12]. It has also been observed that a decreased cortical thickness and an increased medullary diameter are associated with the occurrence of interprosthetic fractures [11]. However, despite these associations, the clinical evidence for the technical implementation of ipsilateral adjacent femoral implants is sparse [13]. In particular, there is a lack of clinical and biomechanical studies investigating the effect of different interprosthetic distances on the resulting risk of interprosthetic fracture. A better understanding of the effect of interprosthetic spacing on the risk of interprosthetic fracture would be a critical step in improving patient care. Reliable biomechanical evidence on the relationship between interprosthetic spacing and fracture risk may lead to clinical recommendations for the correct intraoperative placement of the endoprosthesis or, in cases of fracture, to the correct placement of the osteosynthesis.

The purpose of the present study was to determine the effect of the interprosthetic distance between implants on periprosthetic fracture risk. As a surrogate marker of fracture risk, strain on the bone surface was investigated. We hypothesized that reducing the interprosthetic distance or decreasing the cortical thickness of the femur would increase the maximum strain in the femoral shaft.

2. Materials and Methods

To investigate the strain in the femoral shaft between two ipsilateral implant tips, a simplified physical model consisting of synthetic bone tubes and metallic implant cylinders was built. Subsequently, the physical model was transferred into a finite element model (FE model) to perform a parametric analysis of the effects of interprosthetic distance and cortical thickness on the maximum strain in the femoral shaft.

2.1. Biomechanical Model

As a bone substitute, an epoxy glass laminate tube (Kruelit 750, Krueger & Sohn GmbH, Landshut, Germany) with an outer diameter of 24 mm and a wall thickness of 2 mm was cut to a length of 300 mm. The Young's modulus of the material was investigated in an axial compression test and found to be 20.47 GPa, which matches human cortical bone [14–16]. Two aluminum cylinders were lathe faced to a diameter of 19.95 mm and a length of 170 mm and represented simplified stems of intramedullary implants. Biomechanical tests were carried out on a mechanical testing machine (Zwick Z010, Zwick Roell, Ulm, Germany) using a 10 kN load cell (Serie K, accuracy 0.5, GTM Testing and Metrology, Bickenbach, Germany).

To investigate realistic loading scenarios on the femoral shaft, such as a fall with lateral impact and load induced during activities of daily living, the constructs were tested under 3-point-bending (3PB) and 4-point-bending (4PB), respectively (Figure 1). The distance between the lower supports was 280 mm for both load cases. For 4PB, the upper supports were mounted on a rocker at a distance of 120 mm. The support pads were semicircular with a diameter of 10 mm.

For each bending scenario, a separate bone tube was used and the aluminum cylinders were inserted symmetrically to the defined depth. In both setups the same interprosthetic distances were investigated: 0 mm, 5 mm, 10 mm, 20 mm, 30 mm, 40 mm, 50 mm, 60 mm, 80 mm, 100 mm and without any implants. The constructs were loaded in two consecutive ramps within its linear elastic region at a velocity of 50 N/s, up to a maximum load of 800 N for 3PB, resulting in a bending moment of 56 Nm, and a load of 1600 N for 4PB, resulting in a bending moment of 64 Nm. A preload of 2 N guaranteed reproducible reference conditions.

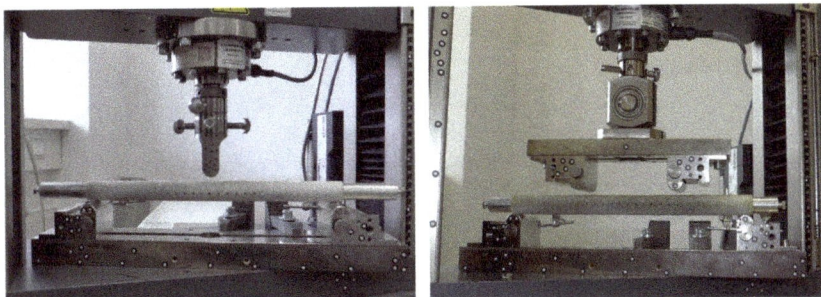

Figure 1. Experimental setup for quasi-static 3-point-bending (**left**) and 4-point-bending (**right**). The load cell is mounted on the machine actuator and a simple semicircular load applicator is used for 3-point-bending and two load applicators on a rocker were used for 4-point-bending.

To investigate strains at the surface of the synthetic bone tubes, the tubes were sprayed with a stochastic pattern that was detected by an optical measurement system (ARAMIS 5M, GOM GmbH, Braunschweig, Germany). For validation of the FE model, ten additional marker points were attached along the tube to measure absolute deformation of the tube (Figure 2). Strain patterns were analyzed by digital image correlation at the maximum loading conditions (GOM Correlate Professional 2020, GOM GmbH, Braunschweig, Germany). The coordinate system was defined with the y-axis aligned along the axis of the bone tube and the z-axis aligned vertically in the direction of the machine actuator. The center of the coordinate system was placed in the center of the bone tube, directly below the load actuator. Only cortical strain on the tension surface of the tube, opposite from the load actuator, was analyzed. Therefore, virtual points were created along an intersection line on the surface. These points were placed at a distance of 0.5 mm and strains in the direction of the bone axis (y-axis) were evaluated over a total length of 110 mm.

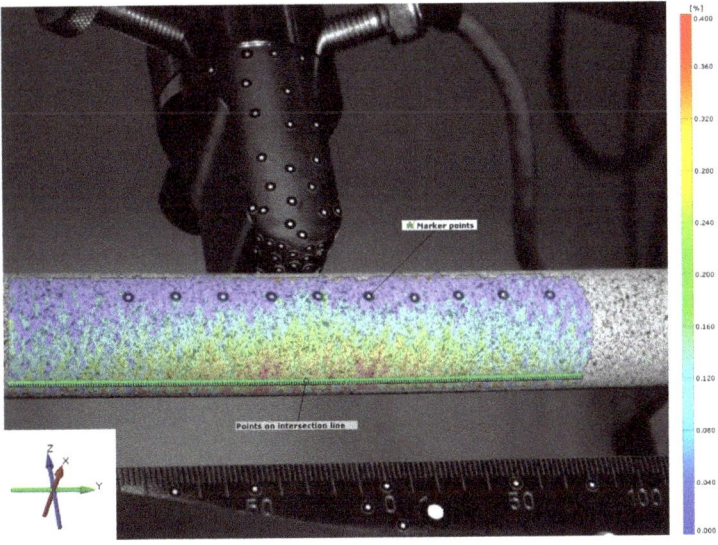

Figure 2. Strain measurement on the stochastic spray pattern based on points along the intersection line. The color coding provides information on the amount and distribution of the tensile strain from 0% strain (blue) to 0.4% strain (red). Attached marker points along the bone tube were used for analysis of the bending curve for FE model validation.

2.2. Finite Element Model

The physical models of the tube and implants were replicated in ANSYS Design Modeler (ANSYS 2022 R1, Canonsburg, PA, USA). Static structural simulations were built with two variations: (a) 3- and 4-point-bending loading case and (b) with and without implants. The load applicator and bearings were modeled as rigid bodies at the same distances as in the experimental part.

ANSYS Mechanical was used to build and calculate the non-linear FE simulations using an implicit solver. To reduce simulation time and resources, a quarter of the model was calculated using two symmetry planes to maintain the mechanical situation (Figure 3). A mesh convergency study resulted in 23,532 (with implant) and 20,882 (without implant) quadratic hexahedral elements. The material properties for simulation were applied according to the manufacturer's information (Table 1). Contacts between the implant and the tube as well as the tube and bearings were modeled as frictional contacts with coefficients of 0.1 and 0.3, respectively. In the parametric analysis, the implant distance to the symmetry axis was varied between 0.5 mm and 60 mm to simulate interprosthetic distances between 1 mm and 120 mm. The thickness of the bone tube was varied between 2, 4 and 6 mm to analyze the effect of varying the cortical bone thickness.

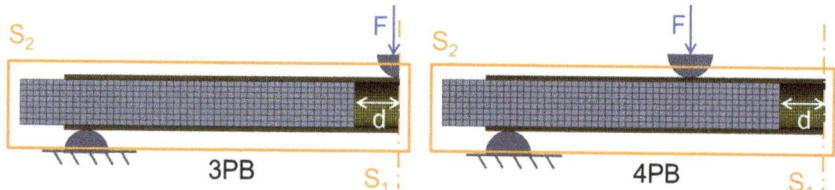

Figure 3. Mechanical specification of the FE model with additional information about the symmetry planes (S1 and S2), definition of the implant distance (d) and the applied force (F) in 3-point-bending (3PB) and 4-point-bending (4PB).

Table 1. Material properties of the bone tube and the aluminum cylinder.

Part	Material	Young's Modulus (MPa)	Poisson's Ratio
Bone tube	HGW 2735.4 (DIN 7735) EP GC 22 (EN 61212)	20,470	0.18
Implant cylinder	Aluminum Alloy	66,530	0.33

Validation was performed by comparing the experimental data with the simulation results. The deformation of attached marker points in the middle of the tube, the strain at the tensile site of the tube at the center, 40 mm off the center and at the implant location were analyzed using the relative deformation of the facets on the spray pattern (Figure 4). The experimental and simulation data were analyzed using a linear fit and Pearson's correlation to judge the quality of prediction. Additionally, the principal strain pattern over the tensile area of the tube was compared at a 20 mm implant distance between experiment and simulation. Data were analyzed and visualized and the root mean square error (RMSE) was calculated in Matlab (R2022b, The MathWorks, Portola Valley, CA, USA).

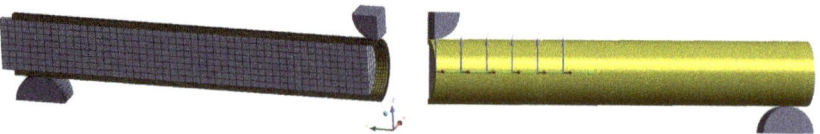

Figure 4. Isometric mesh model (**left**) and 6 points of interests used for comparison with the mechanical tests to validate the bending curve (**right**) of the FE model.

3. Results

Without an implant, the surface strains at the tensile site were 0.32% and 0.41% of the absolute principal strain for 3PB and 4PB, respectively. The presence of the intramedullary implants reduced the overall strain on the surface of the bone tube by about 0.05% of the absolute strain but generated distinct strain peaks at the respective positions of the implant tips. At the implant tips, the strain values were amplified by about 0.2% of the absolute strain. For an interprosthetic distance of 20 mm, peak strains of approximately 0.5% for 3PB and 0.6% for 4PB were identified (Figure 5). The strain patterns and the strain values measured in the experiment were well represented by the numerical calculation with the FE model. The validation showed very good correlations of the measured tube deformation (RMSE: 0.08 mm for 3PB and 0.13 mm for 4PB) and the local strain values (RMSE: 0.04% for 3PB and 4PB) with the respective simulated values (Figure 6).

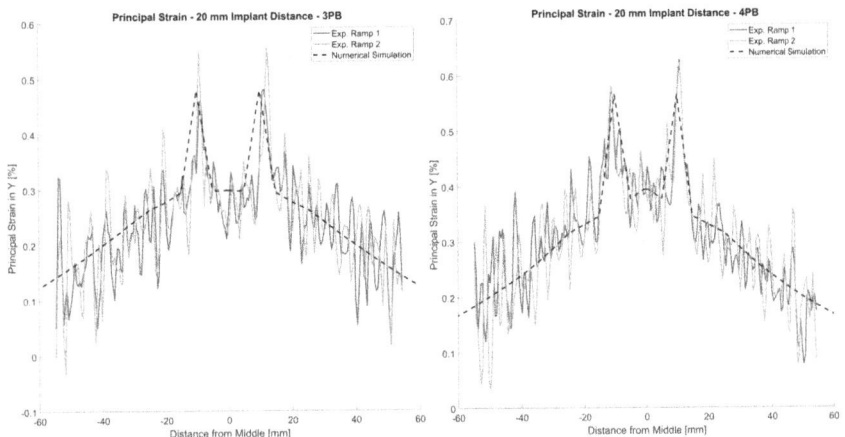

Figure 5. Principal strain for 20 mm interprosthetic distance for 3-point-bending (**left**) and 4-point-bending (**right**). The solid lines show the experimental data for two consecutive loading ramps and the dashed line represents the calculation from the FE model.

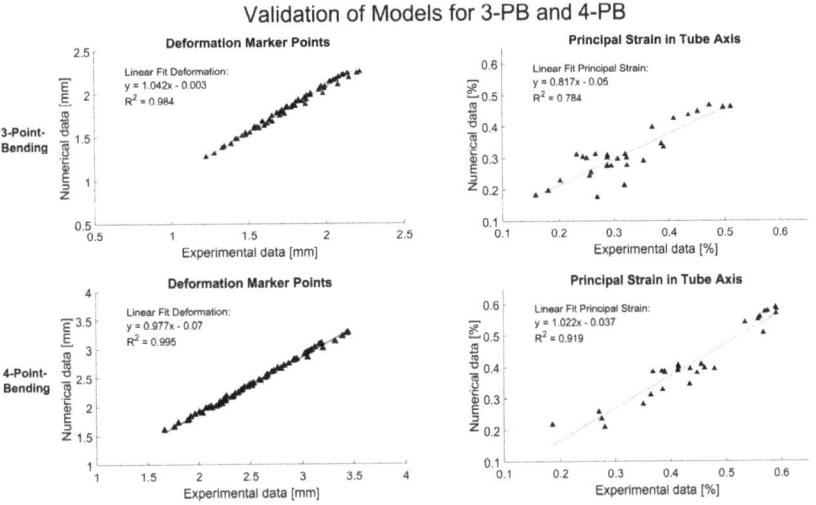

Figure 6. FE model validation over six marker points and principal strain along the tube axis. The model deformations were compared to the experimental data and analyzed using Pearson's correlations.

The FE model was first employed to assess the effect of the distance between the implant tips on the strain values of the tube. Overall, the presence of an implant reduced the principal strain values in the tube over its entire length. However, the change in material properties at the tip of the implant resulted in distinct peaks of the principal strain values of up to 0.55% for 3-point-bending and up to 0.63% for 4-point-bending (Figure 7). These peaks were consistently located at the respective positions of the implant tips. For 4-point-bending, these distinct peaks were found at all investigated implant distances. For 3-point-bending, the strain peak for 80 mm implant distance was reduced to 0.35% and no peak was detected at an implant distance of 120 mm.

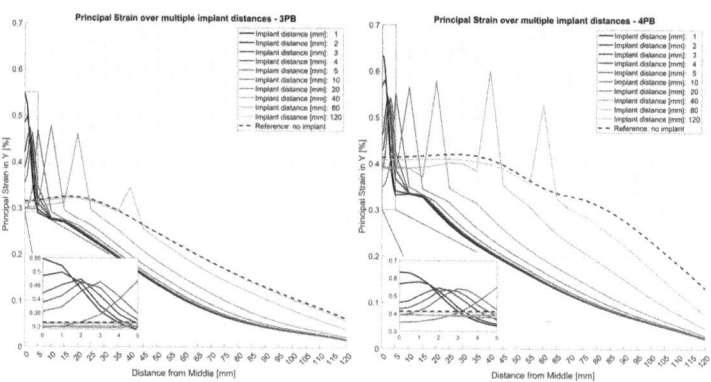

Figure 7. Principal strain analysis of different interprosthetic distances for a 2 mm cortical thickness in 3- and 4-point-bending. Due to the symmetry of the model, a distance of 20 mm represents an interprosthetic distance of 40 mm.

The FE model was further employed to assess the effect of cortical thickness on the surface strain in the presence of an intramedullary implant (Figure 8). The peak strains generally decreased with increasing cortical thickness. The amplification of the strain at the locations of the implant tips was more pronounced with thinner cortices. For a cortical thickness of 6 mm, the strain amplification was less than 0.02% strain for 4-point-bending and almost indiscernible for 3-point-bending. For 3-point-bending, the peak strains remained at a low level of 0.1 to 0.2% for a 4 mm cortical thickness and increased up to 0.5% for a 2 mm cortical thickness. For 4-point-bending, the peak strains were between 0.2% and 0.3% for a 4 mm cortical thickness and up to 0.65% for a 2 mm cortical thickness.

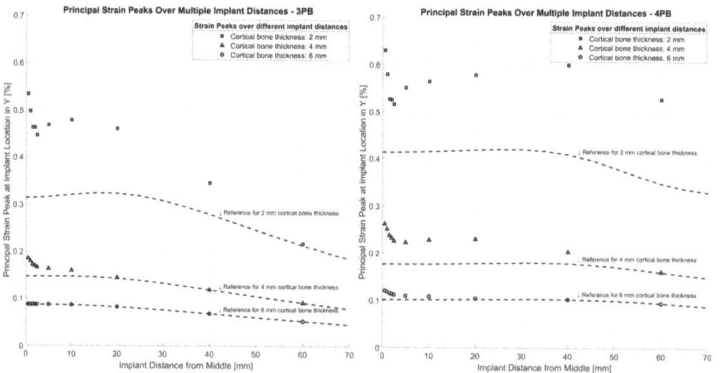

Figure 8. Principal strain peaks at implant position for different cortical bone thicknesses in 3- and 4-point-bending. Due to the symmetry of the model, a distance of 20 mm represents an interprosthetic distance of 40 mm.

4. Discussion

This study provides a valid finite element model to investigate the effect of interprosthetic distances between ipsilateral implants on the strain pattern in femoral shafts. Overall, the presence of an implant reduced the principal strain values in the femoral shaft over its entire length. However, distinct strain peaks were identified at the locations of the implant tips. Depending on the interprosthetic distance and cortical thickness, the strain was magnified by up to 80%. An increased cortical thickness reduced the peak strains at the implant tip position and had a greater effect on overall stiffness than the interprosthetic distance did.

For interprosthetic distances of less than 10 mm, the strain values increased exponentially due to accumulation of the strain peaks of the individual implant tips. This may be one of the reasons for bone failure around implant tips observed in clinical practice. This result is consistent with Sun et al., who described a shift in strain concentration in ipsilateral implants to the area between the two implants [17]. The strain peak pattern across the tube at a 10 mm interprosthetic distance and beyond was different for the two different loading cases. In the case of 3-point-bending, the overall strain values decreased, while in the case of 4-point-bending, the strain values remained relatively constant over the course of the tube. This phenomenon can be explained by the nature of the loading cases, where in 4-point-bending, the applied moment was constant between the load applicators. In contrast, in 3-point-bending, the applied moment decreases along the tube.

Soenen et al. found an increased fracture risk in 4-point-bending scenarios and suggested a minimal interprosthetic distance threshold of 110 mm. However, they did not test interprosthetic distances of less than 50 mm. Thus, the exponential strain peak effect that occurred in the present study at 10 mm or less was not found [12].

Another study by Walcher et al. investigated the effect of plate positioning in periprosthetic or interprosthetic femur fractures and found a strain increase on the bone with a decreasing overlap or gap in the implants. According to the authors, this might not be a similar biomechanical effect as the strain peak effect in the present study analyzing intramedullary implants [18]. Further investigations are necessary to substantiate or contradict this statement.

Clinically, an increase in fracture severity was found by Townsend et al. when a total hip prosthesis and a total knee prosthesis are present in one bone. In one third of the cases, the fracture occurred distal to the hip implant, resulting in unstable bending-type fractures more often than in a group that only had hip implants inserted [19]. These findings suggest a stress increasing effect of adjacent implants and their distances.

In a finite elements analysis study by Plausinis et al., the effect of interprosthetic spacing in the humerus was examined. They claimed that the stresses near the stem tips of the ipsilateral prostheses did not increase above the level seen in single implant cases. In their study, they used pure bending and torsional moments of 10 Nm with tubes of 1.5 mm and 3 mm cortical thicknesses [20]. In the present study, similar results were obtained with the 6 mm thick tube samples. This indicates that the occurrence of strain peaks in ipsilateral settings is strongly dependent on cortical thickness in relation to the amount and type of loading. Patients are postoperatively advised to bear their full weight if tolerated after 2 to 4 months, which increases the bending load on the femur. Thus, a higher load for the test setup seems more suitable [6,21]. Weiser et al. also demonstrated the importance of cortical thickness but rejected a critical effect of interprosthetic distance on strain amplification between implants [22]. In the present study, a constant increase in strain peaks was observed with decreasing cortical thickness. Bone quality is reported as one major factor for interprosthetic fracture risk in the literature, confirming the findings of this study [8,11,23]. The present results suggest that interprosthetic distance has an important effect on the strain pattern when the cortical thickness is 4 mm or less.

The constructs were mechanically loaded in 3-point- and 4-point-bending to cover clinically relevant loading scenarios. Three-point-bending was thought to mimic loading during an unintentional loading event, such as a fall onto the side or onto an obstacle. Four-point-bending, which produces a more homogeneous bending moment along the femoral shaft, was thought to mimic the loading that occurs during walking due to ground reaction and muscle forces. Strain magnification at the implant tips was similar for both loading scenarios when the interprosthetic distance was 40 mm or less. For larger interprosthetic distances, the strain magnification was less pronounced for 3-point-bending compared to 4-point-bending.

The limitations of the study include the simplified representation of a femoral shaft by a cylindrical bone substitute. Human cadaveric specimens demonstrate inter-specimen variability, such as cortical thickness, geometry and mechanical properties. On the other hand, bone surrogates with human anatomy eliminate this problem, but by anatomical nature, the cortical thickness changes over the axial length of the bone [24]. Therefore, a parametrical analysis of the interprosthetic distance in these specimens is not possible to be isolated but is combined with the parameter of cortical thickness. Since the material properties were comparable to those of human bone, the synthetic tube provides a good alternative and allowed to investigate the effect of strain caused by ipsilateral implants. The material was chosen because it represents a homogenous thickness of cortical bone over the tube length; therefore, it is well suited for a parametrical analysis of interprosthetic distance with constant geometric conditions. Furthermore, implant stems for hip and knee arthroplasties typically have conical tips to facilitate easier implant insertion and to reduce strain peaks. The strain values were not evaluated continuously, but at intervals of 0.5 mm for distances below 5 mm distance and in 5 mm intervals for distances larger than 5 mm. Therefore, the spatial resolution could have affected the strain data, but the differences are expected to be minor. In a clinical setting, the implant stems derive their stability through press-fit anchorage or embedding in bone cement. Although the outer diameter of the aluminum cylinders was close to the inner diameter of the tubes, the fit was not perfectly tight to allow for a reproducible and precise manipulation of the implant position. Loose stems have previously been shown to produce larger strain peaks than fixed or embedded stems [25]. Therefore, our boundary conditions without bonding between the implant stem and the outer bone tube may have overestimated the absolute amount of strain magnification.

5. Conclusions

The findings from this study suggest a minimum interprosthetic distance of 10 mm to avoid the accumulation of strain peaks caused by adjacent implant tips. Strain amplification occurred at reduced cortical thicknesses of 4 mm and 2 mm but was not detectable at 6 mm. Therefore, careful interprosthetic management becomes more important in patients with reduced bone quality. Additional clinical and biomechanical studies are needed to further analyze the relationship between interprosthetic distance and strain amplification in the femoral shaft for different implant fixations and to develop an index for interprosthetic fracture risk assessments.

Author Contributions: Conceptualization, S.H. (Sven Hungerer) and C.G.; methodology, all authors; validation and testing, M.M. and S.S.; investigation and data collection, M.M., S.S. and S.H. (Sven Herrmann); resources, P.A. and S.H. (Sven Hungerer); formal analysis and discussion, all authors; writing—original draft preparation, M.M. and S.S.; writing—review and editing, all authors; visualization, M.M., S.S. and S.H. (Sven Herrmann); supervision, P.A., C.G. and S.H. (Sven Hungerer). All authors have read and agreed to the published version of the manuscript.

Funding: This research received no external funding.

Institutional Review Board Statement: Ethical approval is not required for studies not involving human or animal tissue.

Data Availability Statement: Data relating to this study are available upon reasonable request.

Acknowledgments: The authors would like to thank Martin Winkler and Johanna Finkel for their preliminary work in this project.

Conflicts of Interest: The authors declare no conflict of interest.

References

1. Cui, A.; Li, H.; Wang, D.; Zhong, J.; Chen, Y.; Lu, H. Global, regional prevalence, incidence and risk factors of knee osteoarthritis in population-based studies. *EClinicalMedicine* **2020**, *29–30*, 100587. [CrossRef] [PubMed]
2. Turkiewicz, A.; Petersson, I.F.; Bjork, J.; Hawker, G.; Dahlberg, L.E.; Lohmander, L.S.; Englund, M. Current and future impact of osteoarthritis on health care: A population-based study with projections to year 2032. *Osteoarthr. Cartil.* **2014**, *22*, 1826–1832. [CrossRef] [PubMed]
3. Meyer, J.A.; Zhu, M.; Cavadino, A.; Coleman, B.; Munro, J.T.; Young, S.W. Infection and periprosthetic fracture are the leading causes of failure after aseptic revision total knee arthroplasty. *Arch. Orthop. Trauma Surg.* **2021**, *141*, 1373–1383. [CrossRef] [PubMed]
4. Schwartz, A.M.; Farley, K.X.; Guild, G.N.; Bradbury, T.L., Jr. Projections and Epidemiology of Revision Hip and Knee Arthroplasty in the United States to 2030. *J. Arthroplast.* **2020**, *35*, S79–S85. [CrossRef]
5. Tarazi, J.M.; Chen, Z.; Scuderi, G.R.; Mont, M.A. The Epidemiology of Revision Total Knee Arthroplasty. *J. Knee Surg.* **2021**, *34*, 1396–1401. [CrossRef]
6. Kosters, C.; den Toom, D.; Metzlaff, S.; Daniilidis, K.; Barz, L.; Rosslenbroich, S. Peri- and Interprosthetic Femoral Fractures-Current Concepts and New Developments for Internal Fixation. *J. Clin. Med.* **2022**, *11*, 1371. [CrossRef]
7. Loucas, M.; Loucas, R.; Akhavan, N.S.; Fries, P.; Dietrich, M. Interprosthetic Femoral Fractures Surgical Treatment in Geriatric Patients. *Geriatr. Orthop. Surg. Rehabil.* **2021**, *12*, 21514593211013790. [CrossRef]
8. Lehmann, W.; Rupprecht, M.; Nuechtern, J.; Melzner, D.; Sellenschloh, K.; Kolb, J.; Fensky, F.; Hoffmann, M.; Puschel, K.; Morlock, M.; et al. What is the risk of stress risers for interprosthetic fractures of the femur? A biomechanical analysis. *Int. Orthop.* **2012**, *36*, 2441–2446. [CrossRef] [PubMed]
9. Prodinger, P.M.; Harrasser, N.; Scheele, C.; Knebel, C.; Hertel, G.; Suren, C.; von Eisenhart-Rothe, R. Megaimplants of the Proximal Femur: Current Concepts. *Z. Orthop. Unfall.* **2018**, *156*, 685–691. [CrossRef]
10. von Salis-Soglio, M.; Ghanem, M.; Lycke, C.; Roth, A.; Osterhoff, G. Megaendoprostheses in the management of malignant tumors of the lower extremities-risk factors for revision surgery. *J. Orthop. Surg. Res.* **2021**, *16*, 508. [CrossRef]
11. Lipof, J.S.; Amitai, A.D.; Judd, K.T.; Gorczyca, J.T. Radiographic Risk Factors For Interprosthetic Femur Fractures. *Iowa Orthop. J.* **2017**, *37*, 35–39. [PubMed]
12. Soenen, M.; Baracchi, M.; De Corte, R.; Labey, L.; Innocenti, B. Stemmed TKA in a femur with a total hip arthroplasty: Is there a safe distance between the stem tips? *J. Arthroplast.* **2013**, *28*, 1437–1445. [CrossRef] [PubMed]
13. Stoffel, K.; Sommer, C.; Kalampoki, V.; Blumenthal, A.; Joeris, A. The influence of the operation technique and implant used in the treatment of periprosthetic hip and interprosthetic femur fractures: A systematic literature review of 1571 cases. *Arch. Orthop. Trauma Surg.* **2016**, *136*, 553–561. [CrossRef]
14. Bayraktar, H.H.; Morgan, E.F.; Niebur, G.L.; Morris, G.E.; Wong, E.K.; Keaveny, T.M. Comparison of the elastic and yield properties of human femoral trabecular and cortical bone tissue. *J. Biomech.* **2004**, *37*, 27–35. [CrossRef] [PubMed]
15. Dong, X.N.; Acuna, R.L.; Luo, Q.; Wang, X. Orientation dependence of progressive post-yield behavior of human cortical bone in compression. *J. Biomech.* **2012**, *45*, 2829–2834. [CrossRef] [PubMed]
16. Pernelle, K.; Imbert, L.; Bosser, C.; Auregan, J.C.; Cruel, M.; Ogier, A.; Jurdic, P.; Hoc, T. Microscale mechanical and mineral heterogeneity of human cortical bone governs osteoclast activity. *Bone* **2017**, *94*, 42–49. [CrossRef]
17. Sun, Z.H.; Liu, Y.J.; Li, H. Femoral stress and strain changes post-hip, -knee and -ipsilateral hip/knee arthroplasties: A finite element analysis. *Orthop. Surg.* **2014**, *6*, 137–144. [CrossRef]
18. Walcher, M.G.; Giesinger, K.; du Sart, R.; Day, R.E.; Kuster, M.S. Plate Positioning in Periprosthetic or Interprosthetic Femur Fractures With Stable Implants-A Biomechanical Study. *J. Arthroplast.* **2016**, *31*, 2894–2899. [CrossRef]
19. Townsend, O.; Jain, S.; Lamb, J.N.; Scott, C.E.H.; Dunlop, D.G.; Pandit, H.G. Periprosthetic femoral fracture type and location are influenced by the presence of an ipsilateral knee arthroplasty implant: A case-control study of 84 interprosthetic femoral fractures. *Injury* **2022**, *53*, 645–652. [CrossRef]
20. Plausinis, D.; Greaves, C.; Regan, W.D.; Oxland, T.R. Ipsilateral shoulder and elbow replacements: On the risk of periprosthetic fracture. *Clin. Biomech.* **2005**, *20*, 1055–1063. [CrossRef]
21. Rozell, J.C.; Delagrammaticas, D.E.; Schwarzkopf, R. Interprosthetic femoral fractures: Management challenges. *Orthop. Res. Rev.* **2019**, *11*, 119–128. [CrossRef] [PubMed]
22. Weiser, L.; Korecki, M.A.; Sellenschloh, K.; Fensky, F.; Püschel, K.; Morlock, M.M.; Rueger, J.M.; Lehmann, W. The role of inter-prosthetic distance, cortical thickness and bone mineral density in the development of inter-prosthetic fractures of the femur: A biomechanical cadaver study. *Bone Jt. J.* **2014**, *96-B*, 1378–1384. [CrossRef] [PubMed]
23. McMellen, C.J.; Romeo, N.M. Interprosthetic Femur Fractures: A Review Article. *JBJS Rev.* **2022**, *10*, e22. [CrossRef] [PubMed]

24. Gardner, M.J.; Silva, M.J.; Krieg, J.C. Biomechanical testing of fracture fixation constructs: Variability, validity, and clinical applicability. *J. Am. Acad. Orthop. Surg.* **2012**, *20*, 86–93. [CrossRef] [PubMed]
25. Iesaka, K.; Kummer, F.J.; Di Cesare, P.E. Stress risers between two ipsilateral intramedullary stems: A finite-element and biomechanical analysis. *J. Arthroplast.* **2005**, *20*, 386–391. [CrossRef]

Disclaimer/Publisher's Note: The statements, opinions and data contained in all publications are solely those of the individual author(s) and contributor(s) and not of MDPI and/or the editor(s). MDPI and/or the editor(s) disclaim responsibility for any injury to people or property resulting from any ideas, methods, instructions or products referred to in the content.

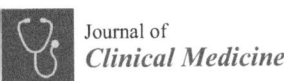

Article

Septic History Limits the Outcome of Tibiotalocalcaneal Arthrodesis

Magalie Meinert [1,†], Christian Colcuc [2,†], Eva Herrmann [3], Johannes Harbering [4], Yves Gramlich [1], Marc Blank [5], Reinhard Hoffmann [1] and Sebastian Fischer [5,*]

1 Department for Trauma and Orthopaedic Surgery, Berufsgenossenschaftliche Unfallklinik Frankfurt am Main, 60389 Frankfurt, Germany
2 Department for Trauma and Orthopaedic Surgery, Evangelical Hospital Bethel Bielefeld, 33611 Bielefeld, Germany
3 Division of Biostatistics and Mathematical Modelling, Goethe-University, Frankfurt am Main, Theodor-Stern-Kai 7, 60596 Frankfurt am Main, Germany
4 Department for Septic Bone Surgery, Berufsgenossenschaftliche Unfallklinik Frankfurt am Main, 60389 Frankfurt, Germany
5 Department of Foot and Ankle Surgery, Berufsgenossenschaftliche Unfallklinik Frankfurt am Main, 60389 Frankfurt, Germany
* Correspondence: sebastian.fischer@bgu-frankfurt.de
† These authors contributed equally to this work.

Abstract: Joint destruction necessitates tibiotalocalcaneal arthrodesis (TTCA) in cases of clinical deficits that cannot be controlled conservatively, possibly leading to sepsis. We aimed to compare the underlying etiology of posttraumatic joint destruction and the outcomes after TTCA in patients with a septic or aseptic history. Between 2010 and 2022, 216 patients with TTCA were retrospectively enrolled (septic TTCA (S-TTCA) = 129; aseptic TTCA (A-TTCA) = 87). Patient demographics, etiology, Olerud and Molander Ankle Scores (OMASs), Foot Function Index (FFI-D) scores, and Short Form-12 Questionnaire (SF-12) scores were recorded. The mean follow-up period was 6.5 years. Tibial plafond and ankle fractures were the most common causes of sepsis. The mean OMAS was 43.0; the mean FFI-D was 76.7; and the mean SF-12 physical component summary score was 35.5. All the scores differed significantly between the groups ($p < 0.001$). With an average of 11 operations until the arthrodesis was achieved, the S-TTCA patients underwent about three times as many operations as the A-TTCA patients ($p < 0.001$), and 41% of S-TTCA patients remained permanently unable to work ($p < 0.001$). The significantly worse results of S-TTCA compared to A-TTCA show the long and stressful ordeal that patients with a septic history suffer. Further attention must be paid to infection prophylaxis and, if necessary, early infection revision.

Keywords: ankle arthrodesis; tibiotalocalcaneal arthrodesis; septic history; hindfoot fusion nail; posttraumatic septic osteoarthritis

1. Introduction

Tibiotalocalcaneal arthrodesis (TTCA) is usually the last resort after severe destruction of the ankle joint to relieve the affected patient's pain and restore stability. However, infections that cannot be controlled after ankle fractures can often only be healed in this way. In this case, freedom from infection and pain relief are preferred to the preservation of ankle function.

Regarding histories of septic TTCA (S-TTCA) and aseptic TTCA (A-TTCA), infections represent S-TTCA due to underlying open fractures or operative fracture treatment [1]. However, elective surgery to address chronic ligament instability, chronic syndesmotic instability, nonunion revisions, lower limb malpositions, and failed total ankle replacements may also result in a septic situation and require a TTCA [2,3]. Primary arthrosis of all ankle arthroses plays only a minor role, as does hematogenous infection [3,4]. It is well

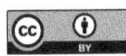

known that TTCA represents an already massive impairment to quality of life and must not be indicated too generously [5,6].

We aimed to determine the level of impairment following TTCA for the treatment of end-stage posttraumatic osteoarthritis of the ankle with a history of sepsis and to compare it with the level of impairment after aseptic TTCA. The selected scores (Olerud and Molander Ankle Score (OMAS), Foot Function Index (FFI-D), and Short Form-12 Questionnaire) were intended to improve the understanding of how to cope with daily life after TTCA and to objectify the influence of the septic history. Our results may assist in the planning and implementation of the surgical procedure with appropriate care and adaption at an early stage to prepare the patient for the expected lengthy treatment.

2. Patients and Methods

2.1. Population

Between 2010 and 2022, 216 patients with TTCA due to posttraumatic osteoarthritis (135 males and 81 females; mean age: 64 years (range: 27–93 years)) were retrospectively enrolled in this comparative monocentric study. In total, 129 patients suffered a septic history (S-TTCA) until the fusion of the arthrodesis; 87 had an aseptic history (A-TTCA). Regarding demographics, both groups were equally distributed (Table 1). All patients were seen at our study center (Figure 1). In line with the focus of the study center, approximately one-third of the patients with septic histories were admitted from other hospitals. All arthrodeses were then performed at our study center, involving five surgeons with the same amount of expertise in this type of surgery.

Table 1. Patient characteristics.

Characteristic		Septic TTCA (n = 129)	Aseptic TTCA (n = 87)	All (n = 216)	p
Follow-up (months)	Mean	85.10	68.87	78.61	0.003
	SEM	3.36	4.42	2.73	
	Minimum	18.00	12.00	12.00	
	Maximum	154.00	151.00	154.00	
Age, years	Mean	63.59	64.68	64.02	0.528
	SEM	1.02	1.47	0.85	
	Minimum	27.00	30.00	27.00	
	Maximum	89.00	93.00	93.00	
BMI, kg/m^2	Mean	30.34	29.95	30.18	0.660
	SEM	0.56	0.68	0.43	
	Minimum	16.40	18.80	16.40	
	Maximum	58.30	49.60	58.30	
Sex, n (%)	Male	84 (65.12)	51 (58.62)	135 (62.50)	0.336
	Female	45 (34.88)	36 (41.38)	81 (37.50)	
Affected side, n (%)	Left	67 (51.94)	44 (50.58)	111 (51.39)	0.845
	Right	62 (48.06)	43 (49.42)	105 (48.61)	
Smoker, n (%)	Yes	34 (26.36)	17 (19.54)	51 (23.61)	0.266
	No	92 (71.32)	67 (77.01)	159 (73.61)	
	n.a.	3 (2.33)	3 (3.45)	6 (2.78)	
Pre-existing conditions (multiple answers), n (%)	Metabolic-syndrome-associated	52 (41.27)	30 (35.71)	82 (37.96)	0.063
	Rheumatism	7 (5.43)	3 (3.45)	10 (4.63)	
	Others	25 (19.38)	19 (21.84)	44 (20.37)	
	None	30 (23.26)	15 (17.24)	45 (20.83)	

BMI, body mass index; SEM, standard error of the mean; TTCA, tibiotalocalcaneal arthrodesis.

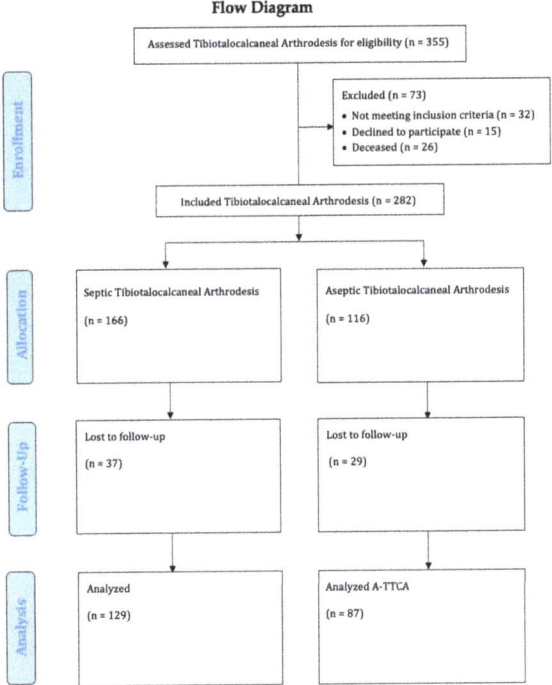

Figure 1. Study flow chart.

The mean follow-up duration for clinical outcomes was 6.5 years (range: 12–154 months). All procedures were performed in accordance with the 1964 Helsinki Declaration and its later amendments. The ethics committee of the institutional review board approved this study.

2.2. Inclusion and Exclusion Criteria

Only patients older than 18 years of age were included. There was no maximum age limit. Written informed consent was required prior to participation. The indication for TTCA was based on underlying painful, end-stage septic or aseptic osteoarthritis of the ankle. Only TTCAs performed at the study center were included.

Destruction of the ankle joint due to malignant neoplasms of bone, such as osteosarcoma, were excluded. Patients who required (partial) amputation of the affected limb as part of the septic history were also excluded.

2.3. Surgical Procedure

The choice of osteosynthetic procedure was based on the experience of the surgeon as well as the intraoperative findings. In the S-TTCA group, approximately 70% of the ankle arthrodesis procedures were performed with a hindfoot fusion nail with 5° of valgus, approximately 20% with an external fixator, and 10% with screws and wires (Figure 2). Procedure changes from nail to fixator or vice versa were often necessary (Figure 3). Depending on the focus of the septic history, all common approaches to the ankle and hindfoot were used, with the lateral approach being the most common at over 60%. For hindfoot nails, the diameter and length of the nail were chosen between 150 and 300 mm according to preoperative planning and intraoperative findings (Figure 4). A shorter nail with a diameter of 12 mm was the most common version.

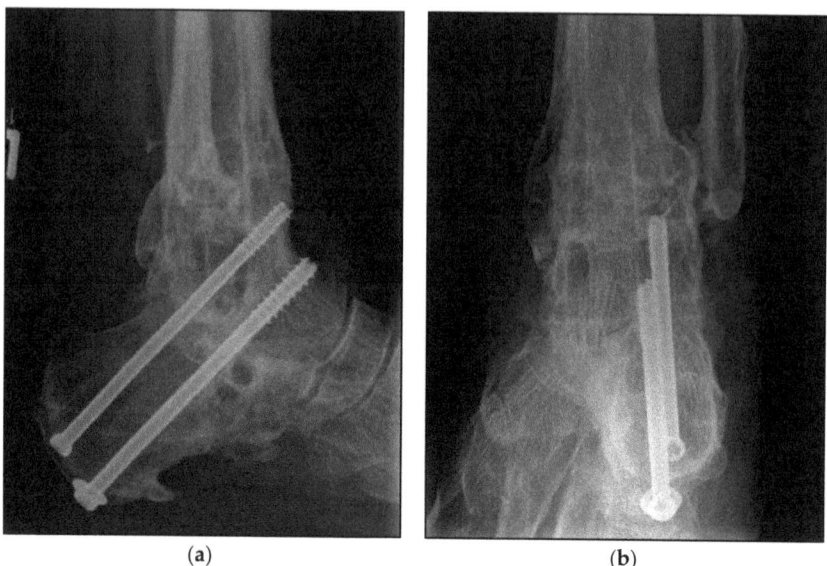

Figure 2. Postoperative radiographic findings of end-stage posttraumatic arthritis of the left ankle with septic history of a 54-year-old male treated with a screw fixation due to nonunion after tibiotalocalcaneal arthrodesis treated with arthrodesis nail. (**a**,**b**) Anteroposterior and lateral view; view, 6 years post operation.

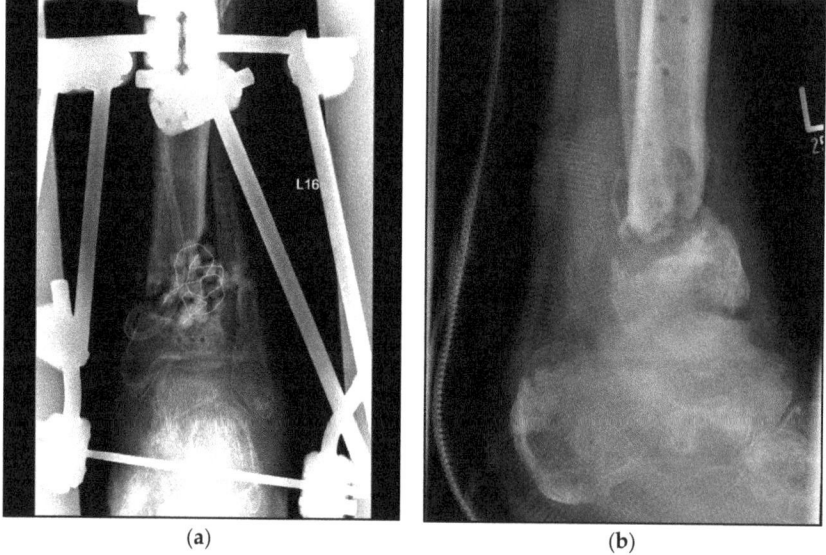

Figure 3. Radiographic findings of the left ankle of a 82-year-old male patient with condition according to open 3° tibial fracture with septic history and treated with external fixator. (**a**) Anteroposterior view; (**b**) lateral view.

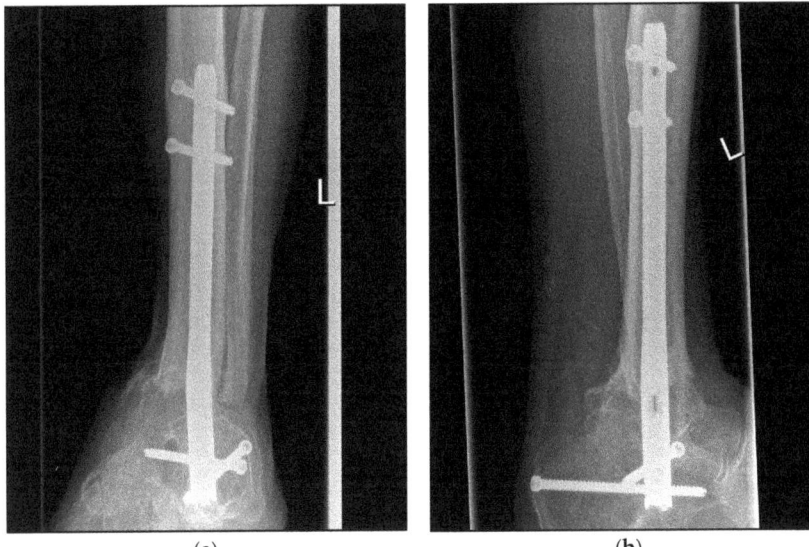

Figure 4. Postoperative radiographic findings of end-stage posttraumatic arthritis of the left ankle with septic history of a 82-year-old male treated with a tibiotalocalcaneal arthrodesis T2™ Ankle Arthrodesis Nail, 200 × 10 mm. (**a**,**b**) Anteroposterior and lateral view; view, 5 years post operation.

In the case of a history of infection, in addition to the surgical treatment of the infection, an accompanying antibiotic therapy was regularly carried out. The antibiotics were discontinued 2–4 weeks after the insertion of the nail during the last revision and the receipt of a negative microbiological result. Individual decisions varied depending on the clinical findings.

In the A-TTCA group, almost all arthrodeses were performed with a hindfoot fusion nail with 5° of valgus (predominantly with a T2™ Ankle Arthrodesis Nail, © Stryker, Kalamazoo, MI, USA). The lateral approach was the most frequent at over 80%, followed by approximately 10% of the ventral approach with the use of a fusion plate at the tibiotalar joint in combination with mini-open arthrodesis using screw fixation at the subtalar joint. The interposition of autogenous or autologous cancellous bone grafting was performed in approximately 15% and 25% of the S-TTCA and A-TTCA procedures, respectively.

2.4. Rehabilitation Protocol

After the last stage of revision for the treatment of infection, the post-treatment scheme involved wearing an orthotic boot (e.g., VACOped™, OPED GmbH, Valley, Germany) for a total of 12 weeks and ambulation on forearm or armpit crutches for all patients. For the first 6 weeks, patients were required to wear the boot for 24 h per day with merely sole contact; the removal of the boot for personal hygiene and physiotherapy was permitted. After X-ray examination, the boot was worn for an additional 6 weeks with gradual weight bearing; during this time, the boot could be removed at night. At 12 weeks post operation, computed tomography was carried out, and the footwear was orthopedically adapted for everyday use.

2.5. Assessment Methods

Demographic data, including age, body mass index (BMI), pre-existing conditions, such as those associated with syndrome-x, and nicotine abuse, were obtained for each patient. Additionally, the underlying etiology of joint destruction, accident mechanism, if applicable, type of fracture and tissue damage according to the Gustilo grade I–III classification, and the outcome using the Olerud and Molander Ankle Score (OMAS), Foot

Function Index in its validated German version (FFI-D), and Short Form-12 Questionnaire (SF-12) were recorded. The type and number of revisions were also recorded as part of the follow-up (Table 2).

Table 2. Etiology of the underlying end-stage posttraumatic osteoarthrosis of the ankle joint.

Predisposing Factors, Multiple Answers		Septic TTCA (n = 129)	Aseptic TTCA (n = 87)	All (n = 216)	p
Mechanism, n (%)	Fall from height	43 (33.33)	26 (29.89)	69 (31.94)	0.697
	Distortion	29 (22.48)	14 (16.09)	43 (19.91)	
	Traffic accident	30 (23.26)	21 (24.14)	51 (23.61)	
	Others	26 (20.63)	26 (29.89)	52 (24.07)	
Ankle fracture, n (%)	Yes	43 (33.33)	25 (28.74)	68 (31.48)	0.478
	No	86 (66.67)	62 (71.27)	148 (68.52)	
Talar fracture, n (%)	Yes	6 (4.65)	18 (20.70)	24 (11.11)	0.001
	No	123 (95.35)	69 (79.30)	192 (88.89)	
Tibial plafond fractures, n (%)	Yes	47 (36.43)	5 (5.75)	52 (24.08)	0.001
	No	82 (63.57)	82 (94.25)	164 (75.92)	
Open fracture, n (%)	Yes	32 (24.81)	7 (8.05)	39 (18.06)	<0.001
	No	97 (75.19)	80 (91.95)	177 (81.94)	
	Gustilo Grade I	2 (1.55)	0 (0.00)	2 (0.93)	
	Gustilo Grade II	12 (9.30)	3 (3.45)	15 (6.94)	
	Gustilo Grade III	18 (13.95)	4 (4.59)	22 (10.19)	
Delayed union tibial, n (%)	Yes	58 (44.96)	17 (19.54)	75 (34.72)	<0.001
	No	71 (55.04)	70 (80.46)	141 (65.28)	
Chronic ankle instability, n (%)	Yes	8 (6.20)	7 (8.05)	15 (6.94)	0.603
	No	121 (93.80)	80 (91.95)	201 (93.06)	
Chronic syndesmotic instability, n (%)	Yes	4 (3.10)	6 (6.90)	10 (4.63)	0.120
	No	125 (96.90)	81 (93.10)	206 (95.37)	
Failed total ankle replacement, n (%)	Yes	17 (13.18)	12 (13.79)	29 (13.43)	0.897
	No	112 (86.82)	75 (86.21)	187 (86.57)	
Deformities of the lower limb, n (%)	Valgus deformity	1 (0.78)	9 (10.35)	10 (4.63)	<0.001
	Varus deformity	6 (4.65)	23 (26.44)	29 (13.43)	<0.001
	No	122 (94.57)	55 (63.21)	177 (81.94)	<0.001
Previous neurological disease, n (%)	Yes	4 (3.10)	6 (6.90)	10 (4.63)	0.195
	No	125 (96.90)	81 (93.10)	206 (95.37)	
Primary arthrosis, n (%)	Yes	3 (2.33)	6 (6.90)	9 (4.17)	0.100
	No	126 (97.67)	81 (93.10)	207 (95.83)	
Others, n (%)	Yes	23 (17.83)	14 (16.01)	37 (17.13)	0.735
	No	106 (82.17)	73 (83.99)	179 (82.87)	

TTCA, tibiotalocalcaneal arthrodesis.

2.6. Statistical Analysis

The primary aim was to compare significant differences in the outcomes of S-TTCA and A-TTCA using a representative number of cases which illustrated the power of the included data with a mean follow-up time of 6.5 years. Due to the retrospective design, there was no case number calculation. So far, monocentric studies with comparable questions have tended to have smaller population groups [7–9]. All the statistical analyses were performed using SPSS, v. 23, software (IBM Dtl. GmbH, Ehningen, Germany). Furthermore, for descriptive and explorative statistical analyses for the queried scores, including within-group means, medians, minima and maxima, and standard deviations, Student's t-test and an ANOVA were used. The power of the study was 0.8, and the significance level was set to $p < 0.05$ with a 95% confidence interval.

3. Results

After an average postoperative follow-up of 6.5 years (range: 12–154 months) the following factors were identified as the causes of the terminal posttraumatic arthritis of the ankle. At 36.4% and 33.3%, tibial plafond fractures and ankle fractures were the most common injuries with septic complications, respectively; in approximately 25% of the cases, the underlying fracture was an open 3° fracture. The proportion of the other causes of end-stage posttraumatic osteoarthritis was 23% in the S-TTCA group, predominantly combined with soft tissue damage; in the A-TTCA group, this proportion was 12% and was due to chronic syndesmotic instability in half of the cases. Multiple answers were possible in both groups.

The mean OMAS was 43.0 (S-TTCA: 39.4, A-TTCA: 48.4); the mean FFI-D was 76.7 (S-TTCA: 81.6, A-TTCA: 69.2); and the mean SF-12 physical component summary score was 35.5 (S-TTCA: 34.1, A-TTCA: 37.7). All the scores differed significantly between the groups ($p < 0.001$). The SF-12 mental component summary, on the other hand, did not show any significant differences (mean: 50.1, S-TTCA: 49.9, A-TTCA: 50.4, $p = 0.783$).

With an average of 11 operations until union of the arthrodesis was achieved, the S-TTCA patients underwent approximately 3 times as many operations as the A-TTCA patients ($p < 0.001$). Approximately 41% of S-TTCA cases remained permanently unable to work, compared to approximately 18% percent of the A-TTCA group ($p < 0.001$) (Table 3).

Table 3. Clinical outcome with subgroups.

Measurements		Septic TTCA (n = 129)	Aseptic TTCA (n = 87)	All (n = 216)	p
Olerud and Molander	Mean	39.40	48.39	43.00	0.008
	SEM	2.08	2.72	1.68	
	Minimum	0.00	0.00	0.00	
	Maximum	100.00	85.00	100.00	
FFI-D	Mean	81.62	69.23	76.64	0.002
	SEM	2.49	3.11	1.98	
	Minimum	19.50	15.00	15.00	
	Maximum	135.00	123.00	135.00	
SF-12 (physical component summary)	Mean	34.09	37.66	35.52	0.019
	SEM	0.96	1.14	35.52	
	Minimum	11.73	14.47	0.75	
	Maximum	55.26	56.63	11.73	
SF-12 (mental component summary)	Mean	49.91	50.36	50.09	0.783
	SEM	1.11	1.19	0.814	
	Minimum	17.10	22.84	17.10	
	Maximum	68.89	65.23	68.89	
Number of operations underwent until union, including fracture treatment, n	Mean	11.23	3.83	8.29	<0.001
	Minimum	1	1	1	
	Maximum	30	25	30	
Complication, revision surgery needed until union (multiple answers), n (%) *	Yes	-	14 (16.09)		
	No	-	73 (83.91)		
	Nonunion	-	8 (9.19)		
	Implant irritation	-	5 (5.74)		
	TTS	-	1 (1.15)		
Footwear (multiple answers), n (%)	Orthotic insoles only	23 (17.83)	18 (20.69)	41 (18.98)	0.012
	Shoe adaption	72 (55.81)	34 (39.08)	106 (49.07)	<0.001
	Other	2 (1.59)	1 (1.19)	3 (1.39)	0.281
	Nothing special	29 (22.48)	31 (35.63)	60 (27.78)	<0.001
Return to learned profession, n (%)	Yes	18 (13.95)	16 (18.39)	34 (15.74)	0.802
Permanently unable to work, n (%)	Yes	52 (41.27)	15 (17.86)	67 (31.02)	<0.001
Retraining, part time, and pension, n (%)	Yes	56 (44.44)	53 (63.09)	109 (50.46)	0.802

SEM, standard error of the mean; SF-12, 12-Item Short Form Health Survey; TTCA, tibiotalocalcaneal arthrodesis; TTS, tarsal tunnel syndrome. * All patients in the septic TTCA group had revisions due to persistent infections with failure of soft tissue healing and pseudarthrosis. Therefore, these procedures were not considered complications.

Complications

Since all patients in the S-TTCA group underwent multiple revisions, including soft tissue debridement as well as nonunion revisions due to persistent infection, these procedures were not listed separately as complications. The overall revision rate of the A-TTCA group was approximately 16%. Revisions had to be performed due to nonunion in eight cases; five revisions were for implant irrigation. Minor complications such as delayed wound healing, swelling, discomfort, and cramps were seen in both treatment groups. Cases not requiring revision were not considered a relevant complication in the present study (Table 3). Another serious difference was found in the time from initial trauma to arthrodesis. This period was 98 months on average in the S-TTCA group and 246 months in the A-TTCA group.

4. Discussion

The data obtained from the validated scores confirm the clinical impression of the authors that the outcome of TTCA with a septic history differs significantly from patients without a history of infection, even after clinically and radiologically confirmed healing of the arthrodesis. Although the patients from the S-TTCA group tended to have more metabolic-syndrome-associated previous diseases, this difference was not significant. All other demographic data, such as age, gender, BMI, and smoking status, were equally distributed.

The proportion of metabolic-syndrome-associated pre-existing conditions was significantly higher than in the normal population, as was the average BMI. It is understandable that patients with a history of infections have an increased risk profile due to their lifestyle [10]. However, this cannot be confirmed based on the available data. The well-known correlation between increased BMI and frequency of ankle injuries was also confirmed [11,12]. The accompanying increased rate of metabolic-syndrome-associated diseases could also be seen in this context.

There were an equal number of men in each group. Men have higher rates than women for all crash types and crash-related injuries, not only for the lower limb [13]. Naturally, this is due to the comparatively higher proportion of male involvement in both traffic accidents and falls from height at construction sites, as can often be inferred from the medical history.

In accordance with the focus of the study center, we found accident- and infection-related joint damage to be the cause of terminal posttraumatic arthrosis of the ankle joint. At approximately 36%, pilon fractures were the leading etiology of ankle joint arthrosis, immediately followed by fractures of the ankle joint and the talus itself. At 24.8%, the proportion of open fractures was approximately four times higher in the S-TTCA group than in the A-TTCA; Gustilo grade III fractures were approximately three times as high (S-TTCA: 13.95%, A-TTCA: 4.59%). The comparative literature confirms this proportion of open fractures in the context of ankle fractures to be approximately 13%, depending on the mechanism and complexity following motor vehicle or motorbike collisions and falls from height [14]. Comparative breakdowns by Gustilo grade I–III injury, as in the present work, are generally difficult to find. However, in the case of smooth transitions between the grades, the data should generally be viewed critically, although there is agreement that all open fractures increase the risk of deep wound infection many times over, with a significantly higher number of reoperations, flap reconstructions, and patients suffering from chronic pain when compared to other grades [14–17].

A remarkable result of our study lies in the period from the first named accident event or ankle osteoarthritis due to rarer causes such as axial malalignment or chronic instability until arthrodesis of the ankle joint or full healing. This period was merely 98 months on average in the S-TTCA group and 246 months in the A-TTCA group. An obvious explanation is that the present infection requires immediate surgical revision but also leads to additional aggressive joint destruction. Studies with comparable questions indicate the period from the designation of septic arthritis to arthrodesis as 30–80 months [18]. For A-TTCA, a period of 8–10 years has been reported [19]. The comparatively longer period, as indicated in the present study, is explained by the designation of the initial trauma and not by the designation of the first evidence of deep infection. Accordingly, the period from the first trauma to the final performance of A-TTCA is significantly longer than is usually stated in comparative studies [20].

The attempt to assess the choice of osteosynthesis procedure led to the following conclusion. The data analysis did not reveal any difference between the individual osteosynthetic procedures, such as nails, screws, and external fixators, which were therefore not presented separately. Again, multiple changes were reported regarding the number of previous operations, from fusion nails to external fixators and vice versa, especially in the S-TTCA group. Therefore, an evaluation of which procedure is superior cannot be made. Again, the data agree with those of the comparative literature and confirm the fusion nail as the method of choice for TTCA in the absence of infection. Furthermore, an external fixator such as the Ilizarov frame is a proven alternative, with comparable results in the presence or after the revision of a deep infection [10,21–24].

The clinical outcome of both the separately presented S-TTCA and the aseptic TTCA, with an average of 33.5 points in the physical component summary (PCS) of the SF-12 Questionnaire and 50.1 points for the mental component summary of the SF-12 Questionnaire, is largely in line with the results of studies with comparable questions [25]. Studies also indicate values above 50 for the PCS of the SF-12 [26]. An obvious explanation is the lack of patients with a history of sepsis. Similarly, studies have evaluated comparatively worse outcomes measured by the OMAS. Fuchs et al. gave a score of 59 points in their 20-year review [27]. In addition to the few representative cases, the proportion of the septic population in that study was just 4/18 (22.2%) and not 129/216 patients (59.7%), as in our present study. There was also no comparison of the two groups. Jonas et al. and Georgiannos et al. present data that appears to be more realistic. Values above 50 points for a purely aseptic population support the original and confirmed assumption of the present study that S-TTCA and A-TTCA differ significantly in outcome [28,29].

In addition to the strength of a large population in this monocentric study, this study had some limitations. First, this was a study with a retrospective design, and the clinical scores and the extent of septic and posttraumatic damage to the tibiotalar and subtalar joints were not collected preoperatively. Based on the retrospectively collected data, it can be determined which cases with septic arthritis would have healed even without arthrodesis or in which cases, viewed retrospectively, the decision was made too early or should have been made earlier. Regardless, all patients equally presented with posttraumatic terminal osteoarthritis of the ankle. Second, regarding the group with a history of sepsis, the complications in the context of the necessary TTCA cannot be reliably distinguished from the multiple revisions for infection treatment and thus provide a direct comparison.

5. Conclusions

The available data, with the significantly worse results of S-TTCA compared to A-TTCA in clinical scores and prolonged downtime or permanent incapacity, show the long and stressful ordeal that patients with a septic history suffer. For that reason, more attention should be paid to infection prophylaxis and, if necessary, early infection revision, especially in the context of tibial plafond fractures and even more so in the case of an open fracture.

Author Contributions: Conceptualization, methodology, S.F. and M.M.; writing—original draft preparation, and writing—review and editing, C.C. and S.F.; software, validation, and formal analysis, J.H. and Y.G.; investigation and data curation, C.C. and M.B.; resources and supervision, E.H. and M.M.; project administration, R.H. and S.F. All authors have read and agreed to the published version of the manuscript.

Funding: This research received no external funding.

Institutional Review Board Statement: All procedures were performed in accordance with the 1964 Helsinki Declaration and its later amendments. This study was approved by the Institutional Review Board of the Hessian Medical Association Germany (DRKS00031612).

Informed Consent Statement: Informed consent was obtained from all subjects involved in the study. Written informed consent has been obtained from the patients to publish this paper.

Data Availability Statement: All data intended for publication are included in the manuscript.

Acknowledgments: Sincere thanks are extended to all co-authors for their excellent cooperation.

Conflicts of Interest: The authors declare no conflict of interest.

References

1. Horisberger, M.; Valderrabano, V.; Hintermann, B. Posttraumatic ankle osteoarthritis after ankle-related fractures. *J. Orthop. Trauma* **2009**, *23*, 60–67. [CrossRef] [PubMed]
2. Fischer, S.; Klug, A.; Faul, P.; Hoffmann, R.; Manegold, S.; Gramlich, Y. Superiority of upper ankle arthrodesis over total ankle replacement in the treatment of end-stage posttraumatic ankle arthrosis. *Arch. Orthop. Trauma Surg.* **2022**, *142*, 435–442. [CrossRef] [PubMed]
3. Saltzman, C.L.; Salamon, M.L.; Blanchard, G.M.; Huff, T.; Hayes, A.; Buckwalter, J.A.; Amendola, A. Epidemiology of ankle arthritis: Report of a consecutive series of 639 patients from a tertiary orthopaedic center. *Iowa Orthop. J.* **2005**, *25*, 44–46. [PubMed]
4. Valderrabano, V.; Horisberger, M.; Russell, I.; Dougall, H.; Hintermann, B. Etiology of ankle osteoarthritis. *Clin. Orthop. Relat. Res.* **2009**, *467*, 1800–1806. [CrossRef]
5. Cibura, C.; Lotzien, S.; Yilmaz, E.; Baecker, H.; Schildhauer, T.A.; Gessmann, J. Simultaneous septic arthrodesis of the tibiotalar and subtalar joints with the Ilizarov external fixator-an analysis of 13 patients. *Eur. J. Orthop. Surg. Traumatol.* **2022**, *32*, 1063–1070. [CrossRef]
6. Easley, M.E.; Montijo, H.E.; Wilson, J.B.; Fitch, R.D.; Nunley, J.A., 2nd. Revision tibiotalar arthrodesis. *J. Bone Jt. Surg. Am.* **2008**, *90*, 1212–1223. [CrossRef]
7. Gross, J.B.; Belleville, R.; Nespola, A.; Poircuitte, J.M.; Coudane, H.; Mainard, D.; Galois, L. Influencing factors of functional result and bone union in tibiotalocalcaneal arthrodesis with intramedullary locking nail: A retrospective series of 30 cases. *Eur. J. Orthop. Surg. Traumatol.* **2014**, *24*, 627–633. [CrossRef]
8. Kappler, C.; Staubach, R.; Abdulazim, A.; Kemmerer, M.; Walter, G.; Hoffmann, R. Hindfoot arthrodesis for post-infectious ankle destruction using an intramedullary retrograde hindfoot nail. *Unfallchirurg* **2014**, *117*, 348–354. [CrossRef]
9. Wang, S.; Li, B.; Yu, X.; Wu, H.; Liu, L. Is Ankle Arthrodesis With an Ilizarov External Fixator an Effective Treatment for Septic Ankle Arthritis? A Study With a Minimum of 6 Years of Follow-up. *Clin. Orthop. Relat. Res.* **2023**, *481*, 717–725. [CrossRef]
10. Suda, A.J.; Richter, A.; Abou-Nouar, G.; Jazzazi, M.; Tinelli, M.; Bischel, O.E. Arthrodesis for septic arthritis of the ankle: Risk factors and complications. *Arch. Orthop. Trauma Surg.* **2016**, *136*, 1343–1348. [CrossRef]
11. Rosen, A.B.; Jaffri, A.; Mitchell, A.; Koldenhoven, R.M.; Powden, C.J.; Fraser, J.J.; Simon, J.E.; Hoch, M.; Burcal, C.J. Association of Ankle Sprain Frequency With Body Mass and Self-Reported Function: A Pooled Multisite Analysis. *J. Sport Rehabil.* **2022**, *31*, 1000–1005. [CrossRef] [PubMed]
12. Vuurberg, G.; Altink, N.; Rajai, M.; Blankevoort, L.; Kerkhoffs, G. Weight, BMI and stability are risk factors associated with lateral ankle sprains and chronic ankle instability: A meta-analysis. *J. ISAKOS* **2019**, *4*, 313–327. [CrossRef] [PubMed]
13. Cullen, P.; Möller, H.; Woodward, M.; Senserrick, T.; Boufous, S.; Rogers, K.; Brown, J.; Ivers, R. Are there sex differences in crash and crash-related injury between men and women? A 13-year cohort study of young drivers in Australia. *SSM Popul. Health* **2021**, *14*, 100816. [CrossRef] [PubMed]
14. Simske, N.M.; Audet, M.A.; Kim, C.Y.; Vallier, H.A. Open ankle fractures are associated with complications and reoperations. *OTA Int.* **2019**, *2*, e042. [CrossRef] [PubMed]
15. Ovaska, M.T.; Madanat, R.; Honkamaa, M.; Makinen, T.J. Contemporary demographics and complications of patients treated for open ankle fractures. *Injury* **2015**, *46*, 1650–1655. [CrossRef] [PubMed]
16. Bugler, K.E.; Clement, N.D.; Duckworth, A.D.; White, T.O.; McQueen, M.M.; Court-Brown, C.M. Open ankle fractures: Who gets them and why? *Arch. Orthop. Trauma Surg.* **2015**, *135*, 297–303. [CrossRef]
17. Herrera-Pérez, M.; González-Martín, D.; Vallejo-Márquez, M.; Godoy-Santos, A.L.; Valderrabano, V.; Tejero, S. Ankle Osteoarthritis Aetiology. *J. Clin. Med.* **2021**, *10*, 4489. [CrossRef]
18. Klouche, S.; El-Masri, F.; Graff, W.; Mamoudy, P. Arthrodesis with internal fixation of the infected ankle. *J. Foot Ankle Surg.* **2011**, *50*, 25–30. [CrossRef]
19. Gaedke, I.E.; Wiebking, U.; O'Loughlin, P.F.; Krettek, C.; Gaulke, R. Clinical and Radiological Mid- to Long-term Outcomes Following Ankle Fusion. *In Vivo* **2018**, *32*, 1463–1471. [CrossRef]
20. Frey, C.; Halikus, N.M.; Vu-Rose, T.; Ebramzadeh, E. A Review of Ankle Arthrodesis: Predisposing Factors to Nonunion. *Foot Ankle Int.* **1994**, *15*, 581–584. [CrossRef]
21. Zak, L.; Wozasek, G.E. Tibio-talo-calcaneal fusion after limb salvage procedures-A retrospective study. *Injury* **2017**, *48*, 1684–1688. [CrossRef]
22. Klaue, K.; Wichelhaus, A.; Maik, P.; Mittlmeier, T. The circular arc shaped nail for fixing the tibiotalocalcaneal arthrodesis. After clinical results. *Injury* **2019**, *50* (Suppl. S3), 23–31. [CrossRef] [PubMed]

23. Popelka, S.; Vavrik, P.; Landor, I.; Bek, J.; Popelka ml, S.; Hromadka, R. [Tibio-talo-calcaneal arthrodesis with the retrograde intramedullary nail MEDIN]. *Acta Chir. Orthop. Traumatol. Cech.* **2013**, *80*, 400–406.
24. Rüschenschmidt, M.; Glombitza, M.; Dahmen, J.; Hax, P.-M.; Lefering, R.; Steinhausen, E. External versus internal fixation for arthrodesis of chronic ankle joint infections—A comparative retrospective study. *Foot Ankle Surg.* **2020**, *26*, 398–404. [CrossRef]
25. Jeng, C.; Campbell, J.; Tang, E.; Cerrato, R.; Myerson, M. Tibiotalocalcaneal Arthrodesis With Bulk Femoral Head Allograft for Salvage of Large Defects in the Ankle. *Foot Ankle Int. Am. Orthop. Foot Ankle Soc. Swiss Foot Ankle Soc.* **2013**, *34*, 1256–1266. [CrossRef]
26. Lee, T.Y.; Wu, C.C.; Yang, K.C.; Yeh, K.T.; Chen, I.H.; Wang, C.C. Midterm outcomes of midfoot and hindfoot arthrodesis with strut allograft for Muller-Weiss disease. *BMC Musculoskelet. Disord.* **2022**, *23*, 715. [CrossRef]
27. Fuchs, S.; Sandmann, C.; Skwara, A.; Chylarecki, C. Quality of life 20 years after arthrodesis of the ankle. A study of adjacent joints. *J. Bone Jt. Surg. Br.* **2003**, *85*, 994–998. [CrossRef]
28. Jonas, S.C.; Young, A.F.; Curwen, C.H.; McCann, P.A. Functional outcome following tibio-talar-calcaneal nailing for unstable osteoporotic ankle fractures. *Injury* **2013**, *44*, 994–997. [CrossRef]
29. Georgiannos, D.; Lampridis, V.; Bisbinas, I. Fragility fractures of the ankle in the elderly: Open reduction and internal fixation versus tibio-talo-calcaneal nailing: Short-term results of a prospective randomized-controlled study. *Injury* **2017**, *48*, 519–524. [CrossRef]

Disclaimer/Publisher's Note: The statements, opinions and data contained in all publications are solely those of the individual author(s) and contributor(s) and not of MDPI and/or the editor(s). MDPI and/or the editor(s) disclaim responsibility for any injury to people or property resulting from any ideas, methods, instructions or products referred to in the content.

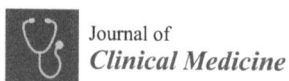

Systematic Review

Arthroscopic vs. Open-Ankle Arthrodesis on Fusion Rate in Ankle Osteoarthritis Patients: A Systematic Review and Meta-Analysis

Alejandro Lorente [1], Leire Pelaz [1], Pablo Palacios [2], Iker J. Bautista [3,4], Gonzalo Mariscal [5,*], Carlos Barrios [5] and Rafael Lorente [6]

[1] Ankle and Foot Surgery Unit, Department of Traumatology and Orthopaedic Surgery, University Hospital Ramón y Cajal, 28034 Madrid, Spain; alejandro.lorentegomez@gmail.com (A.L.); dra_lire@hotmail.com (L.P.)
[2] Department of Traumatology and Orthopaedic Surgery, Sanchinarro University Hospital, 28050 Madrid, Spain; pablopalacios@drpalacios.com
[3] Institute of Sport, Nursing, and Allied Health, University of Chichester, Chichister PO19 6PE, UK; i.bautista@chi.ac.uk
[4] Physiotherapy Department, Valencia Catholic University of Valencia, 46900 Valencia, Spain
[5] Institute for Research on Musculoskeletal Disorders, School of Medicine, Valencia Catholic University, 46001 Valencia, Spain; carlos.barrios@ucv.es
[6] Department of Orthopedic Surgery and Traumatology, University Hospital of Badajoz, 06080 Badajoz, Spain; rafaalelorente@hotmail.com
* Correspondence: gonzalo.mariscal@mail.ucv.es; Tel.: +34-649-6154-89

Abstract: Although open surgery is the conventional option for ankle arthritis, there are some reports in the literature regarding the use of the arthroscopy procedure with outstanding results. The primary purpose of this systematic review and meta-analysis was to analyze the effect of the surgery technique (open-ankle arthrodesis vs. arthroscopy) in patients with ankle osteoarthritis. Three electronic databases (PubMed, Web of Science, and Scopus) were searched until 10 April 2023. The Cochrane Collaboration's risk-of-bias tool was used to assess the risk of bias and grading of the recommendations assessment, development, and evaluation system for each outcome. The between-study variance was estimated using a random-effects model. A total of 13 studies (including n = 994 participants) met the inclusion criteria. The meta-analysis results revealed a nom-significant (p = 0.072) odds ratio (OR) of 0.54 (0.28–1.07) for the fusion rate. Regarding operation time, a non-significant difference (p = 0.573) among both surgical techniques was found (mean differences (MD) = 3.40 min [−11.08 to 17.88]). However, hospital length stay and overall complications revealed significant differences (MD = 2.29 days [0.63 to 3.95], p = 0.017 and OR = 0.47 [0.26 to 0.83], p = 0.016), respectively. Our findings showed a non-statistically significant fusion rate. On the other hand, operation time was similar among both surgical techniques, without significant differences. Nevertheless, lower hospital stay was found in patients that were operated on with arthroscopy. Finally, for the outcome of overall complications, the ankle arthroscopy technique was a protective factor in comparison with open surgery.

Keywords: ankle osteoarthritis; arthroscopic; open surgery; arthrodesis; meta-analysis

1. Introduction

Osteoarthritis (OA) is a common degenerative joint disease that affects the cartilage, bone, and surrounding tissues of joints. It is also known as a degenerative joint disease or wear-and-tear osteoarthritis [1,2]. OA can occur in any joint in the body but commonly affects the knees, hips, spine, and hands [3]. The disease is thought to result from not only the aging process but also from biomechanical and biomechanical change stresses affecting the articular cartilage; however, the exact cause of osteoarthritis is not well known. Indeed, several factors contribute to its development, including age [4], genetics [5], joint injury or overuse [6], and obesity [7,8]. Several studies have identified post-traumatic etiology as the principal cause of ankle arthritis [9]. While the management of OA should be individually guided to satisfy the needs of each patient, the surgical option is reserved for more advanced OA patients and/or for patients where early treatment (i.e., patient education, weight management, and assistive devices) fails [10].

According to the definition of terms in medical subject headings, the surgical fixation of a joint by a procedure designated to accomplish the fusion of the joint surface by promoting the proliferation of the bone cell is called arthrodesis. In this regard, open-surgery arthrodesis represents the traditional option for the treatment of ankle osteoarthritis and related pathologies (i.e., chronic instability and degenerative deformity) due to its effect on pain relief and functional improvements [11]. In recent years, however, ankle replacement has gained more consideration, becoming the preferred treatment for this pathology. A meta-analysis found a greater improvement in function and range of motion when compared to ankle arthrodesis [12]. Nonetheless, the complications following lower-extremity open surgery include infections, wound issues, nerve entrapment, and delayed union and non-union, which could represent an important burden for patient quality of life [13]. On the other hand, the ankle arthroscopic technique represents a valid alternative to open surgery for patients with ankle arthrosis. Although open surgery is the traditional option for ankle osteoarthritis, there are some reports in the literature regarding the use of the arthroscopy procedure with outstanding results, including shorter operative time [14] and hospital stay [15], as well as comparable fusion rates between open vs. arthroscopic interventions [16]. For these reasons, there is still an open debate about the adequacy of which surgical technique (i.e., open vs. arthroscopic) yields better responses in patient outcomes.

The choice of surgical approach, whether arthroscopic or open, may depend on a variety of factors, including the surgeon's preference, the patient's condition, and the extent of the surgery required [11]. These inconsistencies and gaps in the literature establish a need for a systematic review that, with the highest scientific rigor, shows the effect of two surgery techniques (i.e., open-ankle arthrodesis vs. arthroscopy) on several clinical outcomes. To date, there are several systematic reviews and meta-analyses where this question was addressed [13,17]. However, some of them fail in study research design classification and others in the statistical analysis approach [18], which could lead to misinterpreting the conclusions obtained. Therefore, the primary purpose of this systematic review and meta-analysis was to analyze the effect of the surgery technique (open-ankle arthrodesis vs. arthroscopy) on fusion rate in patients with ankle osteoarthritis. On the other hand, the second objective of this systematic review and meta-analysis was to analyze the effect of the surgery technique on operation time and length of hospital stay. Finally, our review described the overall complications after the use of both surgical techniques described above.

2. Materials and Methods

2.1. Study Design

A systematic review and meta-analysis were developed using the Reporting Items for Systematic Reviews and Meta-Analysis (PRISMA) statement guidelines [19]. In addition, the Prisma in Exercise, Rehabilitation, Sport Medicine and Sports Science (PERSiT) was also implemented [20]. The PRISMA checklist is detailed in Supplementary File S1.

2.2. Eligibility Criteria

To be included, studies had to adhere to the following criteria: (1) Type of studies: randomized or non-randomized controlled trial where the effect of the surgery technique was assessed. Only studies in English were considered. Conference abstracts were excluded. (2) Type of participant: studies included patients with osteoarthritis, including post-traumatic osteoarthritis, osteoarthritis, and end-stage osteoarthritis, or patients with ankle instability. (3) Types of interventions: open surgery for the intervention group; meanwhile, arthroscopy was the comparison group. (4) Type of outcome measures: the primary outcome of interest was fusion rate. However, in addition to that variable, operation time and length of hospital stay were collected from studies that provided this information. Finally, overall complications were also collected.

2.3. Search Strategy

A PICO strategy was used to build search criteria for electronic databases (i.e., PubMed, Web of Science, and Scopus). No restrictions were applied concerning the year of publication. The PICO consisted of terms for open-ankle arthrodesis, arthroscopy, fusion rate, and blood loss. The primary search string used for PubMed was: ("open ankle arthrodesis" [All Fields] OR "open ankle" [All Fields] OR "ankle joint/surgery" [MeSH Major Topic]) AND ("arthroscopy" [All Fields] OR "arthroscopy technique" [All Fields] OR "arthrodesis" [All Fields] OR "minimally invasive" [All Fields]) AND ("fusion rate" [All Fields] OR "Visual analogue scale (VAS)" [All Fields] OR "blood loss" [All Fields] OR "American Orthopaedic Foot and Ankle Society (AOFAS)" [All Fields]). The search strings used for other databases were adapted using the Polyglot Search Translator Tool (https://sr-accelerator.com/#/polyglot, accessed on 4 May 2023) [21] and are reported in Supplementary File S2. The final search date was performed on 10 April 2023. Forward and backward citation tracking of articles that met the eligibility criteria was performed using an online tool (citation chaser) [22].

2.4. Methodological Quality and Level of Evidence

Two researchers independently assessed the methodological quality of the studies using a modified version of the Risk of Bias 2 (RoB 2) Cochrane Bias Assessment Tool [23] In the case of disagreement between the scores provided, the primary author made the final decision. RoB 2 was considered in the interpretation of the results by applying the Grading of Recommendations Assessment, Development and Evaluation (GRADE) system. A more extensive description of the risk of bias assessment procedure and the GRADE system is found in Supplementary File S3.

2.5. Data Extraction

The following data were extracted: authors, year of publication, research design (i.e., randomized controlled trial (RCT) and non-randomized controlled trial but intervention study (nRCT)), sample size, sex (i.e., male/female), age (i.e., years), body mass index, fusion rate, follow-up period (i.e., months), hospital stay (i.e., days), and overall complications both arthroscopy and open-surgery groups. Data extraction was manually performed by two researchers. Where data were not available or insufficient information was reported, the corresponding author of the studies was contacted by email, with one reminder after 2 weeks if they did not respond to the first email. If the corresponding authors did not reply, the study was discarded.

2.6. Statistical Analysis

The sample size and means (or events), standard deviation, 95% confidence intervals ($CI_{95\%}$) (if applicable) of fusion rate, complications, hospital stay, and operation time were extracted independently from the included studies. Mean differences (MD) were calculated for hospital stay and operation time since all studies were reported in the same units. We first computed a change score within each group and then determined the difference between the change scores between groups using the following equation:

$$MD = Mean_{arthroscopy} - Mean_{open}$$

Finally, the variance of the MD was computed as follows [22]:

$$S^2_{MD} = \frac{(n_{arthr} - 1)S^2_{arthr} + (n_{open} - 1)S^2_{open}}{n_{arthr} + n_{open} - 2} \left(\frac{1}{n_{arthr}} + \frac{1}{n_{open}} \right)$$

where "S^2_{arthr}" and "S^2_{open}" denote the variance of the change score for the arthroscopy and open-surgery groups, respectively.

On the other hand, for nominal variables (fusion rate and overall complications), odds ratios (ORs) and 95% of confidence intervals were calculated using the following approach [24]:

$$OR = \frac{a(event_{arthr})/b(noevent_{arthr})}{c(event_{open})/d(noevent_{open})}$$

The ORs were transformed to *log-OR* using the natural logarithm:

$$logOR = log_e(OR)$$

Meanwhile, the standard error of the *log-OR* was calculated using the formula:

$$SE_{logOR} = \sqrt{\frac{1}{a} + \frac{1}{b} + \frac{1}{c} + \frac{1}{d}}$$

The consistency of the effects found was assessed using the I^2 and τ^2 tests, with heterogeneity (I^2) being considered small (<25%), moderate (25–49%), and high (>50%). In addition, Tau-square tests (τ^2) and prediction interval (PI) were included, because τ^2 cannot readily point to the clinical implications of the unobserved heterogeneity [25] for ratio variables. The prediction interval allows a better clinical evaluation of the results obtained because it represents the range in which the effect size of a future study conducted on the topic will most likely be. The Egger's test and a representation of the funnel plot were used to assess small study bias. Variance estimations between studies were calculated using a random-effects model (i.e., Hartung–Knapp/Sidik–Jakman adjustment (HKSJ)) with a 95% confidence interval ($CI_{95\%}$). All statistical analyses were performed using statistical software (R version 4.1.9, R Foundation for Statistical Computing, Austria, metaphor and meta-analysis package, general meta-analysis package; risk-of-bias figures were created using Robvis). The standardized mean difference (SMD) was considered trivial (<0.20), small (0.20–0.59), moderate (0.60–1.19), large (1.20–1.99), and very large (>2.00) [26]. RoB 2 figures were created using the Robvis package [26,27].

3. Results

3.1. Search Results

Figure 1 shows the PRISMA flow diagram with the different phases of the search and selection of studies included in this review. The initial search yielded 394 records. None of the records were removed before screening. After the elimination of duplicates (*n* = 32), another 343 studies were excluded based on abstract and another 10 studies based on full-text assessment (see Supplementary File S4 for more information regarding excluding studies). A total of 13 studies [11,14–16,28–36] were therefore included in the present review on the effectiveness of open-ankle arthrodesis vs. arthroscopy on our primary outcome (i.e., fusion rate).

3.2. Risk-of-Bias Results

The risk-of-bias scores of included studies are reported in Figure 2 both traffic light and summary plots. A total of 13 studies were analyzed [11,14–16,28–36]. Figure 2A,B summarizes the risk of bias on fusion rate outcome. From a general point of view, all studies (100%) were at high risk of bias. From the 13 studies analyzed, Domain 1 (randomization procedure) in 13/13 was at high risk of bias, Domain 2 (deviations from the intended intervention) was at high risk of bias in 13/13 (100%), Domain 3 (missing outcome data) was at low risk of bias in 13/13 (100%), Domain 4 (measurement of the outcome) was at low risk of bias in 13/13 (100%), and finally, Domain 5 (selection of the reported results) was 13/13 (100%) at some concerns.

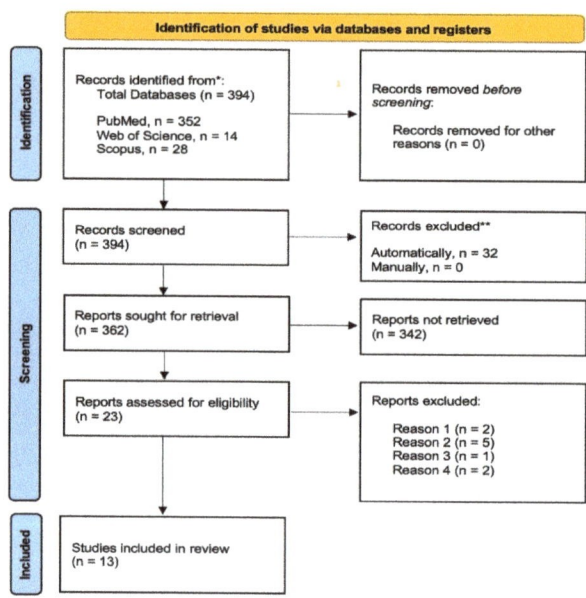

Figure 1. PRISMA flow diagram of the literature search results. * records removed automatically using an online tool (www.sr-accelerator.com, accessed on 4 May 2023). ** records excluded according by reasons.

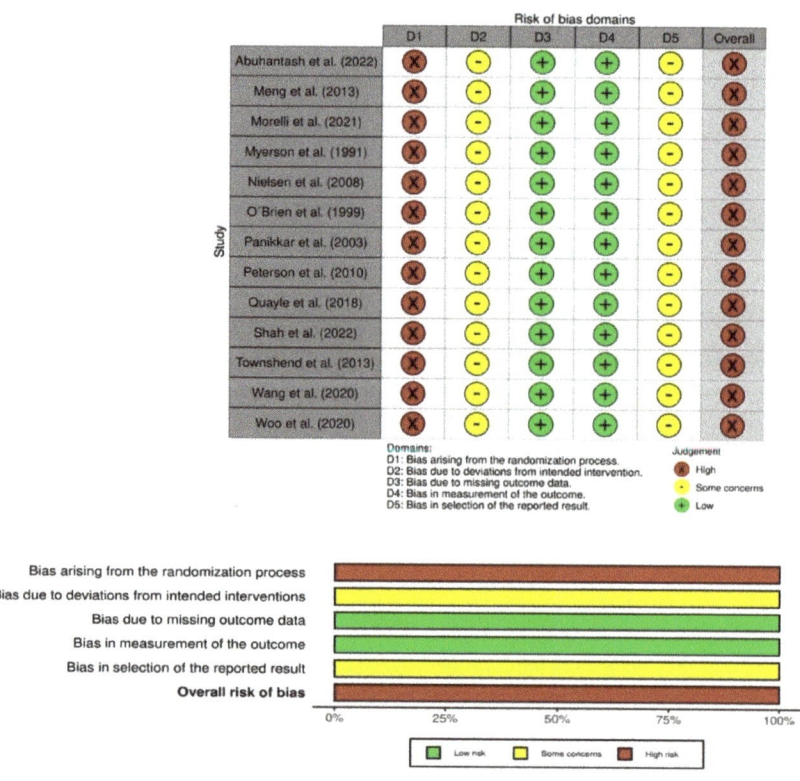

Figure 2. Risk-of-bias assessment for fusion rate traffic light plot and and summary plot [11,14–16,28–36].

3.3. Participants Characteristics

The total sample size across all studies was $n = 994$ participants, where regardless of the operation technique, $n = 23$ (58%) and $n = 383$ (42%) were females and males, respectively. In two studies, the sex was not provided; for that reason, the number of participants was 909. The mean and SD of age were 57.68 ± 6.05 and 57.37 ± 6.49 years for arthroscopy and open surgery, respectively. The body mass index corresponded to 28.07 ± 2.56 and 29.31 ± 4.08 for the arthroscopy and open-surgery groups. A complete description of the patient characteristics is summarized in Table 1.

Table 1. Baseline characteristics of the included studies.

Study	Total, N	Arth N	Open N	Age Art	Age Open	Sex Arth (M/F)	Sex Open (M/F)	BMI Arthr	BMI Open	Follow-Up (Months) Arthr	Follow-Up (Months) Open
Meng et al., (2013) [28]	30	14	16	NR	NR	0/16	0/16	NR	NR	NR	12
O'Brien et al., (1999) [16]	36	19	17	47.3	44.6	9/10	7/10	NR	NR	NR	NR
Nielsen et al., (2008) [31]	107	58	49	51	53	31/27	34/15	NR	NR	12	12
Townshend et al., (2013) [35]	60	30	30	59.4	54.7	20/10	11/19	27.4	29.6	24	24
Myerson et al., (1990) [30]	33	17	16	NR	NR	10/7	9/7	NR	NR	NR	NR
Peterson et al., (2010) [33]	20	10	10	56.2	54.8	6/4	5/5	32.11	37.36	NR	NR
Panikkar et al., (2003) [32]	41	21	20	68	65	12/9	17/3	NR	NR	9	6
Quayle et al., (2018) [15]	79	50	29	57	61.9	37/13	19/10	28.9	28	12	12
Abunhantaash et al., (2022) [11]	351	223	128	57.9	57.1	150/73	81/47	29.1	28.8	39	48
Shah et al., (2022) [34]	87	41	46	NR	NR	NR	NR	NR	NR	4	5
Wang et al., (2020) [14]	43	17	26	54.76	55.35	10/7	16/10	26.55	28.93	32	35
Morelli et al., (2021) [29]	23	12	11	64.6	67	5/7	8/3	23.8	23.6	NR	NR
Woo et al., (2019) [36]	84	28	56	60.6	60.2	9/19	18/38	28.64	28.9	NR	NR

Note: NR = not reported.

3.4. Fusion Rate

A total of 13 studies yielded a non-significant ($p = 0.072$) rate of fusion of 0.54 (0.28–1.07) for arthrodesis compared with open surgery, including 540 (54%) and 454 (46%) patients for arthroscopy and open surgery, respectively. The OR score corresponded to 0.54 (0.28–1.07). The amount of heterogeneity was cataloged as low ($I^2 = 32\%$) (see Figure 3).

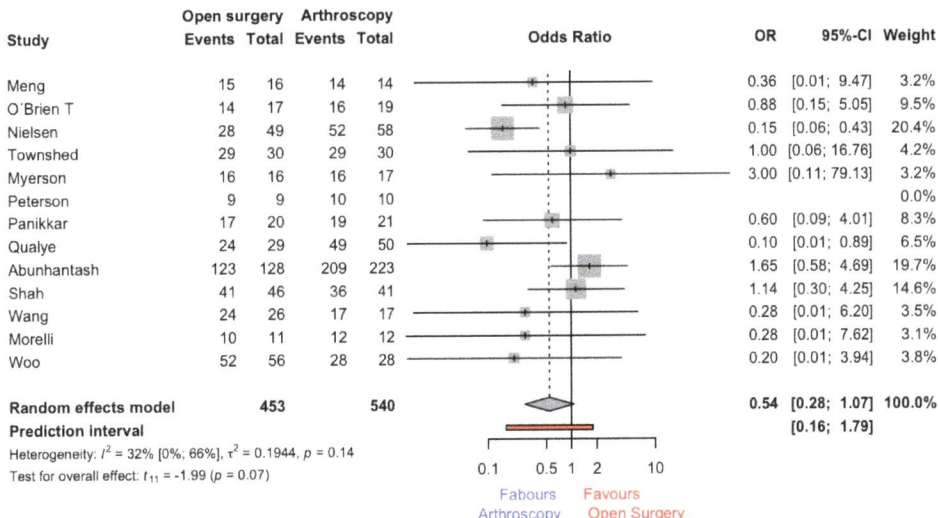

Figure 3. Forest plot for fusion rate outcome [11,14–16,28–36].

3.5. Operation Time

This outcome was reported in a total of eight studies; however, only six studies provided the SD to calculate the MD. The meta-analysis results revealed a non-significant

(p = 0.573) MD and CI$_{95\%}$ of 3.40 min (−11.08 to 17.88) for the open-surgery group. The heterogeneity and prediction interval are shown in Figure 4.

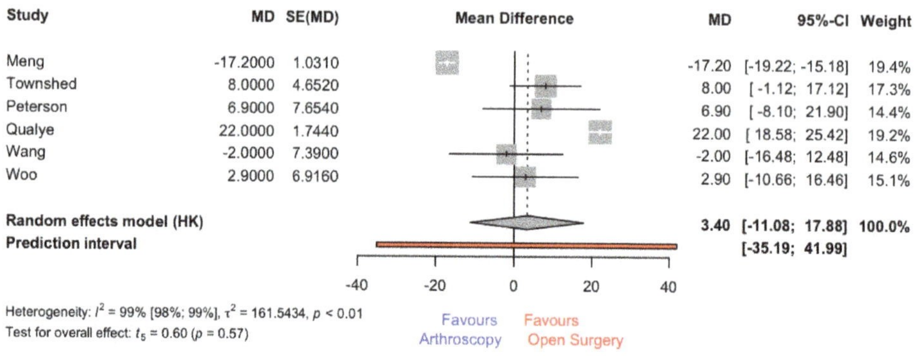

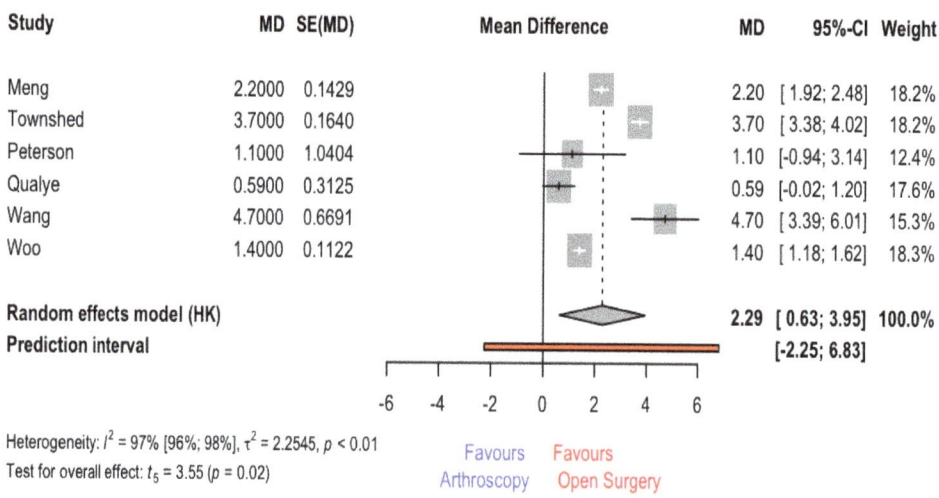

Figure 4. Forest plot for mean difference (MD) (min) for operation time outcome. SE = standard error [14,15,28,33,35,36].

3.6. Length of Hospital Stay

This outcome was reported in a total of 10 studies; however, only 6 studies provided the SD to calculate the MD. The meta-analysis results revealed a significant (p = 0.017) MD and CI$_{95\%}$ of 2.29 days (0.63 to 3.95) for the open-surgery group. The heterogeneity and prediction interval are shown in Figure 5.

Figure 5. Forest plot for hospital length stay [14,15,28,33,35,36].

3.7. Post-Operative Overall Complications

A total of 9 studies, including 43 and 66 patients for arthroscopy and open surgery, respectively, reported the number of complications. The meta-analysis results revealed a statistically significant OR and CI$_{95\%}$ of 0.40 (0.20 to 0.82) (p = 0.012), favoring the arthroscopy surgical technique. The heterogeneity was low (I^2 = 17%) (see Figure 6).

On the one hand, regarding overall complications, the most common complications described were delayed union, wound infection, non-union, deep infection, tibial entrapment, subtalar osteoarthritis, and tarsal tunnel syndrome in the open-surgery group. On the other hand, non-union, malunion, deep infection, and delayed wound healing were reported for the arthroscopy group.

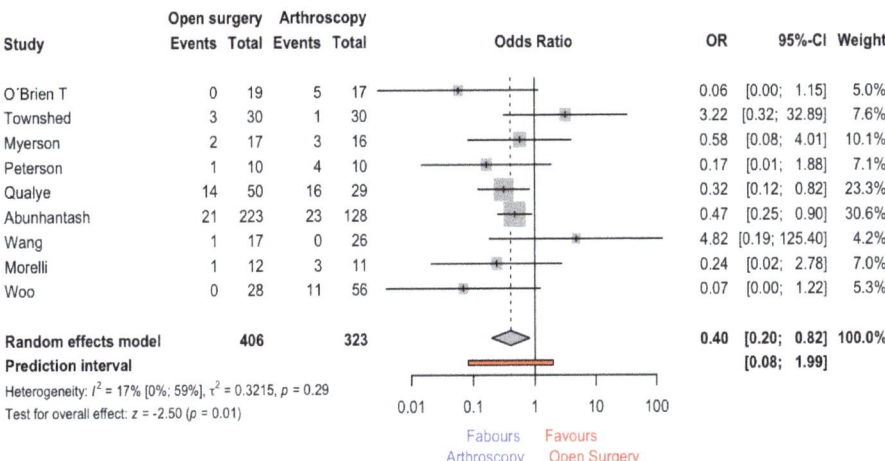

Figure 6. Forest plot for post-operative complications outcome [11,14,16,28–30,33,35,36].

3.8. Heterogeneity Analysis and Publication Bias

Visual analysis of the counter-enhanced funnel plot did not show the presence of publications' bias fusion rate (A) and overall complications (B) (Figure 7). This was confirmed analyzing Egger's test for both outcomes (fusion rate intercept = −0.031, $CI_{95\%}$ = −1.75 to −1.69, t = −0.036, p = 0.972, and overall complications intercept = −0.046, $CI_{95\%}$ = −1.30 to −1.21, t = −0.072, p = 0.944).

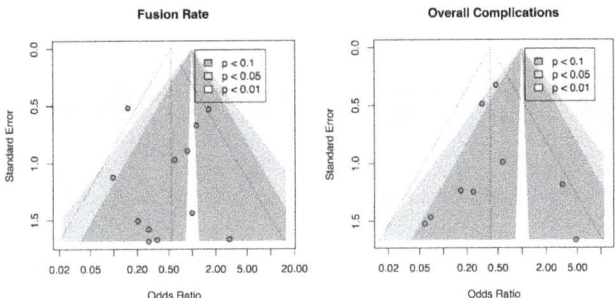

Figure 7. Counter-enhanced funnel plot for fusion rate and overall complications.

Table 2 summarizes the GRADE evaluation system for the outcomes included in the present systematic review and meta-analysis.

Table 2. Grading of Recommendations Assessment, Development and Evaluation system (GRADE) on fusion rate, operation time, hospital stay, and overall complications.

	Summary of Findings				Quality of Evidence Synthesis (GRADE)			
Outcome	k	n	OR (CI$_{95\%}$)	Direction Effect Compared to Control	Imprecision	Inconsistency	Risk of Bias	Overall Quality
Fusion Rate	13	995	0.54 (0.28 to 1.07)	↔	−1	None	−1	●●○○○ Low
Operation Time	6	316	3.40 (−11.08 to 17.88)	↔	−1	−1	−1	●○○○○ Very Low
Hospital Stay	6	316	2.29 (0.63 to 3.95)	↓	−1	−1	−1	●●○○○ Low
Overall Complications	9	413	0.47 (0.26 to 0.84)	↓	None	None	−1	●●●○○ Moderate

Note: CI confidence interval, GRADE Grading of Recommendations Assessment, Development and Evaluation; k, number of studies; n, number of participants; SMD, standardized mean difference.

4. Discussion

The main aim of this systematic review and meta-analysis was to analyze the effect of the surgery technique (i.e., open surgery vs. arthroscopy) on fusion rate in patients with ankle osteoarthritis. Evidence coming from studies with some concerns or high risk of bias showed that the arthroscopy technique had a non-statistical benefit in comparison to open-ankle surgery. The quality of evidence synthesis was rated as low. On the other hand, when operation time was compared among surgical techniques, the meta-analysis results revealed non-significant differences (3.40 min [11.08 to −17.88]). However, significant differences with an MD of 2.29 days (0.63 to 3.95) favoring the open-surgery group were found. In patients that were operated on with the open-surgery technique, the stance in the hospital was higher in comparison to the arthroscopy group. Finally, regarding overall complications, the meta-analysis results revealed that arthroscopy was a protective factor (OR = 0.47 [0.26 to 0.84]) in comparison with open surgery. In the absence of the homogeneity of studies in the outcomes provided, the preferential use of one of these techniques should be guided by other indicators such as patient characteristics or surgical preferences.

Regarding our primary outcome (i.e., fusion rate), the meta-analysis results revealed that although the arthroscopy surgical technique seems to have acted as a protection factor, no significant differences were found when data were compared with the open-ankle surgery technique. In addition, the GRADE evaluation system cataloged fusion rate and operation time as low and very low overall quality, respectively. This result differs from a recent meta-analysis by Bai et al. [17]. On the one hand, new studies were included in our meta-analysis, such as the study by Abuhantash et al. [11], where a total of 351 patients were treated (n = 223 for arthroscopy and n = 128 for open surgery). On the other hand, there are several studies that were included in the study of Bai et al. [17], where it was not possible to find the references (impossible to access Chinese electronic databases), which represents a problem of replicability.

Arthroscopy, in comparison with open surgery, requires only small incisions, which means there is less soft-tissue damage and scarring. This can lead to less pain and a faster recovery time. Our results showed that the use of arthroscopy was more beneficial than open surgery (OR = 0.54), but non-significant differences were found in fusion rate (see Figure 3) and in operation time (see Figure 4). It is important to highlight that these results came from studies with high risk of bias in the first domain (i.e., bias arising from the randomization process). It should be considered that, in all studies included in the present systematic review and meta-analysis, the patient division across groups was made according to a specific criterion (i.e., surgeon preferences or other factors). For example, in the study conducted by Woo et al. [36], the decision of which surgical procedure was performed was based on surgeon preference, as well as the study by Abuhantash et al. [11], which revealed that the surgeon decided on which operation technique to employ on the basis of the anatomy, deformity, and patient comorbidities. These facts could affect the fusion rate and the operation time. The surgeon's expertise could have an effect on operation time and on fusion rate outcomes.

The total number of complications across groups was 43 and 66 for the arthroscopy and open-surgery groups, respectively. However, when this result was adjusted by the total number of patients, the mean and SD of overall complications were 12% ± 0.08 and 27% ± 0.18 (OR = 0.47, see Figure 6). However, deep infection was reported in both surgical techniques; in this sense, Shah et al. [34] concluded that for patients with a remote history of infection, open-ankle arthrodesis may be preferable.

Based on the primary findings of this study, when the fusion rate outcome was analyzed, there was a beneficial use of the arthroscopy surgical technique in comparison with open surgery. However, it is important to highlight that non-significant differences were found between these surgical techniques. Overall, the use of arthroscopy in ankle arthrodesis can provide several advantages over traditional open surgery, resulting in a faster, less painful recovery with fewer complications. However, as with any surgical procedure, the choice of approach should be made in consultation with the patient's surgeon, taking into account individual factors such as the patient's medical history, level of physical activity, and overall health. While arthroscopic ankle arthrodesis offers several advantages over open surgery, there are also some potential disadvantages to consider, for instance, limited visualization; technical difficulty; limited accessibility; risk of complications, such as infection, nerve damage, and blood vessel injury; and limited weight-bearing capacity. However, arthroscopic ankle arthrodesis has demonstrated its advantages, and it is important to highlight that ankle joint replacement is currently the gold standard for ankle osteoarthritis. Ankle arthrodesis is technically less demanding, but patients have limited function. Whereas joint replacement showed better function and range of motion compared with ankle arthrodesis, patient satisfaction showed no difference [12].

There are some limitations in the present systematic review that need to be carefully addressed before interpreting the results obtained. Firstly, there was a large heterogeneity of outcomes across the included studies; meanwhile, some studies included functional scales and pain assessment while other studies did not. The lack of agreement regarding the outcomes assessed creates the necessity for a clinical guideline to be systematic in the outcomes reported. On the other hand, the risk-of-bias analysis of the included studies in this meta-analysis revealed the necessity for studies with a randomization process and an assessor blinded to the patient groups. Finally, arthroscopic ankle arthrodesis is often recommended for well-aligned cases, whereas open fusion is indicated to treat malaligned arthritic ankles. This fact may introduce bias in the interpretation of the results, as the lower complication rate may be attributed to less complex cases and not to the surgical approach itself. In addition, it should be mentioned that the studies do not report on the implants used for fixation, which may also have influenced the results. These major findings could affect the primary outcomes.

5. Conclusions

While both arthroscopic and open surgery can be effective for ankle arthrodesis, the evidence found suggests that arthroscopic surgery may produce similar or even better outcomes with several potential advantages over open surgery (i.e., fewer overall complications). In conclusion, our findings show that studies with some concerns or high risk of bias provided a better but non-statistically significant fusion rate in patients that underwent arthroscopic arthrodesis in comparison with open surgery. The quality of evidence was rated as low. On the other hand, operation time was not different among surgical techniques, although a lower hospital stay was found in patients that were operated on with arthroscopy. Finally, for the outcome of overall complications, the ankle arthroscopy technique was a protective factor in comparison with open surgery. For these reasons, the choice of surgical approach should be based on the careful consideration of the individual patient's condition and the surgeon's experience and preference.

Supplementary Materials: The following are available online at https://www.mdpi.com/article/10.3390/jcm12103574/s1, File S1: Prisma Checklist. File S2: Search strings. File S3: Risk of Bias and Grading of Recommendation Assessment, Development and Evaluation system. File S4: Excluded studies with reasons. References [19,37–46] are cited in Supplementary Materials.

Author Contributions: G.M. is the corresponding author for this article. Contributor roles: conceptualization, A.L., L.P., P.P., I.J.B., G.M., C.B. and R.L.; data curation A.L., L.P., P.P., I.J.B., G.M., C.B. and R.L.; formal analysis, A.L., L.P., P.P., I.J.B., G.M., C.B. and R.L.; investigation, A.L., L.P., P.P., I.J.B., G.M., C.B. and R.L.; methodology, A.L., L.P., P.P., I.J.B., G.M., C.B. and R.L.; project administration, A.L. and R.L.; software, A.L., I.J.B. and G.M.; supervision, R.L.; validation, A.L., L.P., P.P., I.J.B., G.M., C.B. and R.L.; visualization, A.L., L.P., P.P., I.J.B., G.M., C.B. and R.L.; writing original draft, A.L., L.P., P.P., I.J.B., G.M., C.B. and R.L.; writing–review and editing, A.L., L.P., P.P., I.J.B., G.M., C.B. and R.L. All authors have read and agreed to the published version of the manuscript.

Funding: This research received no external funding.

Institutional Review Board Statement: This study is a meta-analysis, and no ethics committee approval is required.

Informed Consent Statement: Not applicable.

Data Availability Statement: All data generated or analyzed during this study are included in this published article (and its Supplementary Materials).

Conflicts of Interest: The authors declare no competing interests.

References

1. Khlopas, H.; Khlopas, A.; Samuel, L.T.; Ohliger, E.; Sultan, A.A.; Chughtai, M.; Mont, M.A. Current concepts in osteoarthritis of the ankle. *Surg. Technol. Int.* **2019**, *35*, 280–294. [PubMed]
2. Glazebrook, M.; Daniels, T.; Younger, A.; Foote, C.J.; Penner, M.; Wing, K.; Lau, J.; Leighton, R.; Dunbar, M. Comparison of health-related quality of life between patients with end-stage ankle and hip arthrosis. *J. Bone Joint Surg. Am.* **2008**, *90*, 499–505. [CrossRef] [PubMed]
3. Migliorini, F.; Torsiello, E.; La Padula, G.; Oliva, F.; Maffulli, N. The Association Between Sex and Osteoarthritis in the Physically Active Population: A Systematic Review. *Sports Med. Arthrosc. Rev.* **2022**, *30*, 87–91. [CrossRef] [PubMed]
4. Baal, J.D.; Cecil, K.L.; Patel, R.; O'Brien, M.; McGill, K.; Link, T.M. Imaging of Overuse Injuries of the Hip. *Radiol. Clin. North Am.* **2023**, *61*, 191–201. [CrossRef]
5. Liu, H.; Yan, L.; Li, X.; Li, D.; Wang, G.; Shen, N.-N.; Li, J.J.; Wang, B. MicroRNA expression in osteoarthritis: A meta-analysis. *Clin. Exp. Med.* **2023**. [CrossRef]
6. Morasiewicz, P.; Dejnek, M.; Kulej, M.; Dragan, S.Ł.; Konieczny, G.; Krawczyk, A.; Urbański, W.; Orzechowski, W.; Dragan, S.F.; Pawik, Ł. Sport and physical activity after ankle arthrodesis with Ilizarov fixation and internal fixation. *Adv. Clin. Exp. Med.* **2019**, *28*, 609–614. [CrossRef]
7. Li, X.; Wang, Y.; Zhang, Y.; Ma, Y.; Pan, F.; Laslett, L.; Cai, G. Longitudinal associations of body mass index and abdominal circumference with back pain among community-dwelling adults: Data from the Osteoarthritis Initiative. *Spine. J.* **2023**, in press. [CrossRef]
8. Kuş, G.; Yasacı, Z.; Boz, C.; Türkmen, E. Association of Osteoarthritis Prevalence with Age and Obesity Factors in OECD Countries: Panel Regression Model. *Am. J. Phys. Med. Rehabil.* **2023**, *2013*, 71. [CrossRef]
9. Weatherall, J.M.; Mroczek, K.; McLaurin, T.; Ding, B.; Tejwani, N. Post-traumatic ankle arthritis. *Bull. Hosp. Jt. Dis.* **2013**, *71*, 104–112.
10. Mann, R.A.; Rongstad, K.M. Arthrodesis of the ankle: A critical analysis. *Foot Ankle. Int.* **1998**, *19*, 3–9. [CrossRef]
11. Abuhantash, M.; Veljkovic, A.; Wing, K.; Gagne, O.; Qian, H.; Wong, H.; Sadr, H.; Penner, M.; Younger, A. Arthroscopic vs. Open Ankle Arthrodesis: A 5-Year Follow Up. *J. Bone Joint Surg. Am.* **2022**, *104*, 1197–1203. [CrossRef] [PubMed]
12. Shih, C.L.; Chen, S.J.; Huang, P.J. Clinical Outcomes of Total Ankle Arthroplasty vs. Ankle Arthrodesis for the Treatment of End-Stage Ankle Arthritis in the Last Decade: A Systematic Review and Meta-analysis. *J. Foot Ankle. Surg.* **2020**, *59*, 1032–1039. [CrossRef] [PubMed]
13. Park, J.H.; Kim, H.J.; Suh, D.H.; Lee, J.W.; Kim, H.J.; Oh, M.J.; Choi, G.W. Arthroscopic vs. Open Ankle Arthrodesis: A Systematic Review. *Arthroscopy.* **2018**, *34*, 988–997. [CrossRef] [PubMed]
14. Wang, C.; Xu, C.; Li, M.; Li, H.; Wang, L.; Zhong, D.; Liu, H. Arthroscopic ankle fusion only has a limited advantage over the open operation if osseous operation type is the same: A retrospective comparative study. *J. Orthop. Surg. Res.* **2020**, *15*, 80. [CrossRef]
15. Quayle, J.; Shafafy, R.; Khan, M.A.; Ghosh, K.; Sakellariou, A.; Gougoulias, N. Arthroscopic vs. open ankle arthrodesis. *Foot Ankle Surg.* **2018**, *24*, 137–142. [CrossRef] [PubMed]
16. O'Brien, T.S.; Hart, T.S.; Shereff, M.J.; Stone, J.; Johnson, J. Open vs. arthroscopic ankle arthrodesis: A comparative study. *Foot Ankle Int.* **1999**, *20*, 368–374. [CrossRef]
17. Bai, Z.; Yang, Y.; Chen, S.; Dong, Y.; Cao, X.; Qin, W.; Sun, W. Clinical effectiveness of arthroscopic vs open ankle arthrodesis for advanced ankle arthritis: A systematic review and meta-analysis. *Medicine* **2021**, *100*, e24998. [CrossRef]
18. Mok, T.N.; He, Q.; Panneerselavam, S.; Wang, H.; Hou, H.; Zheng, X.; Pan, J.; Li, J. Open vs. arthroscopic ankle arthrodesis: A systematic review and meta-analysis. *Orthop. Surg. Res.* **2020**, *15*, 187. [CrossRef]
19. Page, M.J.; McKenzie, J.E.; Bossuyt, P.M.; Boutron, I.; Hoffmann, T.C.; Mulrow, C.D.; Shamseer, L.; Tetzlaff, J.M.; Akl, E.A.; Brennan, S.E.; et al. The PRISMA 2020 statement: An updated guideline for reporting systematic reviews. *BMJ* **2021**, *372*, n71. [CrossRef]
20. Ardern, C.L.; Büttner, F.; Andrade, R.; Weir, A.; Ashe, M.C.; Holden, S.; Impellizzeri, F.M.; Delahunt, E.; Dijkstra, H.P.; Mathieson, S.; et al. Implementing the 27 PRISMA 2020 statement items for systematic reviews in the sport and exercise medicine, musculoskeletal rehabilitation and sports science fields: The persist (implementing Prisma in exercise, rehabilitation, sport medicine and sports science) guidance. *Br. J. Sports Med.* **2022**, *56*, 175–195.
21. Clark, J.M.; Sanders, S.; Carter, M.; Honeyman, D.; Cleo, G.; Auld, Y.; Booth, D.; Condron, P.; Dalais, C.; Bateup, S.; et al. Improving the translation of search strategies using the Polyglot Search Translator: A randomized controlled trial. *J. Med. Libr. Assoc.* **2020**, *108*, 195–207. [CrossRef] [PubMed]
22. Haddaway, N.R.; Grainger, M.J.; Gray, C.T. An R package and Shiny app for forward and backward citations chasing in academic searching. *Zenodo* **2021**, *16*.

23. Higgins, J.P.; Thomas, J.; Chandler, J.; Cumpston, M.; Li, T.; Page, M.J. *Cochrane Handbook for Systematic Reviews of Interventions*; John Wiley & Sons: Hoboken, NJ, USA, 2019.
24. Cooper, H.; Hedges, L.V.; Valentine, J.C. *The Handbook of Research Synthesis and Meta-Analysis*; Russell Sage Foundation: New York, NY, USA, 2019.
25. IntHout, J.; Ioannidis, J.P.; Rovers, M.M.; Goeman, J.J. Plea for routinely presenting prediction intervals in meta-analysis. *BMJ. Open.* **2016**, *6*, e010247. [CrossRef] [PubMed]
26. Hopkins, W.G. A scale of magnitudes for effect statistics. A new view of statistics. *Auckland* **2002**, *502*, 411.
27. McGuinness, L.A.; Higgins, J.P.T. Risk-of-bias VISualization (robvis): An R package and Shiny web app for visualizing risk-of-bias assessments. *Res. Synth. Methods* **2021**, *12*, 55–61. [CrossRef]
28. Meng, Q.; Yu, T.; Yu, L.; Zhao, X.; Qi, C. Effectiveness comparison between arthroscopic and open ankle arthrodeses. *Zhongguo. Xiu. Fu. Chong. Jian. Wai. Ke. Za. Zhi* **2013**, *27*, 288–291.
29. Morelli, F.; Princi, G.; Cantagalli, M.R.; Rossini, M.; Caperna, L.; Mazza, D.; Ferreti, A. Arthroscopic vs open ankle arthrodesis: A prospective case series with seven years follow-up. *World J. Orthop.* **2021**, *12*, 1016–1025. [CrossRef]
30. Myerson, M.S.; Quill, G. Ankle arthrodesis. A comparison of an arthroscopic and an open method of treatment. *Clin. Orthop. Relat. Res.* **1991**, *268*, 84–95.
31. Nielsen, K.K.; Linde, F.; Jensen, N.C. The outcome of arthroscopic and open surgery ankle arthrodesis: A comparative retrospective study on 107 patients. *Foot Ankle Surg.* **2008**, *14*, 153–157. [CrossRef]
32. Panikkar, K.V.; Taylor, A.; Kamath, S.; Henry, A.P.J. A comparison of open and arthroscopic ankle fusion. *Foot Ankle Surg.* **2003**, *9*, 169–172. [CrossRef]
33. Peterson, K.S.; Lee, M.S.; Buddecke, D.E. Arthroscopic vs. open ankle arthrodesis: A retrospective cost analysis. *J. Foot Ankle Surg.* **2010**, *49*, 242–247. [CrossRef] [PubMed]
34. Shah, A.B.; Davis, W.; Littlefield, Z.L.; Young, S.; Alexander, B.; Andrews, N.A.; Khurana, A.; Cage, B.; Sinha, T.; McGwin, G.; et al. Patient and Surgical Factors Affecting Fusion Rates After Arthroscopic and Open Ankle Fusion: A Review of a High-Risk Cohort. *Indian J. Orthop.* **2022**, *56*, 1217–1226. [CrossRef] [PubMed]
35. Townshend, D.; Di Silvestro, M.; Krause, F.; Penner, M.; Younger, A.; Glazebrook, M.; Wing, K. Arthroscopic vs. open ankle arthrodesis: A multicenter comparative case series. *J. Bone Joint Surg. Am.* **2013**, *95*, 98–102. [CrossRef] [PubMed]
36. Woo, B.J.; Lai, M.C.; Ng, S.; Rikhraj, I.S.; Koo, K. Clinical outcomes comparing arthroscopic vs open ankle arthrodesis. *Foot Ankle Surg.* **2020**, *26*, 530–534. [CrossRef]
37. Lopes, R.; Andrieu, M.; Cordier, G.; Molinier, F.; Benoist, J.; Colin, F.; Thès, A.; Elkaïm, M.; Boniface, O.; Guillo, S.; et al. Arthroscopic treatment of chronic ankle instability: Prospective study of outcomes in 286 patients. *Orthop. Traumatol. Surg. Res.* **2018**, *104*, S199–S205. [CrossRef]
38. Murawski, C.D.; Kennedy, J.G. Anteromedial impingement in the ankle joint: Outcomes following arthroscopy. *Am. J. Sport. Med.* **2010**, *38*, 2017–2024. [CrossRef]
39. DeVries, J.G.; Scharer, B.M.; Romdenne, T.A. Ankle stabilization with arthroscopic versus open with suture tape augmentation techniques. *J. Foot Ankle Surg.* **2019**, *58*, 57–61. [CrossRef]
40. Schmid, T.; Krause, F.; Penner, M.J.; Veljkovic, A.; Younger, A.S.; Wing, K. Effect of preoperative deformity on arthroscopic and open ankle fusion outcomes. *Foot Ankle Int.* **2017**, *38*, 1301–1310. [CrossRef]
41. Xu, C.; Li, M.; Wang, C.; Liu, H. A comparison between arthroscopic and open surgery for treatment outcomes of chronic lateral ankle instability accompanied by osteochondral lesions of the talus. *J. Orthop. Surg. Res.* **2020**, *15*, 113. [CrossRef]
42. Cottom, J.M.; Baker, J.; Plemmons, B.S. Analysis of Two Different Arthroscopic Broström Repair Constructs for Treatment of Chronic Lateral Ankle Instability in 110 Patients: A Retrospective Cohort Study. *J. Foot Ankle Surg. Off. Publ. Am. Coll. Foot Ankle Surg.* **2018**, *57*, 31–37. [CrossRef]
43. Rigby, R.B.; Cottom, J.M. A comparison of the 'All-Inside' arthroscopic Broström procedure with the traditional open modified Broström-Gould technique: A review of 62 patients. *Foot Ankle Surg. J. Eur. Soc. Foot Ankle Surg.* **2019**, *25*, 31–36. [CrossRef] [PubMed]
44. Dujela, M.D.; Hyer, C.F. Ankle Arthrodesis: Open Anterior and Arthroscopic Approaches. In *Essential Foot and Ankle Surgical Techniques: A Multidisciplinary Approach*; Springer: Berlin/Heidelberg, Germany, 2016; pp. 275–290.
45. Anderson, T.; Maxander, P.; Rydholm, U.; Besjakov, J.; Carlsson, A. Ankle arthrodesis by compression screws in rheumatoid arthritis: Primary nonunion in 9/35 patients. *Acta Orthop.* **2005**, *76*, 884–890. [CrossRef] [PubMed]
46. Holt, E.S.; Hansen, S.T.; Mayo, K.A.; Sangeorzan, B.J. Ankle arthrodesis using internal screw fixation. *Clin. Orthop. Relat. Res.* **1991**, *268*, 21–28.

Disclaimer/Publisher's Note: The statements, opinions and data contained in all publications are solely those of the individual author(s) and contributor(s) and not of MDPI and/or the editor(s). MDPI and/or the editor(s) disclaim responsibility for any injury to people or property resulting from any ideas, methods, instructions or products referred to in the content.

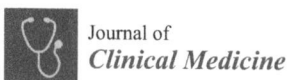

Review

A Systematic Review of the Retrograde Drilling Approach for Osteochondral Lesion of the Talus: Questioning Surgical Approaches, Outcome Evaluation and Gender-Related Differences

Francesca Veronesi [1], Melania Maglio [1,*], Silvia Brogini [1], Antonio Mazzotti [2], Elena Artioli [2] and Gianluca Giavaresi [1]

1. Surgical Sciences and Technologies, IRCCS Istituto Ortopedico Rizzoli, Via di Barbiano 1/10, 40136 Bologna, Italy; francesca.veronesi@ior.it (F.V.); silvia.brogini@ior.it (S.B.); gianluca.giavaresi@ior.it (G.G.)
2. 1st Orthopaedic and Traumatologic Clinic, IRCCS Istituto Ortopedico Rizzoli, Via G.C.Pupilli 1, 40136 Bologna, Italy; antonio.mazzotti@ior.it (A.M.); elena.artioli@ior.it (E.A.)
* Correspondence: melania.maglio@ior.it; Tel.: +39-0516366784

Abstract: Background: Retrograde drilling (RD) is a minimally invasive surgical procedure mainly used for non-displaced osteochondral lesions (OCL) of the talus, dealing with subchondral necrotic sclerotic lesions or subchondral cysts without inducing iatrogenic articular cartilage injury, allowing the revascularization of the subchondral bone and new bone formation. Methods: This systematic review collected and analyzed the clinical studies of the last 10 years of literature, focusing not only on the clinical results but also on patients' related factors (gender, BMI, age and complications). Results: Sixteen clinical studies were retrieved, and differences in the type of study, follow-up, number and age of patients, lesion type, dimensions, grades and comparison groups were observed, making it difficult to draw conclusions. Nevertheless, lesions on which RD showed the best results were those of I–III grades and not exceeding 150 mm^2 in size, showing overall positive results, a good rate of patient satisfaction, improvements in clinical scores, pain reduction and return to daily activities and sports. Conclusions: There are still few studies dealing with the issue of post-surgical complications and gender-related responses. Further clinical or preclinical studies are thus mandatory to underline the success of this technique, also in light of gender differences.

Keywords: retrograde drilling; osteochondral lesions; clinical studies; review; gender; orthopaedic

1. Introduction

The ankle is the most damaged joint of the body because it supports body forces and mass, sustaining the highest weight per unit area compared to all the other joints [1].

Osteochondral lesions (OCL) of the talus are the most common injury occurring in the ankle, especially among athletes at all levels, because of ankle sprains and fractures [2]. OCL affects talar articular cartilage and subchondral bone (SB), and worldwide, 50% of patients with ankle sprains and two out of three patients with chronic lateral ankle instability are affected by OCL [3,4]. Talar dome OCL has an incidence of 0.9% among all talar OCL and can be idiopathic or a consequence of ankle trauma, which can be classified as acute (for trauma that occurred 6 weeks before) or chronic (for trauma that occurred earlier) [5–7]. Usually, OCL is localized in the posteromedial aspect of the talus and, unlike knee OCL, spreads deeper into SB, causing a higher frequency of subchondral cysts [8]. The common clinical symptoms of OCL are chronic ankle pain, swelling, stiffness, instability, increased fall risk and limited functional activity [9].

Regarding management strategies, nonoperative conservative strategies are employed for acute and nondisplaced lesions, while surgical procedures are performed when the lesions are chronic and displaced [10]. More precisely, conservative treatments are indicated for stable lesions with a Berndt–Harty–Loomer (BHL) classification stage $\leq$ III. Such approaches foresee activity modifications (such as low-impact weight-bearing and immobilization) or intra-articular injections of platelet-rich plasma (PRP) or hyaluronic acid [7]. When conservative treatments fail (for 3–6 months), or in the presence of loose bodies, unstable lesions, SB sclerosis or BHL > III, surgical treatments take over [10].

Several different surgical treatments are employed for talus OCL depending on the defect stage and size. Arthroscopic or open surgery techniques primarily aim to revitalize the necrosis of SB. Bone marrow stimulation (BMS) techniques are the most used surgical procedures for the treatment of talus OCL due to their simplicity, low morbidity, low costs and good-to-excellent results. BMS techniques penetrate the SB plate and induce vascular access to SB, forming a clot that fills the defect [11]. This clot is rich in marrow elements, such as mesenchymal stem cells (MSCs), that can differentiate into chondrogenic or osteogenic lineages [12,13]. BMS techniques include abrasion arthroplasty, microfracture or drilling (anterograde and retrograde). The drilling is carried out with a Kirschner wire or a drill bit and through anterograde or retrograde approaches. Unlike microfractures, the drilling technique reaches a deeper part of the subchondral bone, but on the other hand, it induces thermal necrosis [14].

The anterograde drilling (AD) approach, also named the transmalleolar approach, enters the medial malleolus through cartilage and, for this reason, it may cause epiphyseal line injury [15]; in addition, dorsomedial talar dome lesions are frequently inaccessible with AD techniques. Retrograde drilling (RD), also named transtalar drilling, was developed as an alternative approach: it exploits drill guides, intraoperative fluoroscopy, or computer-assisted navigation and allows SB area to be revitalized without damaging the overlayed cartilage [16].

As first reported by Lee and Mercurio in 1981 [17], RD is minimally invasive and does not induce cartilage and epiphyseal line injuries. It is mainly used for undisplaced talus OCL, dealing with subchondral necrotic sclerotic lesions or subchondral cysts without inducing iatrogenic articular cartilage injury [18]. It is useful when the osteochondral fragment is stable with normal or nearly normal overlaying cartilage, inducing the revascularization of the SB, then leading to new bone formation. Although other surgical techniques are highly recommended for the treatment of OCL; however, RD is indicated when the defect is difficult to reach through the usual arthroscopic portals, showing good results in 80–100% of the patients [19]. In the last 10 years, few well-designed clinical studies in the literature reported the results of RD for treating talus OCL.

The present review aimed to systematically revise the literature of the last 10 years to collect all the clinical studies that employed RD as surgical treatment for talus OCL, focusing on the clinical results and complications. The main clinical results were included in this systematic review, with particular attention paid to the possible association between the main results and the gender, body mass index (BMI) or age of the patients.

2. Materials and Methods

2.1. Eligibility Criteria

To select the relevant papers included in this systematic review, a PICO question [population of interest (P), Intervention (I), comparators and outcomes (CO)] statement was formulated.

The "Population" considered was represented by randomized, prospective, retrospective, observational clinical studies and case reports involving patients affected by OCL of the talus. The "Intervention" considered was RD procedures with the specific indication of any augmented treatments. The "Comparator" was any reference group. The considered primary outcome was the main clinical results and complications associated with the RD procedures. In addition, a secondary outcome was represented by the correlation between clinical results and patient gender, BMI or age.

2.2. Search Strategy

The search was performed on 1 November 2022 (from 1 November 2012 to 1 November 2022) according to Preferred Reporting Items for Systematic Reviews and Meta-Analyses (PRISMA) statement (Figure 1). The search was carried out on 3 electronic databases (PubMed, Scopus and Web of Science) to identify relevant papers using the following keywords with boolean operators: "(Retrograde drilling OR transtalar drilling) AND (osteochondral lesion of the ankle)". The limits identified were (1) in PubMed: (i) language (English); (ii) publication date (from 1 November 2012 to 1 November 2022); (2) in Scopus and Web of Science: (i) language (English); (ii) publication date (between 2012 and 2022).

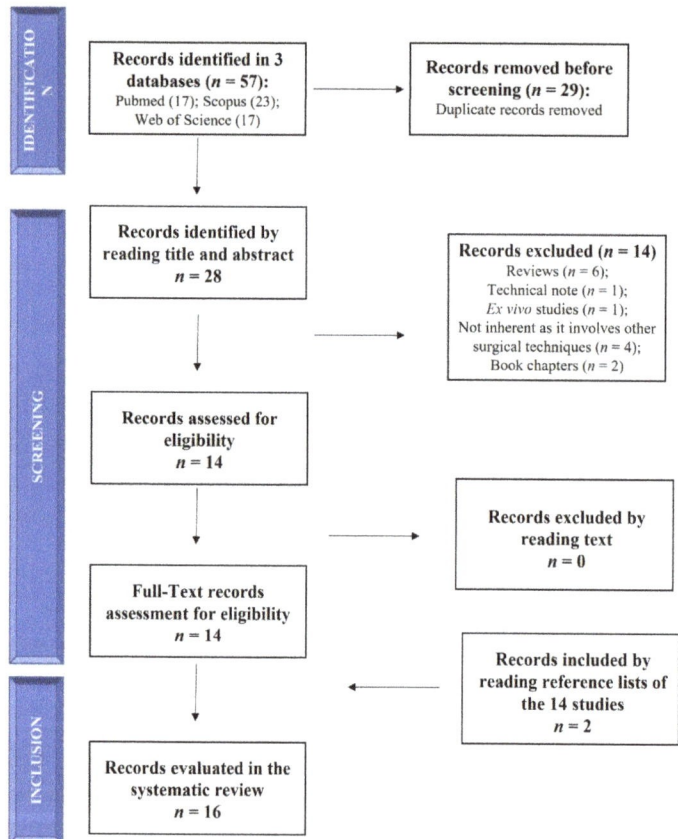

Figure 1. Schematic representation of studies search.

Relevant articles were screened using the title and abstract by 2 authors (FV and MM), and articles that did not meet the inclusion criteria were excluded. Only the clinical studies evaluating RD in OCL of the talus were included in this review and submitted to a public reference manager to eliminate duplicates and manage the references.

2.3. Information Extracted from Articles

The included full-text articles were retrieved and reviewed by the 2 authors (FV and MM), and any disagreement was resolved through discussion until a consensus was reached or with the involvement of a third author (GG). The following information was extracted from each paper and finally tabulated in Table 1 to summarize the evidence reported in each study: (a) References (Ref.); (b) study type; (c) complications; (d) grade/localization of lesion; (e) surgical procedures; (f) Follow-up (FU); (g) evaluations; (h) main results.

Table 1. Summary table of the main findings from the studies included for review.

Ref.	Study Type	Complications	Grade/Localization of Lesion	Surgical Procedure	Fu (mo)	Evaluations	Main Results
Ccrominas 2016 [19]	Case report	n.r.	OCD of the talar head (153 mm^2)	Arthroscopic fluoroscopy-guided RD	>60	AOFAS MRI	At 9 mo: return to former competitive level. At 12 mo: symptom-free. At 24 mo: AOFAS = 90. At 60 mo: AOFAS = 100; MRI evidence of SB healing, with some irregularities at the joint level and a very well-preserved joint space.
Masquijo 2016 [20]	Retrospective chart review	No complications	OCD of the talus: Posteromedial (n = 5); Central (n = 1). Berndt and Harty stage: Grade I (n = 5) and II (n = 1)	Arthroscopic fluoroscopy-guided RD	Mean 37 (16–69)	AOFAS VAS Radiography MRI CT	Progression toward healing Asymptomatic pz Complete healing (50%) ↑AOFAS ↓VAS Satisfaction (100%) 3/6 pz complete radiographic healing at the last follow-up
Ikuta 2020 [21]	Retrospective case series	No complications	Symptomatic stable OCD of the talus: Posteromedial (n = 7); Central (n = 1) Anderson classification: Grade II (n = 3) and III (n = 5)	Arthroscopic fluoroscopy-guided RD	Mean 24 (12–60)	AOFAS Ankle activity score ICRS grade MRI	↑AOFAS score and ankle activity score. At 6 mo: return to former competitive level. ICRS grade 0 = 37.5% ICRS grade I = 62.5% No signs of fragment instability or subsidence. Good fragment incorporation in 6 pz and fair in 2 patients. Good cartilage congruity in 5 pz and slight irregularity with intact cartilage in 3 pz. BML areas ↓, but still detectable at 1 yr.
Jeong 2016 [22]	Case report	Pain (VAS = 9) at 60 mo Subchondral sclerosis and osteophyte formation, cystic lesions, bone marrow edema in talus, thin talar articular cartilage at 60 mo	OCL of the talus with a central subchondral cyst, multiple medial small SB cysts and BME. Anderson classification: 2A	Arthroscopic synovectomy + RD	60	MRI CT	At 12 mo: ↑ depression of the cartilage and no pain. At 60 mo: SB sclerosis and osteophyte formation, multiple cystic lesions, BME in talus, thin talar articular cartilage.
Minokawa 2020 [23]	Retrospective case series	No complications	OCL of the talus: Posteromedial (n = 8); Pritsch Classification System: Grade II (n = 7) and III (n = 1)	RD (n = 6); RD + arthroscopic lateral ankle ligament repair (n = 1); RD + drilling for os subtibiale (n = 1)	Mean 22.8 (8–51)	JSSF scale CT	↑JSSF scale. CT healing: good (50%), fair (37.5%), poor (12.5%). No degenerative changes were noted in the radiographs at the final follow-up.

Table 1. *Cont.*

Ref.	Study Type	Complications	Grade/Localization of Lesion	Surgical Procedure	Fu (mo)	Evaluations	Main Results
Yasui 2014 [24]	Case series	n.r.	CLAI with SB lesion of the talus: Medial ($n = 16$). Nelson classification system: Grade I ($n = 16$). Modified Pritsch classification: Grade I ($n = 16$)	Fluoroscopic guidance RD + AITFL repair with the modified Broström technique ($n = 8$); Fluoroscopic guidance RD + AITFL reconstruction with autologous gracilis tendon ($n = 8$)	Mean 29 (24–46)	AOFAS VAS MRI	↑ mean AOFAS (pain and function). ↓ VAS pain and mean lesion area. Mean lesion area ↓.
Abd_Ella 2017 [25]	Prospective case series	Unsatisfaction with persistent pain and no improvement for 1 yr (1 pz)	Small OCL of the talus (area < 150 mm², cyst depth < 7 mm): Medial ($n = 29$); Lateral ($n = 3$)	Anterior ankle arthroscopy + modified Broström procedures for lateral ankle instability (4/32 pz); Anterior ankle arthroscopy + fluoroscopy-guided RD (5/32 pz)	26 (12–48)	AOFAS Saxena criteria	↑AOFAS Results: Excellent (46.9%), good (37.5%), fair (15.6%) Very satisfied (50%), satisfied (28.1%), satisfied with reservations (18.8%), unsatisfied (3.1%).
Schwartz 2021 [26]	Retrospective series	Secondary procedure (14.0%); AD (62.5%); RD (12.5%); OAT (12.5%); Allograft (12.5%)	OCL of talus (125.2 mm²): Medial (71.9%); Lateral (28.1%)	Lesions with isolated cartilage loss < 150 mm²: AD and/or microfracture ($n = 32$); Intact cartilage cap with a deficient SB plate: RD ($n = 7$); Lesions > 150 mm² or with underlying SB plate defects: OAT ($n = 10$); Uncontained defects: allograft cartilage implantation ($n = 8$)	Mean 79.9 (17–209.8)	VAS SF-12 FADI-sports; Tegner score; Marx activity scores; Naal Sports inventory; Pz satisfaction	Satisfaction = 77.2%. FADI-Sport score = 45.8. Marx activity scale = 2.8. SF-12/PCS = 44.0. SF-12/MCS = 56.3. ↓ Tegner score. AD, OAT, Allograft: ↓ VAS pain; ↑ VAS function Allograft, followed by AD, OAT and RD: ↑ SF-12/MCS.
Korner 2021 [27]	/	Re-operation (25.9%): Arthroscopy + BMS (28.6%); Arthroscopy + RD (57.1%); ACI + ABG (14.3%)	OCL of the talus: Medial (mean 127 mm²) ($n = 17$); Lateral (mean 104 mm²) $n = 10$	Arthroscopy + BMS ($n = 8$); Arthroscopy + RD ($n = 8$); Arthroscopy + BMS + RD ($n = 1$); Arthrotomy + flake fixation ($n = 1$); ACI + ABG ($n = 9$)	42 (6–117)	ICRS grade MOCART score MRI	In re-operated pz: ↑ advanced cartilage damage; ↓ ICRS stage than non-reoperated pz. In re-operated pz: ↑ MOCART score than non-reoperated pz.
Perera 2015 [28]	Case report	n.r.	OCL of the tibia	Step 1): Arthroscopic debridement + chellectomy + microfracture; Step 2) (after 6 mo): Arthroscopic debridement + defect curetted + RD + ABG	2, 6, 12 and 16 wks, 36 mo	Radiography MRI AOFAS MOXFQ FFI	At 6 wks: No pain, AOFAS score = 58. At 12 mo: AOFAS score = 86, MOXFG = 46, FFI = 17 At 16 wks: complete integration of the graft with maintained overlying articular cartilage. At 36 mo: improvements maintained at 36 mo.

Table 1. *Cont.*

Ref.	Study Type	Complications	Grade/Localization of Lesion	Surgical Procedure	Fu (mo)	Evaluations	Main Results
Anders 2012 [29]	/	Ankle swelling up to 3 mo (13.2%); Minor hypesthesia of the forefoot (5.3%); Delayed superficial wound healing (2.6%).	Undisplaced OCL of the talus (7–14 mm): Medial (n = 36); Apical (n = 29); Lateral (n = 4); Central (n = 1) Pritsch classification Grade I (n = 12), II (n = 22) and III (n = 7)	Fluoroscopy-guided RD + ABG	29 ± 13 (12–54)	AOFAS VAS MRI	↑AOFAS and VAS function. ↓VAS pain. 85% satisfaction. Grade I and II lesions: ↑results than grade III lesions. Complete bone remodeling (12.2%).
Sexena 2022 [30]	/	Hardware removal (3.4%), Revision surgery (2%)	OCL of the talar dome "small" (<125 mm^2), "medium" (125–1500 mm^2) and "large" (≥1500 mm^2): Antero-lateral (n = 55); Antero-medial (n = 54); Central-lateral (n = 11); Central-medial (n = 27); Medial-central (n = 6); Postero-medial (n = 30); Postero-lateral (n = 22).	Small lesions without intact cartilage: arthrotomy + microfracture + PRP (n = 112); Lesions with small subchondral cysts and intact cartilage: RD (n = 31); Lesions with large subchondral defect: RD + ABG + PRP (n = 8); Medium lesions: osteotomy + curettage + ABG + PRP (n = 60); Large lesion: allograft + PRP + fixation (n = 7)	Mean 82.5 ± 34.6 (24–132)	AOFAS RM score RTA	RTA = 7.9 ± 5 mo. ↑AOFAS score. RM score = 1.3 ± 0.5. Allograft, autograft and osteotomy: ↓AOFAS. Allograft: ↓activity level.
Kramer 2015 [31]	Retrospective chart review	Re-operation at 20.4 mo (26.6%): Lesions with no change or worse ↑re-operation rate than lesions healed or improved	OCL of the ankle (113 ± 62 mm^2): Medial (n = 22); Lateral (n = 22); Central (n = 5); Tibia (n = 2). Berndt and Harty stage: Grade I (n = 14), II (n = 50), III (n = 16) and IV (n = 3)	Fluoroscopy or not guided RD (n = 59); RD + internal fixation with a bioabsorbable implant (n = 22); Excision of lesion + microfracture (n = 27); RD + ABG (n = 1)	Mean 39.6 (12–129.6)	Radiography Return to sport survey FAOS	Results: Poor (30.3%), fair (21.1%) and good (48.6%). Lesion: healed (16%), improved (64%), unchanged (18%) and worse (3%). Satisfaction (81.8%). At 6 mo: Return to sport (84.1%). FAOS = 77 ± 18.
Mehta 2012 [32]	Retrospective review	Case 1: Achilles tendon pain and symptomatic subsidence at 17 wks. Case 2: No complications	OCL of the talus: Posteromedial lesion of grade I (Case 1); Posteromedial lesion (1 cm) with BME and with grade III (Case 2)	Case 1: RD + rhBMP-2 + PRO-DENSE regenerative graft; Case 2: RD + rhBMP-2 + Hydroset	1 wk–18 mo	Radiography MRI	Case 1: ↑early clinical and radiographic findings. At 17 wks: Consolidation of OCL. Case 2: At 1 mo: ankle motor strength = 5/5, ↑radiographic appearance. At 4 mo: radiographic resolution of the OCL, new bone formation, return to work.
Beck 2015 [33]	Prospective case series	Minor anterior tibial spur removed (28.6%); Partial synovectomy (71.4%)	Undetached OCL of the medial talar dome (≥100 mm^2). Pritsch classification: Grade II (n = 5) and II-III (n = 2)	Arthroscopically-guided RD + CaSO4-CaPO4 bone graft substitute	24.1 (20–28)	AOFAS FADI score Radiography MRI	↑AOFAS and FADI scores. ↓AOFAS pain score. Good restoration of the medial talar dome contour. Bony ingrowth and remodeling of the lesion. Disappearing of bone bruising adjacent to the lesion.

Table 1. Cont.

Ref.	Study Type	Complications	Grade/Localization of Lesion	Surgical Procedure	Fu (mo)	Evaluations	Main Results
Gao 2017 [34]	Retrospective, non-blinded comparative study	Ankle swelling for 12 mo (Group A: 12.2%; Group B: 25%; Hypesthesia of the midfoot (Group B: 2.4%)	Unilateral undisplaced OCL of the talus (mean 110 mm^2, 70–140 mm^2); Medial (n = 61); Lateral (n = 8), Group A (n = 41) and Group B (n = 28). Hepple grade: Grade I (n = 19), II (n = 42) and III (n = 8)	Group A (n = 41): RCD + BMDC + ESWT Group B (n = 28): RCD + BMDC	Mean 49.2 ± 33.6 Group A: 44.4 ± 14.4 Group B: 51.6 ± 26.4	AOFAS MRI	Groups A, B: ↑ overall AOFAS, pain relief, function, daily life function, progressive regression of the lesion. Group A: ↑ AOFAS pain and function, incidence of distinct lesion reduction than group B. Grade I and II: ↑ results than grade III.

Abbreviations: ABG = autologous bone graft; ACI = autologous chondrocyte implantation; AD = anterograde drilling; AOFAS = American Orthopaedic Foot and Ankle Society; ATFL = anterior talofibular ligament; BMDC = bone marrow-derived cells; BML = bone marrow lesion; BME = bone marrow edema; BMS = bone marrow stimulation; CaSO4-CaPO4 = calcium sulfate-calcium phosphate; CLAI = chronic lateral ankle instability; CT = computed tomography; ESWT = extracorporeal shock wave treatment; FADI = Foot and Ankle Disability Index; FAOS = Foot and Ankle Outcome Score; FFI = foot function index; FU = follow-up; ICRS = International Cartilage Repair Society; JSSF = Japanese Society for Surgery of the Foot; mo = months; MOCART = Magnetic Resonance Observation of Cartilage Repair Tissue; MOXFQ = Manchester–Oxford Foot Questionnaire; MRI = magnetic resonance imaging; n.a. = not applicable; n.r. = not reported; OAT = osteochondral autograft transfer; OCD = osteochondritis dissecans; OCL = osteochondral lesions; PRP = platelet rich plasma; pz = patients; RCD = retrograde core drilling; RD = retrograde drilling; Ref. = references; rhBMP-2 = recombinant human bone morphogenetic protein-2; RM = Roles and Maudsley; RTA = return to activity; SB = subchondral bone; SF-12/MCS = Short Form-12/mental component score; SF-12/PCS = Short Form-12/Physical Component Summary; VAS = Visual Analogue Score; wks = weeks.

3. Results

3.1. Search Results

The initial literature search retrieved 17 studies from PubMed, 23 from Scopus and 17 from Web of Science for a total of 57 articles. After removing duplicates (29 papers) using a public reference manager (Mendeley Desktop 1.19.8) software, 28 papers remained. Among these 28 papers, 14 papers were excluded because they were reviews ($n = 6$), a technical note ($n = 1$), an ex vivo study ($n = 1$), non-inherent studies that involved other surgical techniques ($n = 4$) and book chapters ($n = 2$). The remaining 14 articles were reviewed and considered eligible. Two additional studies were found by reading the selected articles' reference lists, so 16 studies were included in this systematic review in agreement with the PICO question and PRISMA methodological tool (Figure 1).

Tables 1 and 2 summarize the highlights of the studies and the characteristics of the patients. Among the 16 studies included in the present systematic review, 9/16 studies (56%) performed only the RD technique, compared or not to other surgical techniques [19–27], while 7/16 (44%) performed RD procedures with the addition of bone substitutes or bone marrow-derived cells (BMDC) [28–34].

3.1.1. Main Results of RD Technique

The main results were evaluated through clinical scores. The most used instruments for measuring the outcome of treatment in patients, who sustained a complex ankle or hindfoot injury, combined a clinician-reported and a patient-reported part, measuring pain and ankle instability, cartilage lesion grades, quality of life and activity in daily life or sports:

- American Orthopaedic Foot and Ankle Society (AOFAS) [19–21,24,25];
- Visual Analogue Score (VAS) [20,24,26];
- Japanese Society for Surgery of the Foot (JSSF) scale [23];
- Ankle activity score [21];
- International Cartilage Repair Society (ICRS) grade [21,27];
- Saxena criteria [25];
- Short Form-12 (SF-12) [26];
- Tegner score [26];
- Marx activity scores [26];
- Naal Sports inventory [26];
- Foot and Ankle Disability Index (FADI) [26].

As for imaging diagnostics, the approaches reported were magnetic resonance imaging (MRI) [19–22,24,27], computed tomography (CT) scans [20,22,23] and radiography [20]. For each study, the grades of OCL were indicated in Table 2 according to radiographic or MRI grading systems.

Table 2. Grading scores employed to classify lesion grades.

	Grading Score Description	Grade	Ref.
Radiographic grading system	Pritsch Classification	II and III	[23]
		I	[24]
		I–III	[29]
		II and III	[33]
	Berndt and Harty clinical grade	I and II	[20]
		I–IV	[31]
MRI grading score	Anderson classification	II and III	[21]
		IIA	[22]
	Nelson classification system	I	[24]
	Hepple grade	I–III	[34]

In three studies, one case report [19] and two retrospective case series [20,21], 1 [19], six [20] and eight [21] patients, respectively, were treated with arthroscopic fluoroscopy-guided RD for ankle osteochondritis dissecans (OCD) of the talar head (14 mm in diameter) [19], posteromedial and central OCD [21], or posteromedial and central OCL of the talus [21]. In adolescent patients, one male of 14 years old [19], one female and five males of a mean of 13 years old [20] and three females and five males of a mean age of 14.9 years [21], AOFAS score improved during 24, 37 and 60 months of follow-up [19–21]. In addition, a return to the previous sport level was observed within 9 months, with symptom-free recovery at 12 months and SB healing [19]. Complete healing was observed in 50% of patients, with reduced VAS scores and 100% satisfaction [20]. Finally, Ikuta et al. showed that all patients return to their previous sport level within 6 months, with a 62.5% of good congruity of cartilage and a reduction of bone marrow lesions (BML) [21].

MRI, CT and radiography showed variable results, with evidence of SB healing with only some irregularities at the joint levels [19], complete healing in half of the patients [20] and good fragment incorporation, good cartilage congruity and reduction of BML [21].

In a case report [22] and a retrospective case series [23], OCL of the talus was treated with RD in association with synovectomy in one male of 53 years old [22] or with lateral ankle ligament repair or drilling for os subtibiale in two females and four males' children of a mean age of 11.1 years [23].

Jeong et al. observed that even if cartilage depression gradually increased during 60 months of follow-up, no pain was registered after 12 months [22]. After 60 months, SB sclerosis and osteophyte formation, multiple cysts and BME were observed [22]. On the other hand, Minokawa et al. showed that the JSSF scale improved with good healing in 50% of patients after a mean of 22.8 months [23]. No degenerative changes were noted [23].

In the case series [24] and prospective case series [25], 16 young patients with a mean of 25 years of age, were affected by chronic lateral ankle instability (CLAI) with SB lesions of the talus in the medial position [24], and 32 patients with a mean of 32 years old suffered of symptomatic medial or lateral talus OCL [25]. In the study by Yasui et al., RD was associated with anterior talofibular ligament (ATFL) repair with modified Brostrom technique or ATFL reconstruction with autologous gracilis tendon [24], while Abd-Ella et al., performed anterior ankle arthroplasty with simultaneous modified Brostrom procedures for CLAI or RD [25]. After a mean of 26 and 29 months, AOFAS pain and function improved [24,25], VAS pain reduced, as well as the mean lesion area [24], with excellent results in 46.9% of patients and very satisfaction in 50% of patients [25]. MRI images showed that the mean lesion area decreased over time [24].

Finally, two studies compared the RD technique with other ones in 57 (21 females and 36 males) patients with a mean age of 37.1 years [26] and in 27 (17 females and 10 males) patients with a mean age of 16.9 years [28] affected by medial or lateral OCL of the talus [26,27]. Schwartz et al. compared RD with AD or microfracture for small lesions with cartilage loss, osteochondral autograft transfer (OAT) in larger lesions with subchondral plate defects and allograft cartilage implantation in uncontained defects [26]. After a mean of 79.9 months, in all the procedures, patient satisfaction was 77.2%, the FADI-sport score was 45.8, the Marx activity scale was 2.8, SF-12/PCS was 44, SF-12/MCS was 56.3, the Tegner score decreased and 85.7% of patients participated in some sport activities. However, RD showed the highest VAS pain, lowest VAS function and SF-12/MCS [26].

Korner et al. compared RD with bone marrow stimulation (BMS) and/or RD, flake fixation or autologous cartilage implantation (ACI) followed by autologous bone graft (ABG) implantation. The primary outcome was re-operation, showing that, after a mean of 42 months of follow-up, 25.9% of the patients underwent re-operation. Among them, the highest percentage of re-operation was observed for RD procedures. Re-operated patients had higher cartilage damage and lower ICRS stage than no re-operated ones [27]. In addition, MRI showed that in re-operated patients MOCART score was slightly higher than non-reoperated ones [27].

3.1.2. Complications

No complications relating to RD techniques were reported in two studies [19,24], and no complications were found in the other three studies [20,21,23]. In one study, patients' pain was high (VAS = 9), and SB sclerosis, osteophyte formation, cystic lesions, BME and thin articular cartilage were observed 60 months after the RD procedure [22]. Unsatisfaction, with associated persistent pain and no improvement after 12 months, was experienced by one patient [25], or secondary surgeries were required [26].

3.1.3. Main Results of RD Technique Associated with Bone Substitutes or Cells

The main scores employed were the same as those from the previous studies, such as AOFAS [28–30,33,34], FADI and VAS [29]. The other scores evaluated (1) the impact that foot pathologies have on the patient's perceived state of health in terms of pain, disability and activity limitations, such as foot function index (FFI) [28], (2) subjective and objective assessment of pain and discomfort, such as Roles and Maudsley (RM) scores [30], (3) the return to activity (RTA) [30] and the return to sport survey [31]. Finally, the Foot and Ankle Outcome Score (FAOS) [33] considers pain, other symptoms, activities of daily living, sport and recreational function and foot- and ankle-related quality of life. In addition, radiography [28,31–33] and MRI [28,29,32–34] were used to evaluate the results and the lesion grades, as indicated in Table 2.

After RD procedures, ABG was used to fill the tibia OCL of the talar dome and OCD of the ankle [28–31]. Perera et al. treated one male of 46 years old with arthroscopic debridement, cheilectomy and microfracture, followed, after 6 months, by arthroscopic debridement defect curettage, RD and ABG. No pain was observed after 6 weeks, and AOFAS increased from 3 to 12 months with MOXFG of 46 and FFI of 17. The complete integration of the graft and overlying cartilage was observed, and clinical improvements were maintained for 36 months [28]. Fluoroscopy-guided RD with ABG was employed in 38 patients (16 females and 22 males) with a mean age of 33.2 years. During a mean follow-up of 29 months, AOFAS pain and function improved, and VAS pain and VAS function scores were respectively reduced and increased, with 85% of satisfaction and 12.2% of complete bone remodeling, showing that grade I and II lesions had better results than grade III ones [29]. Saxena et al. treated small OCL lesions without intact cartilage with microfracture and PRP, while those with intact cartilage with RD, ABG and PRP in 204 patients (85 females and 119 males) with a mean age of 37.9 and 39.7 years for females and males, respectively. After a mean of 82.5 months, the RTA was 7.9, the RM score was 1.3 and AOFAS increased [30]. Finally, Kramer et al. performed RD with a bioabsorbable implant or ABG in 100 patients (75 females and 25 males) with a mean age of 14.3 years. After a mean of 39.6 months, lesions improved in 64% of cases, satisfaction was 81.8%, the rate of return to sport after 6 months was 84.1% and FAOS was 77 [31].

In two studies, RD was followed by the implantation of a biodegradable orthopedic biocomposite (composed of calcium sulfate and/or calcium phosphate) with [32] or without recombinant human bone morphogenetic protein 2 (rhBMP2) [33]. Two males, 44 and 31 years old, showed an OCL consolidation after 17 weeks and clinical and radiographic improvement after 2 months [32]. In seven patients (four females and three males) of a mean of 36 years old, after a mean of 29 months, AOFAS total score and FADI increased, AOFAS pain decreased, and good restoration of the medial talar dome contour, bony ingrowth and remodeling of the lesion were shown [33].

Finally, Gao et al. treated 69 patients (32 females and 37 males; mean age 46.2 years) affected by talus OCL with an injection of BMDC after RD, with or without focused extracorporeal shock wave treatment (ESWT) applied after the injection. After a mean of 49.2 months, this procedure increased AOFAS, daily life function and the regression of the lesion. The use of ESWT increased AOFAS pain and function and the reduction of lesions more than the absence of ESWT. In addition, lesions of grades I and II showed significantly better results than those of grade III [34].

3.1.4. Complications

One study did not report complications [28]. In the studies that employed ABG, ankle swelling for up to 3 months, minor hypesthesia of the forefoot and delayed superficial wound healing in 13.2%, 5.3% and 2.6% of cases [29], hardware removal (3.4%) and revision surgery (2%) [30] and re-operation after a mean of 20.4 months in 26.6% of cases [31] were reported. Achilles tendon pain and symptomatic subsidence after 17 weeks in one patient and minor anterior tibial spur removal (28.6%) and partial synovectomy (71.4%) were shown with the use of calcium sulfate and/or calcium phosphate biocomposite [32,33]. Finally, ankle swelling for 12 months was observed in 12.2% of patients treated with BMDC and ESWT and in 25% of patients that did not use ESWT, while hypesthesia of the midfoot in 2.4% of patients with BMDC alone [34].

3.2. Association between Main Results and Gender, BMI or Age

Table 3 summarizes the gender, age and BMI of patients of the studies and, as observed in Table 4, in most of the studies (75%), the associations between main results and gender, BMI or age were not evaluated [19–26,28,32–34]. Andersen et al. showed that gender, BMI and age did not influence the outcomes of the surgical procedure [29]. Similarly, another study did not observe a significant association between re-operated patients and gender, BMI and age [27]. One study did not find significant differences between males and females as regards mean RTA ($p = 0.08$), postoperative AOFAS ($p = 0.52$) and post-RM score ($p = 0.41$). The association between BMI and age with outcomes was not evaluated [30]. Only one study showed that females had worse FAOS than males ($p < 0.01$), and a BMI over 30 induced worse FAOS than BMIs of 16–24 and 25–30, even if no association was evaluated between FAOS and age [31].

Table 3. Gender, age and BMI of patients of the studies included in the review.

Ref.	Pz (n°) (F vs. M)	Age (yrs)	BMI (Kg/m^2)
Corominas 2016 [19]	1 M	14	n.r.
Masquijo 2016 [20]	6 (1 F, 5 M)	Mean 13 (11–15)	n.r.
Ikuta 2020 [21]	8 (3 F, 5 M)	Mean 14.9 (11–19)	20.0 (17.2–23.9)
Jeong 2016 [22]	1 M	53	23.6
Minokawa 2020 [23]	6 (2 F, 4 M)	Mean 11.1 (9–12)	19.2 (15.6–31.0)
Yasui 2014 [24]	16 (11 F, 5 M)	Mean 25 (14–49)	n.r.
Abd_Ella 2017 [25]	32 (10 F, 22 M)	Mean 32 ± 8 (18–50)	n.r.
Schwartz 2021 [26]	57 (21 F, 36 M)	Mean 37.1 (15–62)	27.7 (27.2–28.3)
Korner 2021 [27]	27 (17 F, 10 M)	Mean 16.9 ± 2.2	22.64 (18.0–39.3)
Perera 2015 [28]	1 M	46	n.r.
Anders 2012 [29]	38 (16 F, 22 M)	Mean 33.2 (11–56)	24.8 ± 3.6
Saxena 2022 [30]	204 (85 F, 119 M)	F mean 37.9 ± 17.4 (range 12–74); M mean 39.7 ± 15.2 (range 5–68)	n.r.
Kramer 2015 [31]	100 (75 F, 25 M)	Mean 14.3 (7–18)	23.6 ± 4.5 (16.6–38.9)
Mehta 2012 [32]	Case 1: 1 M; Case 2: 1 M	Case 1: 44 yrs; Case 2: 31 yrs	n.r.
Beck 2015 [33]	7 (4 F, 3 M)	Mean 36 (18–69)	n.r.
Gao 2017 [34]	69 (32 F, 37 M)	Mean 46.2 (19–62)	25.1 ± 4.9

BMI = body mass index; F = female; M = male; pz = patients.

Table 4. Correlation between main results and gender, BMI and age of the patients of the studies included in the review.

Ref	Gender	BMI	Age
Corominas 2016 [19]	n.a.	n.a.	n.a.
Masquijo 2016 [20]	n.r.	n.r.	n.r.
Ikuta 2020 [21]	n.r.	n.r.	n.r.
Jeong 2016 [22]	n.a.	n.a.	n.a.
Minokawa 2020 [23]	n.r.	n.r.	n.r.
Yasui 2014 [24]	n.r.	n.r.	n.r.
Abd_Ella 2017 [25]	n.r.	n.r.	n.r.
Schwartz 2021 [26]	n.r.	n.r.	n.r.
Korner 2021 [27]	Re-operated pz (males = 2 vs. females = 5); No re-operated pz (males = 8 vs. females = 12). No significant differences were detected for gender.	Re-operated pz (21.7 kg/m^2); No re-operated pz (23.6 kg/m^2). No significant differences were detected for BMI.	Re-operated pz (16.3 ± 1.6 yrs); No re-operated pz (17.1 ± 2.4 yrs). No significant differences were detected for age.
Perera 2015 [28]	n.a.	n.a.	n.a.
Anders 2012 [29]	No significant differences were detected for gender.	No significant differences were detected for BMI.	No significant differences were detected for age.
Saxena 2022 [30]	Mean RTA (males = 8.0 ± 4.9 mo vs. females = 7.8 ± 5.1 mo; $p = 0.08$); Postoperative AOFAS (males = 96 ± 3.3 vs. females = 96.3 ± 3.7; $p = 0.52$); Post-RM scores (males = 1.3 ± 0.5 vs. females = 1.2 ± 0.5; $p = 0.41$). No significant differences were detected for gender.	n.r.	n.r.
Kramer 2015 [31]	Total FAOS (males = 444 ± 44 vs. females = 368 ± 93; $p < 0.01$). Females showed worse FAOS than males.	BMI >30 showed worse FAOS outcomes than 16–24 and 25–30 BMI.	n.r.
Mehta 2012 [32]	n.a.	n.a.	n.a.
Beck 2015 [33]	n.r.	n.r.	n.r.
Gao 2017 [34]	n.r.	n.r.	n.r.

AOFAS = American Orthopaedic Foot and Ankle Society; BMI = body mass index; F = female; FAOS = Foot and Ankle Outcome Score; M = male; yrs = years; pz = patients; RM = Roles and Maudsley; RTA = return to activity.

4. Discussion

The literature analysis performed in the present systematic review returned a heterogeneous scenario of clinical applications of RD technique for treating talus OCL. In 10 years of published literature, 16 clinical studies were obtained and discussed, and several differences were found regarding the types of study, follow-up, number and age of patients, lesion type, dimensions and grade and comparison groups.

Most of the included studies were retrospective (44%), three were case reports (19%) [19,22,28], two were prospective (12%) [25,33], one was a case series (6%) [24] and three studies did not specify the typology (19%) [27,29,35]. In nine studies, the RD technique was performed alone without the addition of bone substitutes [19–27], while seven studies filled talus lesions with ABG [28,29,31], ABG added with PRP [30], biodegradable calcium sulfate/calcium phosphate biocomposites [32,33] and BMDC with or without physical stimulation [34].

The follow-up varied among the studies, ranging from a minimum of 1 week [32] to a mean of 7 years [26,30]. The other studies have interim follow-ups of 2 [21,23–25,29,33], 3 [20,27,28,31], 4 [34] and 5 [19,22] years.

The clinical relevance of the topic is corroborated by the young age at which patients were present for treatment: in about 80% of evaluated studies, patients' age was under 40 years old, and just under half involved pediatric patients (Figure 2). The presentation is often with painful symptoms, which therefore require an approach that is as decisive as possible and which allows them to resume daily activities as expected for a young adult or to address skeletal development in developing-age patients.

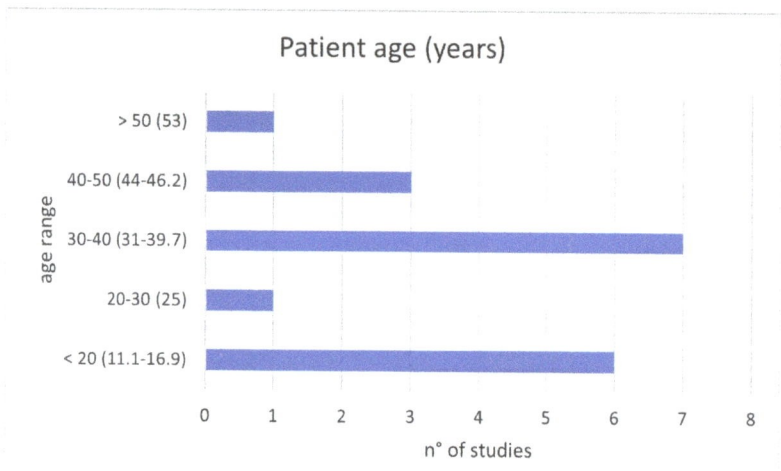

Figure 2. Patient ages of the included studies divided by age range: <20, 20–30, 30–40, 40–50 and >50 years old.

Also, the number of patients treated in each study varied from a minimum of one patient (19% of the studies) to a maximum of >100 patients (12% of the studies). As observed in Figure 3, most of the studies enrolled 1–10 patients (31% of the studies).

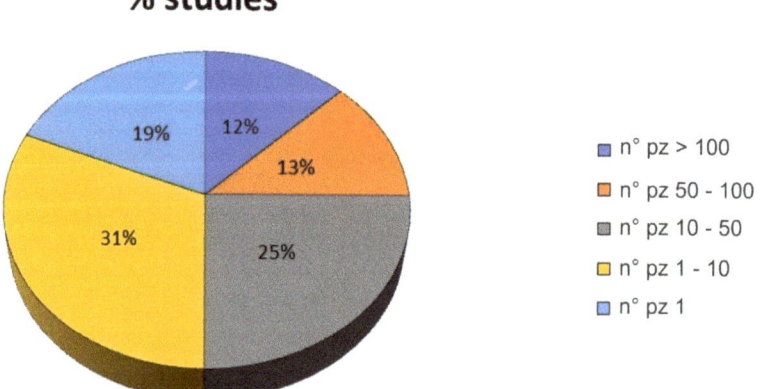

Figure 3. Pie chart of the percentage of studies grouped by the number (n°) of patients involved in the study: >100, 50–100, 10–50, 1–10 and 1.

Lesion dimensions were not always reported, while the position in the talus was usually specified; in most cases, these were posteromedial or medial lesions [20,21,23–27,29,30,32–34]; some cases involved further surgery following a previous one which had not improved the patient's clinical condition.

Dimensions of the lesions, when reported, were around 125–150 mm^2 [19,25–27,30], or <125 mm^2 [27,30,31,33,34] and only one study treated lesions > 1500 mm^2 [30]. The authors did not find a correlation between lesion dimensions and the outcomes. Almost all the studies used the same treatment for any type of lesion size, while two studies treated the lesions differently based on the size. More precisely, Korner et al. treated lesions < 150 mm^2 with AD and/or microfracture and lesions > 150 mm^2 with OAT [26], Saxena et al., employed arthrotomy, microfracture and PRP in lesions of 125 mm^2, osteotomy, curettage, ABG and PRP in 125–1500 mm^2 lesions, and allograft, PRP and fixation in >1500 mm^2 lesions [30]. All these authors found that the treatments performed in the smaller lesions showed higher improvement, as regards pain, activity level and patient satisfaction, probably due to the small dimensions of the lesions.

Heterogeneous classification systems were reported to classify the grade of the lesions: the Pritsch Classification System [23,24,29,33], Berndt and Harty stage [20,31], Anderson classification [21,22], Nelson classification system [24] and Hepple Grade [34]. As reported in Table 5, they are radiographic or MRI grading systems and consider more or less the same parameters. Some scores are more oriented towards the evaluation of cartilage and SB (Pritsch Classification, Nelson classification system and Hepple grade), and the others of only SB (Berndt and Harty clinical grade and Anderson classification).

Table 5. Description of the different grading scores employed to grade lesion types.

Grading Score	Description
Pritsch Classification (radiographic grading system) [36]	0 = normal cartilage with abnormal bone
	I = cartilage fibrillation
	II = fraying cartilage
	III = bone fragmentation detached remaining in the defect
	IV = bone fragment detached and loose
Berndt and Harty clinical grade (radiographic grading score) [37,38]	I = localized area of SB compression
	II = separated bone fragments
	III = undisplaced bone fragments
	IIIA = detached and rotated bone fragments
	IV = bone fragments displaced and inverted in its fracture bed
Anderson classification (MRI grading score) [38]	I = SB compression
	II = incomplete separation of bone fragment
	IIA = presence of subchondral cyst
	III = undisplaced bone fragment
	IV = displaced bone fragment
Nelson classification system (MRI grading score) [39]	0 = normal cartilage
	I = intact cartilage with soft changes
	II = high-signal breach of the cartilage
	III = thin, high-signal rim extending behind the osteochondral fragment
	IV = mixed- or low-signal loose body in the center of the lesion or free within the joint

Table 5. Cont.

Grading Score	Description
Hepple grade (MRI grading score) [35]	I = only cartilage damage
	IIa = cartilage injury, SB fracture and bone edema
	IIb = cartilage injury, SB fracture without bone edema
	III = detached but undisplaced fragments
	IV = detached and displaced bone fragments
	V = detached and displaced bone fragments with SB cysts

The authors that applied the first group of scores [23,24,29,33] treated lesions with fraying or fibrillated cartilage [23,24,29,33,34] and with bone fragments that had detached and remained in the defect [23,29,33] and no lesions of grade IV or V were treated. The studies that employed the second group of scores [20–22,31] treated OCL with localized SB compression [20], separated bone fragments [20,21], undisplaced bone fragments [21], SB cysts [22] and only in one study lesions of all grades were treated [31]. However, all the studies found that the RD technique improved all lesion types, although the initial lesion grade of the defect, for the most part, never exceeded grade 3.

However, the differences in the location and grade of lesions in the present studies make it difficult to uniformly compare studies based on lesion grades.

Regarding comparison groups of treatment, some studies performed only RD in all patients without comparing different techniques or treatments [19–22,29,33], allowing us to monitor the success of the RD technique during the follow-up. All these studies showed increasingly positive results up to several months after RD.

One study that compared RD with other techniques, such as AD, OAT and the use of allografts, observed that RD reduced VAS pain and improved VAS function and SF-12/MCS score to a lesser extent than other techniques [26]. Similarly, in another study, the use of allograft remained the best treatment [30]. Finally, one study compared the results of two patient groups treated with RD, and BMDC was stimulated or not with ESWT. It was observed that stimulation improved AOFAS pain and function and reduced the lesion area more than the not-stimulated one [34]. The other studies, although having different groups of patients treated with different techniques, reported the results in their entirety without highlighting differences between groups [23–25,27,28,31,32], making it difficult to compare RD with other treatments.

Gender and BMI correlation to the outcomes and complications remain underestimated and critical aspects.

The gender-related response to treatments, when indicated, showed very close numbers between males and females who undergo this surgery. Overall, considering all studies, the numbers of females and males were 277 ± 28.15 and 301 ± 29.42, respectively, without significant differences.

In the literature, there is a growing awareness of the difference between gender in talus OCL presentation and in the outcomes from treatments such as autologous osteochondral transplantation or BMS [40,41]. It might be of great interest to differentiate the results obtained from the reported studies based on patient gender to reveal any difference in the clinical presentation or the results or to eventually highlight the comparable effectiveness of RD in the outcomes regardless of gender.

In the present review, most studies did not evaluate the association between clinical outcomes and gender [19–26,28,32–34]. In two studies, the authors observed no differences between males and females as regards clinical scores [29,30] or re-operation rate [27]. Only one study underlined that females had worse FAOS than males [31].

Similarly, the correlation between the BMI and age of the patients was investigated. Furthermore, in this case, most studies did not evaluate this aspect [19–26,28,32,32–34], while one study showed that BMI > 30 induced worse FAOS outcomes than 16–24 and 25–30 BMI [31].

Another critical aspect is related to complications, which were not always reported or described in detail [19–21,23,24,28], making comparing study results difficult and generally complicating the global evaluation of the treatment outcomes. When reported, complications mainly regarded persistent pain [22,27,32], presence of SB sclerosis, osteophyte formation, cystic lesions and BME [22] and no improvement after 1 year from treatment [25]. Re-operation was a complication of some studies [26,27,30,31], and other minor complications regarded ankle swelling and hypesthesia of the forefoot [29,34], delayed superficial wound healing [29], minor anterior tibial spur removal and partial synovectomy [33].

On the other hand, alongside all the aforementioned heterogeneous aspects in the studies, instead, there was a great uniformity in the choice of diagnostic and monitoring tools (mainly radiological imaging, MRI or CT scan) [19–24,27–29,31–34], as well as in the choice of clinical scores to be applied, among which the most common remain the VAS [20,24,26,29] and AOFAS [19–21,24,25,28–30,33,34], which allows the easy and direct comparison of patient's outcomes.

However, despite the scarcity of works and the heterogeneity of several different aspects of the included studies, the results tended to be positive. In fact, it was usually observed a good rate of satisfaction from patients and improvement in clinical scores, with a reduction of pain and a return to daily activities and sports at 3–12 months from surgery; imaging investigations showed new bone formation and, when present, integration of grafts employed during surgery.

5. Conclusions

To conclude, RD has proved to be an advantageous technique in situations where an osteochondral defect of the talus still has the superficial cartilage intact. Although it is a long-standing surgical technique, introduced in 1981, there are still few clinical data produced in the last 10 years in that regard. This systematic review showed the most employed clinical scores and treatments performed in literature to treat OCL with RD technique, alone or in combination with cells, other bone substitutes, or other surgical techniques. In addition, it underlines that lesions on which RD shows the best results are of I-III grades and do not exceed 150 mm^2 in size.

Future studies are necessary to investigate which patient and lesion characteristics are associated with persistent symptoms that eventually require surgical intervention. The clinical studies analyzed in this review are different in terms of type, number and age of patients treated, follow-up and patient comparison groups, making it difficult to draw conclusions. Further clinical or preclinical studies are mandatory to underline the success of this technique, especially related to gender differences if they exist. Gender differences are still a debated topic in the literature for a variety of musculoskeletal diseases, indicating the necessity to perform more preclinical and clinical studies to elucidate the gender-based determinants and mechanisms at the base of these pathologies, also in the view of developing gender-specific protocols and tailored drugs.

Author Contributions: Conceptualization, F.V. and G.G.; methodology, S.B. and M.M.; software, F.V.; validation, A.M. and E.A.; formal analysis, G.G.; investigation, S.B. and M.M.; resources, F.V.; data curation, G.G.; writing—original draft preparation, F.V. and M.M.; writing—review and editing, G.G.; visualization, F.V.; supervision, G.G.; project administration, G.G.; funding acquisition, G.G. All authors have read and agreed to the published version of the manuscript.

Funding: The study was supported by the Italian Ministry of Health "Ricerca Corrente" and by 5x1000 2020 "Fattori legati al paziente e ruolo del microambiente patologico nel potenziale rigenerativo/riparativo di terapie cellulari ed acellulari in medicina rigenerativa muscoloscheletrica".

Institutional Review Board Statement: Not applicable.

Informed Consent Statement: Not applicable

Data Availability Statement: The data that support the findings of this study are available from the corresponding author upon reasonable request.

Conflicts of Interest: The authors declare no conflict of interest.

References

1. O'Loughlin, P.F.; Heyworth, B.E.; Kennedy, J.G. Current concepts in the diagnosis and treatment of osteochondral lesions of the ankle. *Am. J. Sports Med.* **2010**, *38*, 392–404. [CrossRef]
2. Waterman, B.R.; Belmont, P.J., Jr.; Cameron, K.L.; Deberardino, T.M.; Owens, B.D. Epidemiology of ankle sprain at the United States Military Academy. *Am. J. Sports Med.* **2010**, *38*, 797–803. [CrossRef]
3. Saxena, A.; Eakin, C. Articular talar injuries in athletes: Results of microfracture and autogenous bone graft. *Am. J. Sports Med.* **2007**, *35*, 1680–1687. [CrossRef]
4. Leontaritis, N.; Hinojosa, L.; Panchbhavi, V.K. Arthroscopically detected intra-articular lesions associated with acute ankle fractures. *J. Bone Joint Surg. Am.* **2009**, *91*, 333–339. [CrossRef]
5. Schreiner, M.M.; Raudner, M.; Marlovits, S.; Bohndorf, K.; Weber, M.; Zalaudek, M.; Röhrich, S.; Szomolanyi, P.; Filardo, G.; Windhager, R.; et al. The MOCART (magnetic resonance observation of cartilage repair tissue) 2.0 Knee Score and Atlas. *Cartilage* **2021**, *13*, 571S–587S. [CrossRef]
6. Savage-Elliott, I.; Ross, K.A.; Smyth, N.A.; Murawski, C.D.; Kennedy, J.G. Osteochondral lesions of the talus: A current concepts review and evidence-based treatment paradigm. *Foot Ankle Spec.* **2014**, *7*, 414–422. [CrossRef]
7. Buda, R.; Pagliazzi, G.; Castagnini, F.; Cavallo, M.; Giannini, S. Treatment of Osteochondritis dissecans of the talus in skeletally immature population: A critical analysis of the available evidence. *Foot Ankle Spec.* **2016**, *9*, 265–270. [CrossRef]
8. Leumann, A.; Valderrabano, V.; Wiewiorski, M.; Hintermann, B.; Pagenstert, G. Bony periosteum-covered iliac crest plug transplantation for severe osteochondral lesions of the talus: A modified mosaicplasty procedure. *Knee Surg. Sports Traumatol. Arthrosc.* **2014**, *22*, 1304–1310. [CrossRef]
9. Klammaer, G.; Maquieira, G.J.; Spahn, S.; Vigfusson, V.; Zanetti, M.; Espinosa, N. Natural history of nonoperatively treated osteochondral lesions of the talus. *Foot Ankle Int.* **2015**, *36*, 24–31. [CrossRef]
10. Dekker, P.K.; Tainter, D.M.; Easley, M.E.; Adams, S.B. Treatment of osteochondral lesions of the talus. *JBJS Rev.* **2017**, *5*, e4. [CrossRef]
11. Nakasa, T.; Ikuta, Y.; Sumii, J.; Nekomoto, A.; Kawabata, S.; Adachi, N. Clinical Outcomes of Osteochondral Fragment Fixation Versus Microfracture Even for Small Osteochondral Lesions of the Talus. *Am. J. Sports Med.* **2022**, *50*, 3019–3027. [CrossRef]
12. Yoshimura, I.; Kanazawa, K.; Takeyama, A.; Angthong, C.; Ida, T.; Hagio, T.; Hanada, H.; Naito, M. Prognostic factors for small lesions arthroscopic bone marrow stimulation techniques for osteochondral lesions of the talus. *Am. J. Sports Med.* **2013**, *41*, 528–534. [CrossRef]
13. Chen, H.; Hoemann, C.D.; Sun, J.; Chevrier, A.; McKee, M.D.; Shive, M.S.; Hurtig, M.; Buschmann, M.D. Depth of subchondral perforation influences the outcome of bone marrow stimulation cartilage repair. *J. Orthop. Res.* **2011**, *29*, 1178–1184. [CrossRef]
14. Zengerink, M.; Struijs, P.A.; Tol, J.L.; van Dijk, C.N. Treatment of osteochondral lesions of the talus: A systematic review. *Knee Surg. Sports Traumatol. Arthrosc.* **2009**, *18*, 238–246. [CrossRef]
15. Vannini, F.; Cavallo, M.; Baldassarri, M.; Castagnini, F.; Olivieri, A.; Ferranti, E.; Buda, R.; Giannini, S. Treatment of juvenile osteochondritis dissecans of the talus: Current concepts review. *Joints* **2015**, *2*, 188–191. [CrossRef]
16. Conti, S.F.; Taranow, W.S. Transtalar retrograde drilling of medial osteochondral lesions of the talar dome. *Operat. Tech. Orthop.* **1996**, *6*, 226–230. [CrossRef]
17. Lee, C.K.; Mercurio, C. Operative treatment of osteochondritis dissecans in situ by retrograde drilling and cancellous bone graft: A preliminary report. *Clin. Orthop. Relat. Res.* **1981**, *158*, 129–136. [CrossRef]
18. Dahmen, J.; Lambers, K.T.A.; Reilingh, M.L.; van Bergen, C.J.A.; Stufkens, S.A.S.; Kerkhoffs, G. No superior treatment for primary osteochondral defects of the talus. *Knee Surg. Sports Traumatol. Arthrosc.* **2018**, *26*, 2142. [CrossRef]
19. Corominas, L.; Sanpera, I., Jr.; Masrouha, K.; Sanpera-Iglesias, J. Retrograde Percutaneous Drilling for Osteochondritis Dissecans of the Head of the Talus: Case Report and Review of the Literature. *J. Foot Ankle Surg.* **2016**, *55*, 328–332. [CrossRef]
20. Masquijo, J.J.; Ferreyra, A.; Baroni, E. Arthroscopic Retrograde Drilling in Juvenile Osteochondritis Dissecans of the Talus. *J. Pediatr. Orthop.* **2016**, *36*, 589–593. [CrossRef]
21. Ikuta, Y.; Nakasa, T.; Ota, Y.; Kanemitsu, M.; Sumii, J.; Nekomoto, A.; Adachi, N. Retrograde Drilling for Osteochondral Lesion of the Talus in Juvenile Patients. *Foot Ankle Orthop.* **2020**, *5*, 2473011420916139. [CrossRef]
22. Jeong, S.Y.; Kim, J.K.; Lee, K.B. Is retrograde drilling really useful for osteochondral lesion of talus with subchondral cyst? A case report. *Medicine* **2016**, *95*, 49. [CrossRef]
23. Minokawa, S.; Yoshimura, I.; Kanazawa, K.; Hagio, T.; Nagatomo, M.; Sugino, Y.; Shibata, Y.; Yamamoto, T. Retrograde Drilling for Osteochondral Lesions of the Talus in Skeletally Immature Children. *Foot Ankle Int.* **2020**, *41*, 827–833. [CrossRef]
24. Yasui, Y.; Takao, M.; Miyamoto, W.; Matsushita, T. Simultaneous surgery for chronic lateral ankle instability accompanied by only subchondral bone lesion of talus. *Arch. Orthop. Trauma Surg.* **2014**, *134*, 821–827. [CrossRef]
25. Abd-Ella, M.M.; Fayyad, T.; Elzahlawy, H.; Abdeldayem, S.M.; Abdel Rahman, A.F. Arthroscopic management of small osteochondral lesions of the talus: Drilling revisited. *Curr. Orthop. Pract.* **2017**, *28*, 200–207. [CrossRef]

26. Schwartz, A.M.; Niu, S.; Mirza, F.A.; Thomas, A.R.; Labib, S.A. Surgical Treatment of Talus OCL: Mid- to Long-Term Clinical Outcome with Detailed Analyses of Return to Sport. *J. Foot Ankle Surg.* **2021**, *60*, 1188–1192. [CrossRef]
27. Körner, D.; Gonser, C.E.; Döbele, S.; Konrads, C.; Springer, F.; Keller, G. Re-operation rate after surgical treatment of osteochondral lesions of the talus in paediatric and adolescent patients. *J. Orthop. Surg. Res.* **2021**, *16*, 187. [CrossRef]
28. Perera, A.; Beddard, L.; Curran, S.; Robertson, A. Osteochondral Grafting of the Distal Tibia without a Malleolar Osteotomy: An All-Arthroscopic Antegrade Approach. *Tech. Foot Ankle* **2015**, *14*, 120–127. [CrossRef]
29. Anders, S.; Lechler, P.; Rackl, W.; Grifka, J.; Schaumburger, J. Fluoroscopy-guided retrograde core drilling and cancellous bone grafting in osteochondral defects of the talus. *Int. Orthop.* **2012**, *36*, 1635–1640. [CrossRef]
30. Saxena, A.; Maffulli, N.; Jin, A.; Isa, E.; Jaswal, J.; Allen, R. Outcomes of Talar Osteochondral and Transchondral Lesions Using an Algorithmic Approach Based on Size, Location, and Subchondral Plate Integrity: A 10-Year Study on 204 Lesions. *J. Foot Ankle Surg.* **2022**, *61*, 442–447. [CrossRef]
31. Kramer, D.E.; Glotzbecker, M.P.; Shore, B.J.; Zurakowski, D.; Yen, Y.M.; Kocher, M.S.; Micheli, L.J. Results of Surgical Management of Osteochondritis Dissecans of the Ankle in the Pediatric and Adolescent Population. *J. Pediatr. Orthop.* **2015**, *35*, 725–733. [CrossRef]
32. Mehta, S.K.; Chirichella, P.S.; Wey, H.; Lin, S.S. Novel Technique: Retrograde Drilling for Osteochondral Lesions of the Talus Using a Cannulated Screw for the Treatment and Local Delivery of Orthobiologics. *Tech. Foot Ankle* **2012**, *11*, 26–33. [CrossRef]
33. Beck, S.; Claßen, T.; Haversath, M.; Jäger, M.; Landgraeber, S. Operative Technique and Clinical Outcome in Endoscopic Core Decompression of Osteochondral Lesions of the Talus: A Pilot Study. *Med. Sci. Monit.* **2016**, *22*, 2278–2283. [CrossRef]
34. Gao, F.; Chen, N.; Sun, W.; Wang, B.; Shi, Z.; Cheng, L.; Li, Z.; Guo, W. Combined Therapy with Shock Wave and Retrograde Bone Marrow-Derived Cell Transplantation for Osteochondral Lesions of the Talus. *Sci. Rep.* **2017**, *7*, 2106. [CrossRef]
35. Hepple, S.; Winson, I.G.; Glew, D. Osteochondral lesions of the talus: A revised classification. *Foot Ankle Int.* **1999**, *20*, 789–793. [CrossRef]
36. Pritsch, M.; Horoshovski, H.; Farine, I. Arthroscopic treatment of osteochondral lesions of the talus. *J. Bone Joint Surg. Am.* **1986**, *85*, 989–993. [CrossRef]
37. Berndt, A.L.; Harty, M. Transchondral fractures (osteochondritis dissecans) of the talus. *J. Bone Joint Surg. Am.* **1959**, *41*, 988–1020. [CrossRef]
38. Anderson, I.F.; Crichton, K.J.; Grattan-Smith, T.; Cooper, R.A.; Brazier, D. Osteochondral fractures of the dome of the talus. *J. Bone Joint Surg. Am.* **1989**, *71*, 1143–1152. [CrossRef] [PubMed]
39. Nelson, D.W.; DiPaola, J.; Colville, M.; Schmidgall, J. Osteochondritis dissecans of the talus and knee: Prospective comparison of MR and arthroscopic classification. *J. Comput. Assist Tomogr.* **1990**, *14*, 804–808. [CrossRef] [PubMed]
40. Gianakos, A.L.; Okedele, O.; Flynn, S.; Mulcahey, M.K.; Kennedy, J.G. Autologous Osteochondral Transplantation for Osteochondral Lesions of the Talus: Does Gender Impact Outcomes? *Foot Ankle Orthop.* **2022**, *7*, 2473011421S00204. [CrossRef]
41. Gianakos, A.L.; Williamson, E.R.C.; Mercer, N.; Kerkhoffs, G.M.; Kennedy, J.G. Gender Differences May Exist in the Presentation, Mechanism of Injury and Outcomes Following Bone Marrow Stimulation for Osteochondral Lesions of the Talus. *J. Foot Ankle Surg.* **2023**, *62*, 75–79. [CrossRef] [PubMed]

Disclaimer/Publisher's Note: The statements, opinions and data contained in all publications are solely those of the individual author(s) and contributor(s) and not of MDPI and/or the editor(s). MDPI and/or the editor(s) disclaim responsibility for any injury to people or property resulting from any ideas, methods, instructions or products referred to in the content.

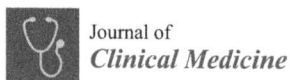

Article

An Easy-To-Use External Fixator for All Hostile Environments, from Space to War Medicine: Is It Meant for Everyone's Hands?

Julie Manon [1,2,3,4,5,*], Vladimir Pletser [6], Michael Saint-Guillain [1], Jean Vanderdonckt [1], Cyril Wain [5], Jean Jacobs [1,5], Audrey Comein [1,5], Sirga Drouet [1,5], Julien Meert [1,5], Ignacio Jose Sanchez Casla [1,5], Olivier Cartiaux [7] and Olivier Cornu [1,3,4]

1 Université Catholique de Louvain (UCLouvain), 1348 Louvain-la-Neuve, Belgium
2 Morphology Lab (MORF), UCLouvain—IREC, 1200 Brussels, Belgium
3 Neuromusculoskeletal Lab (NMSK), UCLouvain—IREC, 1200 Brussels, Belgium
4 Orthopedic Surgery Department, Cliniques Universitaires Saint-Luc, 1200 Brussels, Belgium
5 Crew 227—Mission Analog Research Simulation (M.A.R.S. UCLouvain), Mars Desert Research Station (MDRS), Hanksville, UT 84734, USA
6 European Space Agency, Blue Abyss, Newquay TR8 4RZ, UK
7 Department of Health Engineering, ECAM Brussels Engineering School, Haute Ecole "ICHEC-ECAM-ISFSC", 1200 Brussels, Belgium
* Correspondence: julie.manon@uclouvain.be

Abstract: Long bone fractures in hostile environments pose unique challenges due to limited resources, restricted access to healthcare facilities, and absence of surgical expertise. While external fixation has shown promise, the availability of trained surgeons is limited, and the procedure may frighten unexperienced personnel. Therefore, an easy-to-use external fixator (EZExFix) that can be performed by nonsurgeon individuals could provide timely and life-saving treatment in hostile environments; however, its efficacy and accuracy remain to be demonstrated. This study tested the learning curve and surgical performance of nonsurgeon analog astronauts ($n = 6$) in managing tibial shaft fractures by the EZExFix during a simulated Mars inhabited mission, at the Mars Desert Research Station (Hanksville, UT, USA). The reduction was achievable in the different 3D axis, although rotational reductions were more challenging. Astronauts reached similar bone-to-bone contact compared to the surgical control, indicating potential for successful fracture healing. The learning curve was not significant within the limited timeframe of the study (N = 4 surgeries lasting <1 h), but the performance was similar to surgical control. The results of this study could have important implications for fracture treatment in challenging or hostile conditions on Earth, such as war or natural disaster zones, developing countries, or settings with limited resources.

Keywords: tibial shaft fracture; external fixator; hostile environments; learning curve; space; developing countries; war medicine

Citation: Manon, J.; Pletser, V.; Saint-Guillain, M.; Vanderdonckt, J.; Wain, C.; Jacobs, J.; Comein, A.; Drouet, S.; Meert, J.; Sanchez Casla, I.J.; et al. An Easy-To-Use External Fixator for All Hostile Environments, from Space to War Medicine: Is It Meant for Everyone's Hands? *J. Clin. Med.* **2023**, *12*, 4764. https://doi.org/10.3390/jcm12144764

Academic Editor: Christian von Rüden

Received: 27 June 2023
Revised: 15 July 2023
Accepted: 16 July 2023
Published: 19 July 2023

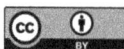

Copyright: © 2023 by the authors. Licensee MDPI, Basel, Switzerland. This article is an open access article distributed under the terms and conditions of the Creative Commons Attribution (CC BY) license (https:// creativecommons.org/licenses/by/ 4.0/).

1. Introduction

Long bone fractures are common musculoskeletal injuries that, while they can be easily managed in developed countries, can become a whole different story when they occur in hostile or uncommon conditions. Fractures may have increased risks of complications such as bleeding, infection, and delayed healing due to the unique conditions present in those environments, such as space, war or natural disaster zones, developing countries, or settings with limited resources. The problem of having a long bone fracture in hostile or uncommon and challenging environments is that traditional methods of fracture repair may not be feasible or effective due to various challenges. These challenges may include weightlessness, restricted resources, absence of healthcare facilities, difficulties in soft tissue and wound management, challenges in anesthesia administration, and, above all, limited access to surgical expertise [1]. Therefore, finding appropriate and effective methods for fracture repair in hostile environments is crucial to ensure successful healing, functional recovery, patient outcomes, and survival, while not compromising all other activities that depend on that injured person.

As a first step, the external fixator can already solve some of these challenges. External fixation allows preservation of fracture hematoma and management of soft tissues, is less invasive, reduces bleeding and infection risk, and could require only a local or locoregional anesthesia [2–4]. A correctly executed procedure could potentially allow immediate weight-bearing, which is crucial for mission success, soldier autonomy, and faster consolidation compared to casts.

However, a major limitation in hostile environments is the restricted availability of trained surgeons to set up the fixator despite the huge need [1]. For example, more than 21% of the surgical activities of Médecins Sans Frontières (MSF) are orthopedic surgeries, including external fixators [1–5], but are not usually performed by a specialized surgeon. The fixator can decrease the rate of amputation and enhance limb salvage and life in humanitarian contexts [5]. Nonsurgeon individuals may need to be self-sufficient and autonomous in managing fractures in such situations, like during space missions, on the battlefield of war or natural disaster, or in remote areas with limited access to medical care. Fractures may also occur as part of emergency situations where immediate intervention is needed to stabilize the fracture and prevent further life-threatening complications. Nonsurgeon individuals who would be trained in using fracture fixation methods could provide timely and life-saving treatment in such situations, even in the absence of skilled surgical personnel. Therefore, having an easy-to-use external fixator (EZExFix) that can be performed by nonsurgeon individuals could allow for prompt, effective, and self-sufficient treatment of fractures without relying solely on surgical expertise.

In this study, our newly developed EZExFix [6,7] is designed to be easy, quick to learn, and accessible to nonsurgeon individuals as a solution for stabilizing tibial shaft fractures, which are one of the most common types of long bone fractures [8–10].

Space was chosen as the ultimate hostile environment to test the efficacy and accuracy of the management of tibial shaft fractures by nonsurgical astronauts. With space exploration missions extending beyond Earth orbit, such as potential travel to Mars, the health and safety of astronauts become critical [2,11–16]. The absence of an orthopedic surgeon in space, combined with the occurrence of a long bone fracture, poses serious risks to the health and life of the injured astronaut and may jeopardize the entire mission. Repatriation for timely surgical treatment is unfeasible due to the vast distance between Mars and Earth. Telesurgery has limitations due to significant transmission delay [2,13,17–19]. Therefore, it is crucial to enhance the autonomy of astronauts, empowering them with the skills and resources necessary to effectively manage medical emergencies on their own and to achieve enough medical outcomes.

Analog astronauts had to quickly learn how to assemble the EZExFix in order to fix tibial shaft fractures during a simulated inhabited mission at the Mars Desert Research Station (MDRS) lasting 2 weeks. This station is a simulated Martian habitat located in the Utah desert, USA [20]. Every year since 2002, from November through April, it serves as a research facility for studying human factors and conducting experiments relevant to future Mars missions [21]. The station provides a Mars-like environment and allows scientists and astronauts to simulate living and working conditions on the Red Planet [22]. The effectiveness and accuracy of fracture reduction, i.e., the medical performance of nonsurgeon astronauts, are evaluated independently without relying on Earth support or extensive surgical skills. This assessment includes analyzing the learning curve based on four surgical sessions (Sessions S_1, S_2, S_3, S_4) and whether some extreme conditions such as simulated extravehicular activities (S_{EVA}) or at an unexpected moment (S_{stress}) can alter their performance. The final objective is to utilize these findings to draw conclusions that can be extrapolated to Earth for the treatment of fractures in challenging or hostile conditions.

2. Materials and Methods

2.1. Fractured Leg Model

The fractured leg model was already described in a previous article [4]. Briefly, the leg model was made from a left tibia with a hard cortical and cancellous intramedullary bone structure (LSH1385, Synbone SDN BHD, Kulai, Malaysia). The AO/OTA 42A2 fracture type was always created by marking a simple oblique fracture line in the middle of the tibial diaphysis using a laser and three vertical benchmarks for references (Figure 1). The leg model was shaped with foam rubber sheet (22320, Komprex®, Lohmann & Rauscher, Neuwied, Germany), covered with a sock to mimic the skin, and fixed onto a foot prosthesis to provide an axis for realignment maneuvers. A new leg model was used for each new surgery. The removal of soft tissues from the bone was possible without having to remove the EZExFix and allowed measurement of the quality of reduction.

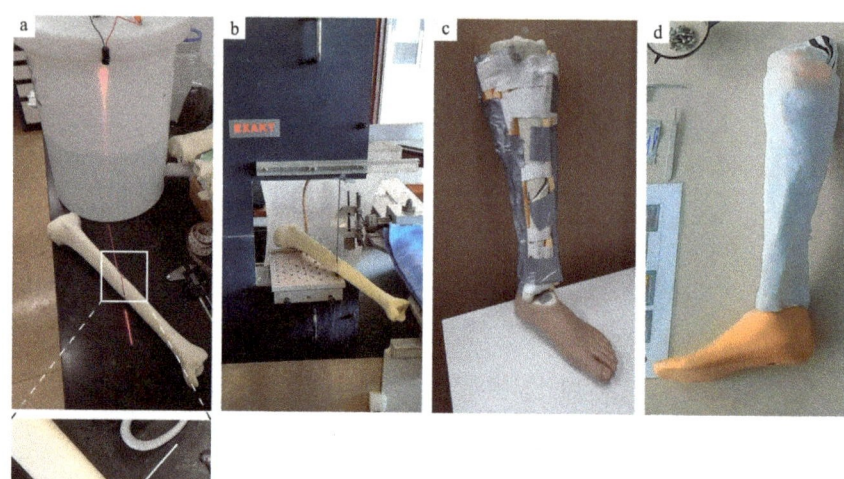

Figure 1. Creation of the fractured leg model. Landmark of the fracture line with a laser ((**a**) above—red line) and vertical benchmarks to further evaluate fracture reduction ((**a**) below—white arrows). Bone cutting by the diamond bandsaw following the fracture landmark (**b**). Soft tissues assembly and fixation around the fractured bone, mounted on a foot prosthesis (**c**). Final fractured leg model (**d**). Adapted from Manon et al. [4].

2.2. External Fixator (EZExFix)

The EZExFix is a newly developed fixator designed to stabilize tibial fractures with an emphasis on the ease of use, the price, and the accessibility in hostile and challenging environments [6]. This device can fix all types of tibial shaft fractures, including complex or comminuted fractures with significant soft tissue lesions. It has been validated to have mechanical properties similar to the Hoffmann® 3 fixator, which is a reference device [7]. The EZExFix consists of various spare parts that can be assembled into a final construct, which is illustrated in Figure 2.

2.4.3. Percentage of Bone Contact

In order to evaluate the surface of bone-to-bone contact, the minimal and maximal distances in mm between the proximal and distal parts of the fracture were calculated following the guidelines for an ISO1101-based assessment of the location parameter (Figure 5) [29]. Because it is widely accepted that the maximal gap to lead to direct bone healing through intramembranous ossification is 2 mm [30,31], this threshold was considered to describe the "bone-to-bone contact". Larger gaps between bone ends may result in the formation of fibrous tissue instead of bone, leading to delayed healing or nonunion [32]. To refine the accuracy, a bone-to-bone contact under 1.5 mm was also assessed. The results are expressed as the percentage of bone-to-bone contact on all the tibial fracture circumference.

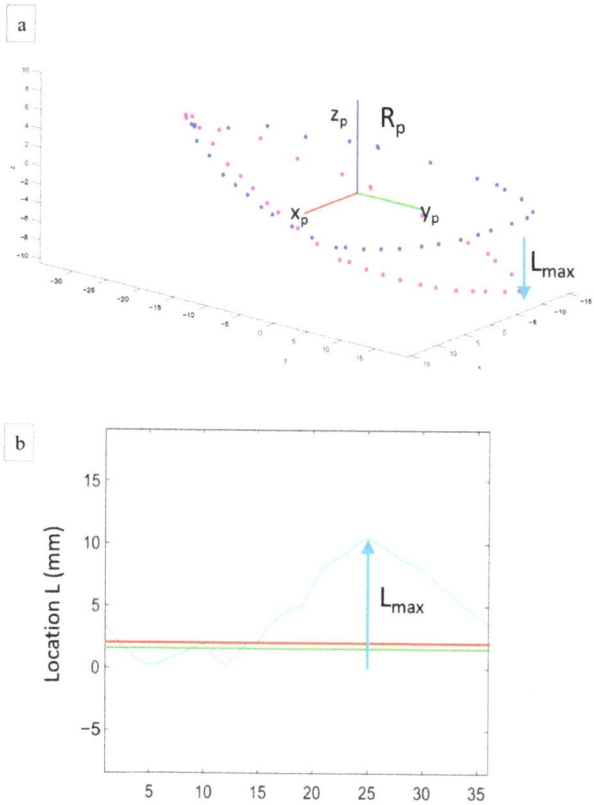

Figure 5. Example of proximal (blue dots) and distal (magenta dots) parts of the fracture registered in the global reference frame R_{world} (**a**). The local reference frame R_p is fixed to the centroid of the blue dots. As an illustration, L_{max} is the maximum distance between proximal and distal parts of the fracture, measured in mm along the axis z_p. Example of results for the calculation of the location parameter between proximal and distal parts of the fracture (**b**). The blue curve represents the evolution of the location of the distal part along the circumference of the proximal part of the fracture. The horizontal red line is the 2 mm threshold. The horizontal green line the 1.5 mm threshold. The 2 mm and 1.5 mm bone-to-bone contacts are computed as the part of the blue curve lying under the red and green horizontal lines, respectively.

After the break, the proximal part, above the fracture line, was considered as the reference in the pathologic world, i.e., fixed part that will be transposed in the anatomical world using the iterative closest point (ICP) registration algorithm using numerical computation software (MATLAB®, R2020b, The MathWorks, Natick, MA, USA). The distal part, below the fracture line, was seen as the moving part of the tibia which had to be reduced. Two local reference frames, R_p and R_d, were defined on the proximal and distal parts of the fracture, respectively, using the 3D points encoded with the CMM (Figure 4). The result of the ICP registration between the proximal and distal parts of the fracture expressed in the pathologic world and the fracture line expressed in the anatomical world is the geometrical transformation that enables expression of the local frames R_p and R_d in the global frame R_{world} in terms of both position and orientation. After fixation, the same data were taken on each side of the fracture line and the residual shift between both could be calculated and compared with the anatomical world to translate into the six initial displacements, divided into three translational displacements and three rotational displacements. Translational displacements included sagittal translation or anteroposterior displacement (A/P), frontal translation or lateromedial displacement (L/M), and axial translation or shortening/lengthening (L−/L+). The rotational displacements included frontal rotation or varus/valgus (VR/VL), sagittal rotation or flessum/recurvatum (FL/RC), and axial rotation or external/internal rotation (ER/IR). Mathematically, those six parameters were calculated as follows. The A/P, L/M, and L−/L+ translational displacements were calculated as the distances in mm, along the X, Y, and Z axes of R_{world}, respectively, between the positions of R_p and R_d. The VR/VL, FL/RC, and ER/IR rotational displacements were calculated as the differences in orientation, in degrees, between R_p and R_d around the X, Y, and Z axes of R_{world}, respectively.

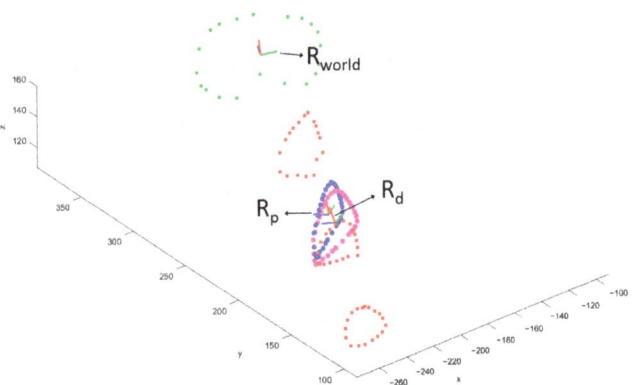

Figure 4. Examples of points of interest (in green, red, blue, and magenta) encoded with the coordinate measuring machine and used to construct the global reference frame R_{world} fixed to the tibial plateau (green dots), the local reference frame R_p fixed to the proximal part of the fracture (blue dots), and the local reference frame R_d fixed to the distal part of the fracture (magenta dots).

2.4.2. Quality Assessment of Fracture Reduction

All of the six displacements were considered pathologic above or below specific thresholds. The A/P, the L/M, and the L−/L+ displacements were pathologic outside the range of −5 to +5 mm of displacement. The VR/VL and FL/RC deformation were pathologic outside the range of −5° to +5° of rotation [27,28]. The ER/IR displacement were pathologic outside the range of −10° to +10° of rotation [27,28]. Outcomes are expressed by the mean of quantitative continuous variables and/or by a binary value if the astronaut reached the physiologic acceptable range or if he stayed in the pathologic one following the previous respective thresholds.

2.3.3. Surgical Control

Meanwhile, an experienced orthopedic surgeon also participated in the study as a surgical control, performing the same experiment as astronauts in standard conditions three times in order to compare astronauts' surgeries to this reference point. The surgeon was experienced in using classical Hoffmann® external fixators [23–25], but not the new EZExFix device, and received the same theoretical information as astronauts.

2.3.4. Operating Schedule

Programming the surgeries for the EZExFix project among the eight different scientific projects of the analog mission was a complex combinatorial problem due to limited time and resources. To solve this, an artificial intelligence system called Romie was used to create a schedule for the entire mission and adapt it based on the progress of the mission in order to maximize the probability of mission success [26].

2.4. Analysis Parameters

2.4.1. Data Collection for Fracture Reduction Positioning

Six main vectors are needed to characterize displacements between two fractured edges after reduction and fixation: three axes of translation following Cartesian coordinates (X, Y, and Z axes) and three of rotation (around each axis) (Figure 3a). In order to quantify them, a coordinate measuring machine (CMM) (Microscribe G2X, Immersion Corporation, San José, CA, USA) encoded the 3D position of a tip laying on points of interest with a precision of 0.2 mm (Figure 3b). First of all, baseline data of unbroken tibias were collected to model the "anatomical world" in order to allow the comparison with the "pathologic world" on fixed broken legs. To perform this, 20 points of tibial plateau were localized in the three Cartesian coordinates, including four cardinal points and 16 secondary points (Figure 3c; green dots). Then, three circumferences were added thanks to measuring three main points on the three tibial rims and 15 additional points in between on three different heights of the tibia (proximal, near the fracture, and distal) (Figure 3c; red dots). All those points allowed fitting of a cylinder approximating the correct tibial axis and which defined the Z axis. X and Y axes were then determined as orthogonal and according to main cardinal points. The X, Y, and Z axes define the world reference frame R_{world} with X the anteroposterior axis, Y the lateromedial axis, and Z the proximodistal axis. The fracture line was also measured in the anatomical position, before creating the fracture, described by three main points and 11 secondary points, and was used to separate the tibia into two parts (Figure 3c; blue dots).

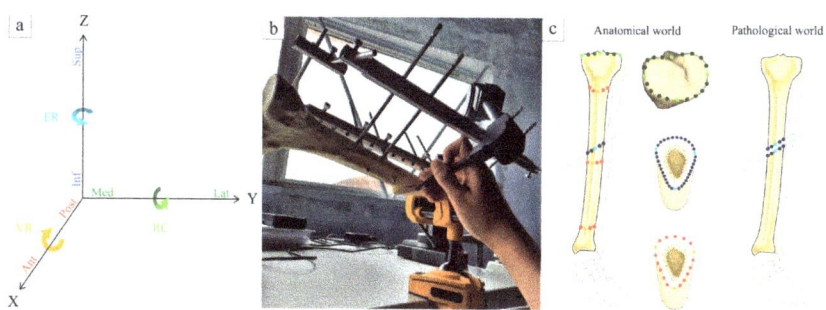

Figure 3. Measurement following six vectors (three translations and three rotations) into Cartesian coordinates (**a**). Ant: anterior, Post: posterior, Inf: inferior, Sup: superior, Med: medial, Lat: lateral, ER: external rotation, VR: varus, RC: recurvatum. For the procedure to harvest points position with the coordinate measuring machine, the pin has to point to the desired localization and a computer registers it (**b**). Points of interest to take measurements of anatomical world and pathologic world (**c**). The green and red dots are used to approximate the correct tibial axis and the blue ones are used to describe the fracture position.

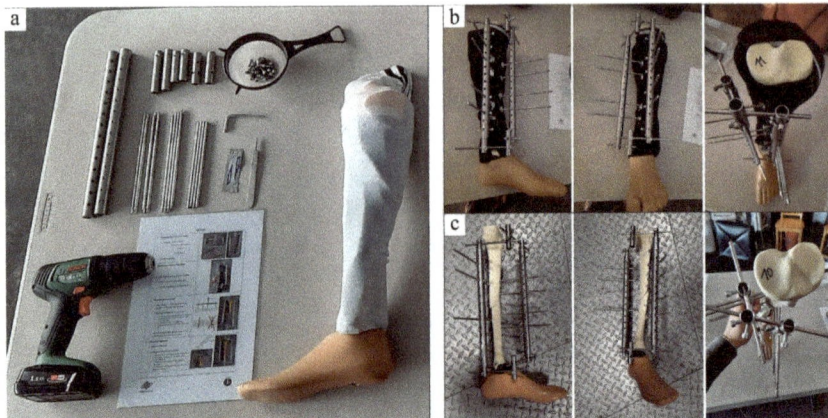

Figure 2. Material needed to build the EZExFix (**a**). Final construct mounted on a broken artificial leg on a sagittal, frontal, and upper view, respectively (**b**). Broken artificial leg after removing soft tissues ready to measure analysis parameters on a sagittal, frontal, and upper view, respectively (**c**). Adapted from Manon et al. [4].

2.3. Study Design

2.3.1. Analog Surgeons

Six analog astronauts participating in the Tharsis mission (2022) at the MDRS were recruited for a study conducted in accordance with the hospital–faculty ethics committee of the Cliniques Universitaires Saint-Luc, Belgium (N°B403201523492). None of the analog astronauts was trained as surgeon, and none of them had experience treating long bone fractures before.

2.3.2. Surgeries

At the early beginning of the mission, the analog astronauts received a brief theoretical training session lasting for one hour and a practical demonstration, during which they were taught about the indications, anatomical landmarks, and steps involved in using the EZExFix device.

The analog astronauts then competed with each other in a series of small timed runs where they had to set up the device on an artificial broken leg in the most efficient way, four times as operator who placed the EZExFix on the broken leg (Sessions S_1, S_2, S_3, S_4), and four times as assistant who helped to maintain the fracture reduction. The whole surgeries were performed without fluoroscopic control, the reduction being guided by the prosthetic foot and palpation of the anterior tibial crest. Each astronaut took turns being the operator or assistant in 12 rounds of runs, with each person being evaluated on four self-achievements (N = 24 experimentations) and on its learning curve. The timed runs were designed to simulate potential increasing stress levels in a challenging spatial environment where fractures may occur. To determine if stress levels could affect the performance, different learning conditions were used to induce stress. Each surgery was timed and carried out as a competitive trial between two operators. The surgeries were performed under three different conditions: standard, where all equipment was already prepared; stressful, which involved performing the surgery during an extravehicular activity (S_{EVA}), or at an unexpected moment with no preparation (S_{stress}). Each astronaut performed the surgeries twice under standard conditions and twice under stress conditions. This study design was already described in more detail previously [4].

2.4.4. Objective Learning Curve

The learning curve of nonmedical astronauts is essential to assess because of the significant impact on patient outcomes, surgical efficiency, and healthcare costs. This could also highlight the time needed for nonsurgeon personnel to handle the EZExFix. The four consecutive sessions allowed us to gain an idea of this short learning curve.

2.5. Statistical Analyses

A descriptive analysis was first performed to summarize and characterize data using boxplots. In the text, central tendencies are expressed by means, and dispersion by standard deviation (+/−SD) and by the ranges (min–max) where appropriate because of small datasets. Inferential statistics were used to make inferences and draw conclusions about population parameters. The normality of all data was evaluated by QQ plots. The comparisons between astronauts and the surgical control were assessed by nonparametric two-tailed Mann–Whitney tests. Nonparametric Friedman tests for repeated measures were computed to analyze differences among all sessions for each shift, followed by multiple Wilcoxon's tests with Bonferroni correction if needed. The threshold for significance was set at 0.05, indicating that the null hypothesis would be rejected if the p-value was below. All statistical analyses were conducted using SPSS software (version 27, IBM SPSS, Inc., Chicago, IL, USA).

3. Results

3.1. Fracture Reduction—Translational displacement

Over the four sessions, translational mean shifts after analog astronauts' surgeries were observed as follows: A posterior shift of −1.048 mm (+/−1.971; range −4.16–+2.25), a lateral shift of 3.247 mm (+/−3.119; range −2.33–+11.44), and a lengthening of −3.094 mm (+/−3.885; range −11.65–+5.16) (Figure 6). All the three translations had the same orientation as those of the surgeon, and none of these displacements were statistically different than that observed after the control surgeries: posterior shift of −1.320 mm (+/−3.750; range −4.74–+2.69) ($p = 0.763$), lateral shift of 0.420 mm (+/−2.909; range −2.83–+2.78) ($p = 0.166$), and a lengthening of −3.617 mm (+/−4.210; range −7.81–+0.61) ($p = 0.966$). None of the astronaut mean shifts was considered pathologic.

3.2. Fracture Reduction—Rotational Displacement

After the four surgeries, astronauts made an average varus displacement of 4.302° (+/−3.872; range −2.70–+10.05), a recurvatum of −12.284° (+/−11.479; range −34.80–+3.03), and an internal rotation of −9.860° (+/−8.078; range −24.51–+1.74) (Figure 7). The surgical control also ended with statistically indistinct varus of 3.340° (+/−3.873; range +0.82–+7.80) ($p = 0.698$) and recurvatum of −1.230° (+/−7.389; range −9.76–+3.20) ($p = 0.094$). However, the surgeon tended to place the foot in an external rotation of 2.920° (+/−4.179; range −0.27–+7.65), which was significantly different from the internal rotation created by astronauts ($p = 0.008$). While none of the residual displacements among the surgeon surgeries was clinically pathologic, the recurvatum was clearly pathologic for astronaut surgeries.

During the four sessions, each astronaut succeeded in reaching an average of almost four physiological axes (mean of 3.95 axes, +/−0.597). Translational reductions were easier to obtain than rotational ones. While the A/P physiologic range was systematically achieved (100% of astronauts), the L−/L+ and the L−/L+ were obtained by 85 and 75% of astronauts, respectively. The VR/VL and the ER/IR success dropped down to 55 and 50%, respectively, but the biggest difficulty was obtaining a physiological range in the FL/RC (only 30% of astronauts reached the normal range on average over the four sessions).

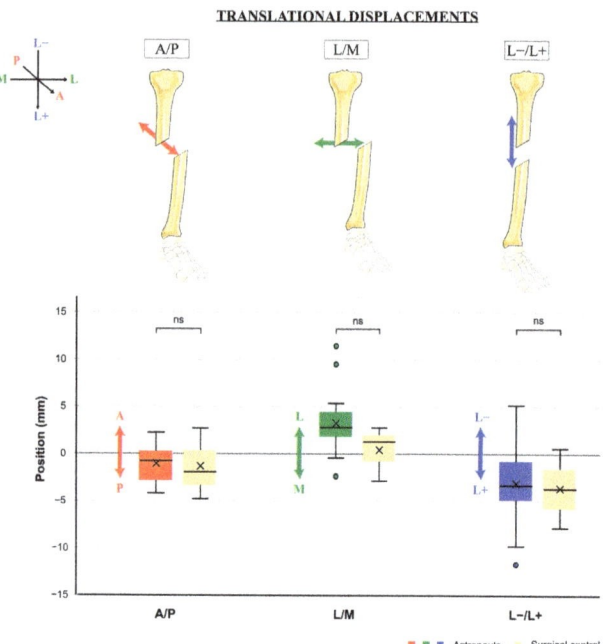

Figure 6. Average translational displacements of analog astronauts' surgeries comparing to surgeon ones. A: anterior, P: posterior, M: medial, L: lateral, L+: lengthening, L−: shortening, ×: mean, °: outliers, ns: nonsignificant.

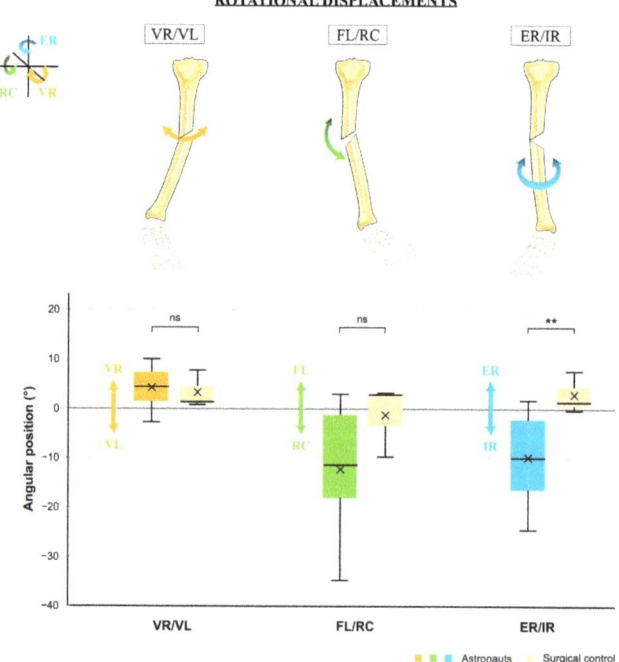

Figure 7. Average angular displacements of analog astronauts' surgeries compared to surgeon ones. VR: varus, VL: valgus, FL: flessum, RC: recurvatum, ER: external rotation, IR: internal rotation, ×: mean, ns: nonsignificant, **: $p < 0.01$.

3.3. Bone-to-Bone Contact

Concerning the cortical contact, the two bone ends were less than 2 mm from each other over 13.47% of the total tibial circumference for astronauts and over 20.60% for the surgeon (Figure 8). Despite this discrepancy, the difference was not significant ($p = 0.60$). However, when considering a bone-to-bone contact less than 1.5 mm apart, both surgeon and astronauts reached approximately 10% contact over the whole circumference ($p = 0.166$). Astronauts were able to successfully perform 60% of all the surgeries, with a minimal portion of 5% of the whole tibial circumference having contact less than 2 mm between the bones.

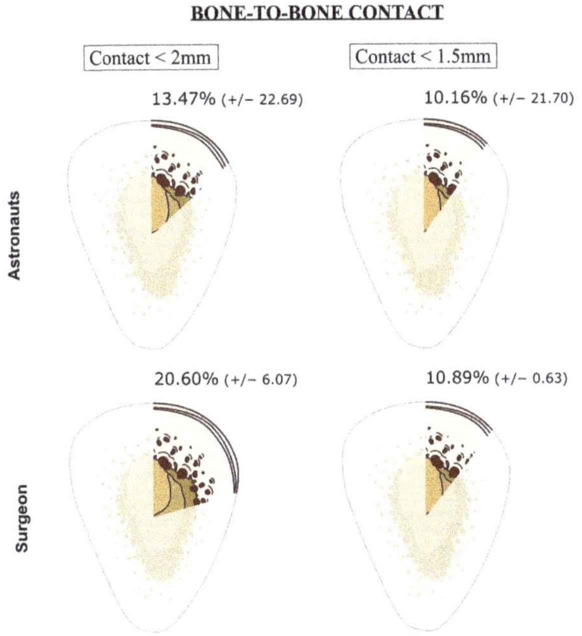

BONE-TO-BONE CONTACT

Astronauts:
- Contact < 2mm: 13.47% (+/− 22.69)
- Contact < 1.5mm: 10.16% (+/− 21.70)

Surgeon:
- Contact < 2mm: 20.60% (+/− 6.07)
- Contact < 1.5mm: 10.89% (+/− 0.63)

Figure 8. Bone-to-bone contact less than 2 and 1.5 mm for astronauts and the surgeon, represented on axial cross sections of the mid-shaft tibial fractures. The opaque surface corresponds to the bone contact percentage under the respective threshold. This contact zone is purely theoretical, not anatomical. Outcomes are expressed as the mean percentage over the total tibial circumference (+/−standard deviation).

3.4. Objective Learning Curve

Figure 9 shows that across the four sessions, the A/P, the L−/L+, and the VR/VL tended to end with a better mean at S_4 (closer to the zero baseline) but none of the six shifts showed a significant improvement ($p > 0.05$). The bony contact started to really improve at S_4 but the difference with S_1 was not yet significant ($p = 0.109$ both for contact < 2 and 1.5 mm). For half of the displacements (i.e., A/P, FL/RC, and ER/IR), the average data during EVA were better than that of S_{stress} and the opposite was seen for the remaining shifts (i.e., L/M, L−/L+, and VR/VL). The mean at S_4 ended three times closer to the zero baselines than that of both S_{EVA} and S_{stress}, suggesting that these conditions did not affect the performance of astronauts. The best clinical outcome at the end of S_4 was the A/P reduction (0.51 mm +/−1.58; range −1.75−+2.25) and the worst one was the FL/RC reduction (−14.29° +/−13.74; range −34.80−+2.38).

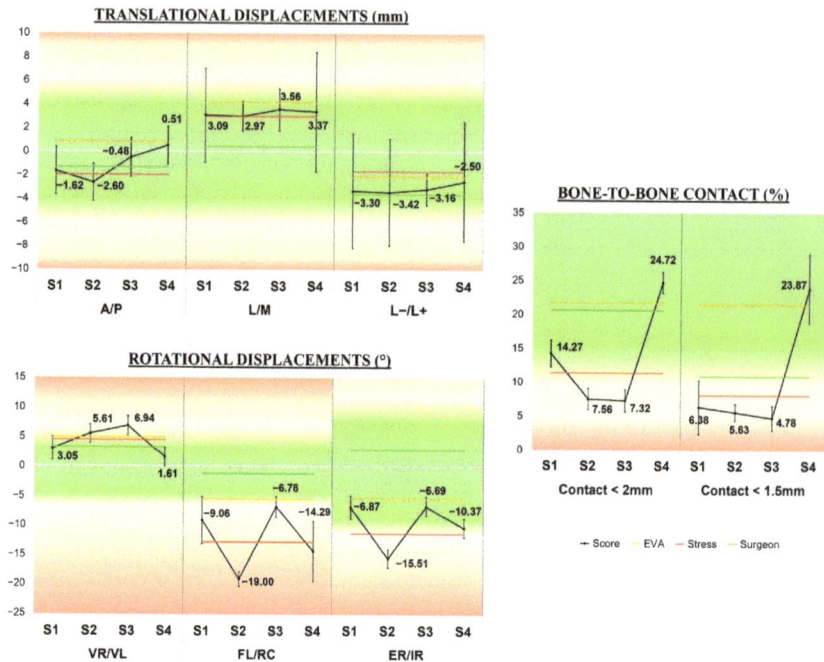

Figure 9. Panel chart of the six different displacements and the bone-to-bone contacts expressed as mean scores (black bold straight lines) across the four successive sessions (Sessions S_1, S_2, S_3, S_4). As a reference, S_{EVA} and S_{stress} are represented by yellow and red lines, respectively, as a horizontal bar calibrated on the corresponding mean scores. Error bars show the standard deviation. Green area shows physiologic range and red warns about the pathologic one. A: anterior, P: posterior, M: medial, L: lateral, L+: lengthening, L−: shortening, VR: varus, VL: valgus, FL: flessum, RC: recurvatum, ER: external rotation, IR: internal rotation.

4. Discussion

Having a reliable and effective fixation method for tibial fractures that can be handled by nonsurgeon astronauts is crucial to ensure proper bone healing and functional recovery in a hostile and challenging environment with limited access to medical facilities and resources.

The EZExFix succeeded in reaching these objectives and the reduction performance was relatively acceptable, although it needs to be discussed.

Reduction displacements. Translational reductions were easy to obtain, with an A/P reduction always obtained, probably due to the ease of palpation of the anterior tibial crest through very thin soft tissues, a true-to-life situation. However, the rotational ones were more complicated, with the FL/RC being the least successful one. Despite the apparent discrepancy in recurvatum between astronauts and surgeon, the difference was not significant ($p = 0.094$) because of the wide dispersion of data. This means that some surgeries were much better than others with non-negligible variability. The excessive variation resulted sometimes in pathologic recurvatum, which is clinically unacceptable. Although there is debate about the occurrence of osteoarthritis and functional outcomes after tibial malunion, a long follow-up study showed that even the malunion can increase the radiological osteoarthritis incidence, and it was not correlated with the patient joint symptomatology [28]. The only significant displacement was the axial rotation. The astronauts fixed the foot in IR while the surgeon fixed it more in ER ($p = 0.008$). Even if the IR remains in the physiologic range above $-10°$ of rotation, the average value is quite borderline ($-9.86°$ of IR). This can be viewed as clinically relevant also, because a residual ER is much more functional as residual IR [33,34]. Nevertheless, the general surgical residency (nonorthopedic surgery) does not give a predisposition to achieve direct correct alignment, because only two teams (2/6) succeeded in realigning a leg after a 2-day course [1].

Bone-to-bone contact. The improvement in bone-to-bone contact became noticeable at S_4, but the difference compared to S_1 was not statistically significant ($p = 0.109$). The bony contact is not significantly different between the surgeon and astronauts, which is a very good aspect of the healing prospect. The degree of contact is an important factor in fracture healing, as greater contact between the two bone ends facilitates bone growth and union. A higher percentage of contact generally indicates a better prognosis for healing, while a lower percentage of contact may increase the risk of delayed or nonunion [32].

Objective learning curve. Assessing the learning curve can aid in determining the number of cases required to become proficient and achieve consistent outcomes. This information can help to guide training programs and establish appropriate benchmarks for evaluating surgical proficiency [35], especially when the training time is restricted. It is also important for ensuring patient safety and optimizing the use of healthcare resources. Another study showed a rapid improvement for senior surgical residents who had never set up an external fixation before, but had some previous surgical knowledge [1]. Astronauts did not show any significant improvement in fracture reduction over the four sessions, suggesting that the number of surgeries may not have been sufficient to see a significant impact on the learning. However, despite the absence of a visible learning curve, the performance was similar to the surgical control for four displacements, meaning that perhaps there is no need for a long-duration learning curve. For the axial (ER/IR) and sagittal (FL/RC) rotation, there would be a real interest to repeat the study with more numerous sessions to see if astronauts could improve their learning curve on these rotational displacements that are more difficult to obtain, and to see how long it would take to meet physiological goals. Stressful conditions did not affect the astronauts' performance, and a subjective learning curve was also assessed. The eight scales (i.e., attractiveness, efficiency, perspicuity, trust, adaptability, usefulness, intuitive use, and haptics) were consistently and continuously assessed over multiple sessions, indicating a pattern similar to a hype cycle curve.

Patient safety, procedure, and time. The fracture-related factors are needed to drive bone healing but patient safety, respect for the procedure, and the duration of execution are also three criteria important to maximize the treatment and were analyzed in a previous study [4]. As a brief reminder, in nearly all cases, safe zones, including arterial and nerve areas, were rigorously maintained to ensure the safety of patients during surgery. The steps of the procedure, the avoidance of skin compression, and the stability of the assembly were achieved in 80% of the surgeries. The average surgical time for an astronaut to apply an EZExFix (52.19 min +/− 11.08) was comparable to the surgical control and aligned with the mean operating time reported in the literature [36–38]. Significantly longer times were observed for reduction and fixation steps among astronauts, and the positioning step showed the most prominent difference comparing to the surgeon. Astronauts allocated more time to precise placement of the EZExFix and avoidance of skin compression, while surgeons prioritized the reduction step, possibly due to their experience. This indicates that astronauts quickly grasped the significance of these criteria, whereas surgeons may rely on their surgical expertise for the EZExFix positioning.

Limits. Tibial shaft fracture was used as a common long bone model and for its ease of handling because it allowed us to replicate exactly same fracture pattern and soft tissue condition. Consequently, the tibial crest is really easy to palpate and facilitates the self-monitoring of the reduction. This experience should be extended to other types or other bone fractures with more soft tissues around the bone and fewer direct benchmarks for reduction, such as femoral fractures. The small number of subjects due to the incompatibility of the space analog habitat with a large cohort is also a limit of this study. To address this, repeating the experiments in subsequent missions or in other hostile conditions on Earth could support the results obtained. The interpretation of all these results is also limited due to differences in variance between the surgical group, which was reduced to within-operator variance, and the astronaut group, which comprised both within- and between-operator variances. Therefore, caution should be exercised when comparing the astronauts' performance with that of the surgeon, as it provides only an approximate idea of expected astronauts' potential achievements. Additionally, future studies could include sterility evaluation. Although the EFORT (European Federation of National Associations of Orthopedics and Traumatology) open reviews have permitted the use of external fixators in emergency rooms for life-threatening patients with pelvic, humeral, femoral, or tibial instability [39], the EZExFix remains an aseptic surgical procedure that needs to be properly executed and assessed.

Improvement and perspectives. While the treatment of fractures in hostile and challenging environments is difficult, the diagnosis can be just as challenging too; however, the latter has to be firm before thinking about repairing a long bone fracture. Ultrasound has a well-established track record of accuracy in diagnosing abdominal and thoracic trauma, and it may be a valuable tool for diagnosing extremity injuries by trained nonphysician personnel in situations where radiography is not readily available, such as in military or space applications [40]. Once the diagnosis has been made, nonsurgeon individuals could be ready to use the EZExFix by having attended just one theoretical session lasting one hour, along with a single demonstration. However, in cases where there is any doubt about the reduction, the teacher should emphasize fixation of the leg in flexion and external rotation to counteract the average opposite tendency.

Impacts on Earth medicine. The parallelism between space and hostile environments on Earth is evident. War or natural disaster zones, developing countries, or settings with limited resources are facing the same challenges as previously described and need the same adaptations of the usual medicine or surgery. On the one side, medicine on Earth can help spatial medicine. For example, there is a wealth of collective maritime and naval experience, with a long-standing history of practices during times of war and peace, that could offer valuable insights on what actions to take and what to avoid when formulating space medicine policies [13]. But on the other side, the opposite is also valuable; space medicine or hurdles can help to improve Earth's medicine in this kind of challenging situation. For example, some doctors from Médecins Sans Frontières (MSF) could be sometimes afraid about using external fixators to fix a fracture because it sounds like a complex procedure reserved for experienced surgeons, and they did not have sufficient exposure during their general surgery curriculum [1]. However, this study highlights the simplicity of the EZExFix and the possibility to achieve medical requirements without any medical background. This would encourage general practitioners, general trauma surgeons, or even nurses or personnel in the field to use the EZExFix in case of life-threatening emergencies or critical situations because of resource constraints. The medical evacuation procedures commonly used on Earth typically involve the application of a leg splint and transferring patients to healthcare facilities on the same day or within a short timeframe for appropriate medical care. This evacuation procedure could be optimized with this EZExFix in terms of fracture reduction and damage control surgery. However, immediate transportation is not always feasible, and relying solely on a splint in these cases does not address the need for definitive treatment, such as stable fixation of complex fractures with multiple fragments or dislocation, soft tissue management, or infection prevention in cases of open fractures. In situations where timely repatriation to a hospital is not possible, such as in developing countries, (sub)marines, or space missions, the lack of access to healthcare facilities can result in dire consequences. The implementation of the EZExFix provides a solution to these challenges, eliminating the dependency on healthcare facilities altogether. The EZExFix is made with materials that reduce the cost and allow local production in order to increase accessibility also for developing countries that are in need of easy accessible stabilization methods [41–43]. The EZExFix could be also considered for inclusion in a medical kit because it is compact, portable (requires only a battery for the drill; no external power supply needed), lightweight (1 kg without the drill), and takes up minimal space

(35 × 20 × 10 cm, maximum of a shoebox) in the limited resources available such as on a spacecraft. This device could be readily available and could facilitate a rapid response in case of emergency, just like a defibrillator kit. The ultimate goal is to simplify the learning and utilization of the external fixator to alleviate apprehensions, reduce fears and preconceptions, and make it accessible and user-friendly, so that anyone can utilize it and save patients in challenging environments.

In conclusion, the EZExFix is a single device that offers the ability for nonsurgeon individuals to handle fracture fixation in hostile environments and to overcome challenges related to limited access to surgical expertise, emergency situations, resource constraints, self-sufficiency, and mission success or patient's fate. Even if all the axes are not perfectly reduced, the consolidation should be achieved and the patient's life saved by nonsurgeon people. The EZExFix combines nearly all the benefits needed to face challenging conditions, making it a promising orthopedic therapy for space applications as well as in settings with limited resources on Earth.

Author Contributions: Conceptualization, J.M. (Julie Manon), O.C. (Olivier Cornu) and O.C. (Olivier Cartiaux); methodology, J.M. (Julie Manon) and O.C. (Olivier Cornu); software (scheduling), M.S.-G.; validation, J.M. (Julie Manon), O.C. (Olivier Cornu) and O.C. (Olivier Cartiaux); formal analysis, J.M. (Julie Manon) and O.C. (Olivier Cartiaux); investigation, J.M. (Julie Manon); data curation, J.M. (Julie Manon), C.W., J.J., A.C., S.D., J.M. (Julien Meert) and I.J.S.C.; writing—original draft preparation, J.M. (Julie Manon) and O.C. (Olivier Cartiaux); writing—review and editing, O.C. (Olivier Cornu), O.C. (Olivier Cartiaux), V.P., J.V. and M.S.-G.; visualization, J.M. (Julie Manon); supervision, O.C. (Olivier Cornu) and O.C. (Olivier Cartiaux); funding acquisition, J.M. (Julie Manon), C.W., J.J., A.C., S.D., J.M. (Julien Meert) and I.J.S.C. All authors have read and agreed to the published version of the manuscript.

Funding: This research was funded by the F.S.R. Fund («Fonds Spéciaux de Recherche», Belgium), a «Student Angel Fund» (Ref. 304907648 val-31.05.) granted by M.A.R.S. UCLouvain crew 2022, and a Fund for Scientific Research—FNRS granted by Dr. Julie Manon («Fonds de la Recherche Scientifique—FNRS », Research Fellow, Application ID 40004991, Belgium).

Institutional Review Board Statement: The study was conducted in accordance with the Declaration of Helsinki, and approved by the Institutional Ethics Committee of the Cliniques Universitaires Saint-Luc, Belgium (N°B403201523492).

Informed Consent Statement: Informed consent was obtained from all subjects involved in the study.

Data Availability Statement: All data analyzed during the study are included in this published article. The complete original datasets generated during the current study are available from the corresponding author on reasonable request.

Acknowledgments: The authors would like to deeply thank Shannon Rupert as well as the Mars Desert Research Station committee and the Mars Society for having welcomed them in the Utah desert for the simulation and for the opportunity to execute this research in a Mars analog environment. They would like to express their special gratitude to Benoît Lengelé and Catherine Behets for allowing them to carry out this project in parallel with other projects, and Lies Fiévé and Christine de Ville de Goyet for their help to create artificial broken legs. Figures 3 and 6–8 were partly generated using a modified template provided by Servier Medical Art (http://smart.servier.com/, accessed and downloaded on the 14 July 2022), licensed under a Creative Commons Attribution 3.0 unported license (https://creativecommons.org/licenses/by/3.0/, accessed on the 14 July 2022). Although this research did not receive direct funding from specific grant agencies in the public, commercial, or not-for-profit sectors, it was made possible thanks to the participation in the Mars analog mission, which was funded by various sponsors, including Louvain4space, Sabca, Aerospacelab, B12 consulting, Oscar, UDH (Urgence Depollution Hydrocarbures), UCLouvain Fipe, SBIM (Société Belge d'Informatique Médicale), Space Application, SPW (Service Public de Wallonie), Ludovic de Meuus, Fonds Jeremy, and WBI (Wallonie-Bruxelles International), whom the authors would like to express their gratitude towards. These funding sources were not involved in the study design, data collection, analysis, interpretation, or outcomes.

Conflicts of Interest: The authors declare no conflict of interest. The funders had no role in the design of this study; in the collection, analyses, or interpretation of the data; in the writing of the manuscript; or in the decision to publish the results.

References

1. Coleman, J.R.; Lin, Y.; Shaw, B.; Kuwayama, D. A Cadaver-Based Course for Humanitarian Surgery Improves Manual Skill in Powerless External Fixation. *J. Surg. Res.* **2019**, *242*, 270–275. [CrossRef] [PubMed]
2. Swaffield, T.P.; Neviaser, A.S.; Lehnhardt, K. Fracture Risk in Spaceflight and Potential Treatment Options. *Aerosp. Med. Hum. Perform.* **2018**, *89*, 1060–1067. [CrossRef] [PubMed]
3. Kirkpatrick, A.W.; Ball, C.G.; Campbell, M.; Williams, D.R.; Parazynski, S.E.; Mattox, K.L.; Broderick, T.J. Severe Traumatic Injury during Long Duration Spaceflight: Light Years beyond ATLS. *J. Trauma Manag. Outcomes* **2009**, *3*, 4. [CrossRef] [PubMed]
4. Manon, J.; Saint-Guillain, M.; Pletser, V.; Buckland, D.M.; Vico, L.; Dobney, W.; Baatout, S.; Wain, C.; Jacobs, J.; Comein, A. Adequacy of In-Mission Training to Treat Tibial Shaft Fractures in Mars Analog Testing. 2023. Available online: https://www.researchsquare.com/article/rs-2967843/v1 (accessed on 25 June 2023).
5. Bertol, M.J.; Van den Bergh, R.; Trelles Centurion, M.; Kenslor Ralph, D.H.; Basimuoneye Kahutsi, J.-P.; Qayeum Qasemy, A.; Jean, J.; Majuste, A.; Kubuya Hangi, T.; Safi, S.; et al. Saving Life and Limb: Limb Salvage Using External Fixation, a Multi-Centre Review of Orthopaedic Surgical Activities in Médecins Sans Frontières. *Int. Orthop.* **2014**, *38*, 1555–1561. [CrossRef]
6. Kouassi, K.J.-E.; Akobé, J.R.; Kouassi, A.A.; Fonkoué, L.; Detrembleur, C.; Kodo, M.; Cornu, O. Locally Developed External Fixators as Definitive Treatment of Open Tibia Diaphyseal Fractures: A Clinical Prospective Study Conducted in Ivory Coast. *Int. Orthop.* **2022**, *46*, 79–87. [CrossRef]
7. Kouassi, K.J.-E.; Cartiaux, O.; Fonkoué, L.; Detrembleur, C.; Cornu, O. Biomechanical Study of a Low-Cost External Fixator for Diaphyseal Fractures of Long Bones. *J. Orthop. Surg. Res.* **2020**, *15*, 247. [CrossRef]
8. Manon, J.; Detrembleur, C.; Van de Veyver, S.; Tribak, K.; Cornu, O.; Putineanu, D. Predictors of Mechanical Complications after Intramedullary Nailing of Tibial Fractures. *Orthop. Traumatol. Surg. Res.* **2019**, *105*, 523–527. [CrossRef]
9. Tzioupis, C.; Giannoudis, P.V. Prevalence of Long-Bone Non-Unions. *Injury* **2007**, *38*, S3–S9. [CrossRef]
10. Manon, J.; Detrembleur, C.; Van de Veyver, S.; Tribak, K.; Cornu, O.; Putineanu, D. Quels Sont Les Facteurs Prédictifs d'une Complication Mécanique Après Enclouage Centromédullaire d'une Fracture Diaphysaire Du Tibia? *Rev. De Chir. Orthopédique Et Traumatol.* **2019**, *105*, 353–357. [CrossRef]
11. Vico, L.; Collet, P.; Guignandon, A.; Lafage-Proust, M.-H.; Thomas, T.; Rehailia, M.; Alexandre, C. Effects of Long-Term Microgravity Exposure on Cancellous and Cortical Weight-Bearing Bones of Cosmonauts. *Lancet* **2000**, *355*, 1607–1611. [CrossRef]
12. LeBlanc, A.D.; Spector, E.R.; Evans, H.J.; Sibonga, J.D. Skeletal Responses to Space Flight and the Bed Rest Analog: A Review. *J. Musculoskelet. Neuronal Interact.* **2007**, *7*, 33–47. [PubMed]
13. John, R.B.; Charles, H.E., Jr. *Safe Passage: Astronaut Care for Exploration Missions*; National Academies Press: Cambridge, MA, USA, 2001; ISBN 978-0-309-50009-8.
14. Sibonga, J. Risk of Bone Fracture Due to Spaceflight-Induced Changes to Bone. In *Human Health Countermeasures (HHC)*; National Aeronautics and Space Administration: Houston, TX, USA, 2022.
15. Lang, T.F. What Do We Know about Fracture Risk in Long-Duration Spaceflight? *J. Musculoskelet. Neuronal Interact.* **2006**, *6*, 319–321.
16. Nelson, E.S.; Lewandowski, B.; Licata, A.; Myers, J.G. Development and Validation of a Predictive Bone Fracture Risk Model for Astronauts. *Ann. Biomed. Eng.* **2009**, *37*, 2337–2359. [CrossRef]
17. Thirsk, R.B. Health Care for Deep Space Explorers. *Ann. Biomed. Eng.* **2020**, *49*, 182–184. [CrossRef] [PubMed]
18. Saluja, I.S.; Williams, D.R.; Woodard, D.; Kaczorowski, J.; Douglas, B.; Scarpa, P.J.; Comtois, J.-M. Survey of Astronaut Opinions on Medical Crewmembers for a Mission to Mars. *Acta Astronaut.* **2008**, *63*, 586–593. [CrossRef]
19. Kirkpatrick, A.W.; Campbell, M.R.; Novinkov, O.L.; Goncharov, I.B.; Kovachevich, I.V. Blunt Trauma and Operative Care in Microgravity: A Review of Microgravity Physiology and Surgical Investigations with Implications for Critical Care and Operative Treatment in Space. *J. Am. Coll. Surg.* **1997**, *184*, 441–453. [PubMed]
20. Mars Desert Research Station. Available online: http://mdrs.marssociety.org/ (accessed on 4 June 2023).
21. Pletser, V.; Foing, B. European Contribution to Human Aspect Investigations for Future Planetary Habitat Definition Studies: Field Tests at MDRS on Crew Time Utilisation and Habitat Interfaces. *Microgravity Sci. Technol.* **2011**, *23*, 199–214. [CrossRef]
22. Terhorst, A.; Dowling, J.A. Terrestrial Analogue Research to Support Human Performance on Mars: A Review and Bibliographic Analysis. *Space Sci. Technol.* **2022**, *2022*, 9841785. [CrossRef]
23. Seligson, D. Evolution of the Hoffmann Fixators. *Injury* **2015**, *46*, S3–S6. [CrossRef]
24. Schwechter, E.M.; Swan, K.G. Raoul Hoffmann and His External Fixator. *J. Bone Jt. Surg.* **2007**, *89*, 672–678. [CrossRef]
25. Carroll, E.A.; Koman, L.A. External Fixation and Temporary Stabilization of Femoral and Tibial Trauma. *J. Surg. Orthop. Adv.* **2011**, *20*, 74–81.
26. Saint-Guillain, M.; Vanderdonckt, J.; Burny, N.; Pletser, V.; Vaquero, T.; Chien, S.; Karl, A.; Marquez, J.; Wain, C.; Comein, A.; et al. Enabling Astronaut Self-Scheduling Using a Robust Advanced Modelling and Scheduling System: An Assessment during a Mars Analogue Mission. *Adv. Space Res.* **2023**, *72*, 1378–1398. [CrossRef]

27. The SPRINT Investigators. Study to Prospectively Evaluate Reamed Intramedually Nails in Patients with Tibial Fractures (S.P.R.I.N.T.): Study Rationale and Design. *BMC Musculoskelet. Disord.* **2008**, *9*, 91. [CrossRef]
28. Milner, S.A.; Davis, T.R.C.; Muir, K.R.; Greenwood, D.C.; Doherty, M. Long-Term Outcome After Tibial Shaft Fracture: Is Malunion Important? *JBJS* **2002**, *84*, 971. [CrossRef] [PubMed]
29. Cartiaux, O.; Paul, L.; Docquier, P.-L.; Francq, B.G.; Raucent, B.; Dombre, E.; Banse, X. Accuracy in Planar Cutting of Bones: An ISO-based Evaluation. *Int. J. Med. Robot. Comput. Assist. Surg.* **2009**, *5*, 77–84. [CrossRef]
30. Claes, L.; Augat, P.; Suger, G.; Wilke, H.-J. Influence of Size and Stability of the Osteotomy Gap on the Success of Fracture Healing. *J. Orthop. Res.* **1997**, *15*, 577–584. [CrossRef] [PubMed]
31. Marsell, R.; Einhorn, T.A. The Biology of Fracture Healing. *Injury* **2011**, *42*, 551–555. [CrossRef] [PubMed]
32. Green, D.P. *Rockwood and Green's Fractures in Adults*; Lippincott Williams & Wilkins: Philadelphia, PA, USA, 2010; Volume 1, ISBN 1-60547-677-3.
33. Fang, C.; Luan, Y.; Wang, Z.; Shao, L.; Qu, T.; Cheng, C.-K. Moderate External Rotation of Tibial Component Generates More Natural Kinematics Than Internal Rotation After Total Knee Arthroplasty. *Front. Bioeng. Biotechnol.* **2022**, *10*, 910311. [CrossRef]
34. Heinrich, S.D.; Mooney, J.F.; Beaty, J.H.; Kasser, J.R. Fractures of the Shaft of the Tibia and Fibula. In *Rockwood Wilkin's Fractures in Children*, 6th ed.; Lippincott Williams & Wilkins: Philadelphia, PA, USA, 2006; pp. 1033–1076.
35. Egol, K.A.; Phillips, D.; Vongbandith, T.; Szyld, D.; Strauss, E.J. Do Orthopaedic Fracture Skills Courses Improve Resident Performance? *Injury* **2015**, *46*, 547–551. [CrossRef]
36. Scalea, T.M.; Boswell, S.A.; Scott, J.D.; Mitchell, K.A.; Kramer, M.E.; Pollak, A.N. External Fixation as a Bridge to Intramedullary Nailing for Patients with Multiple Injuries and with Femur Fractures: Damage Control Orthopedics. *J. Trauma Inj. Infect. Crit. Care* **2000**, *48*, 613–623. [CrossRef]
37. Bayrak, A.; Polat, Ö.; Ursavaş, H.T.; Gözügül, K.; Öztürk, V.; Duramaz, A. Which External Fixation Method Is Better for the Treatment of Tibial Shaft Fractures Due to Gunshot Injury? *Orthop. Traumatol. Surg. Res.* **2021**, *108*, 102948. [CrossRef]
38. Haonga, B.T.; Areu, M.M.M.; Challa, S.T.; Liu, M.B.; Elieza, E.; Morshed, S.; Shearer, D. Early Treatment of Open Diaphyseal Tibia Fracture with Intramedullary Nail versus External Fixator in Tanzania: Cost Effectiveness Analysis Using Preliminary Data from Muhimbili Orthopaedic Institute. *SICOT-J* **2019**, *5*, 20. [CrossRef] [PubMed]
39. Encinas-Ullán, C.A.; Martínez-Diez, J.M.; Rodríguez-Merchán, E.C. The Use of External Fixation in the Emergency Department: Applications, Common Errors, Complications and Their Treatment. *EFORT Open Rev.* **2020**, *5*, 204–214. [CrossRef] [PubMed]
40. Dulchavsky, S.A.; Henry, S.E.; Moed, B.R.; Diebel, L.N.; Marshburn, T.; Hamilton, D.R.; Logan, J.; Kirkpatrick, A.W.; Williams, D.R. Advanced Ultrasonic Diagnosis of Extremity Trauma: The FASTER Examination. *J. Trauma Acute Care Surg.* **2002**, *53*, 28. [CrossRef] [PubMed]
41. Kouassi, K.J.-E.; Manon, J.; Fonkoue, L.; Detrembleur, C.; Cornu, O. Treatment of Open Tibia Fractures in Sub-Saharan African Countries: A Systematic Review. *Acta Orthop. Belg.* **2021**, *87*, 85–92. [CrossRef]
42. Kouassi, K.J.-E.; Manon, J.; Fonkoue, L.; Kodo, M.; Detrembleur, C.; Cornu, O. La prise en charge des fractures ouvertes de jambe dans une structure hospitalière en Côte d'Ivoire pose-t-elle problème et pourquoi ? *Rev. De Chir. Orthopédique Et Traumatol.* **2019**, *105*, 654–658. [CrossRef]
43. Kouassi, K.J.E.; Manon, J.; Fonkoue, L.; Kodo, M.; Detrembleur, C.; Cornu, O. Is the Management of Open Leg Fractures in a Hospital Facility in Ivory Coast a Problem and Why? In Proceedings of the 38th Annual Meeting of the European Bone and Joint Infection Society (EBJIS), Antwerp, Belgium, 12–24 September 2019.

Disclaimer/Publisher's Note: The statements, opinions and data contained in all publications are solely those of the individual author(s) and contributor(s) and not of MDPI and/or the editor(s). MDPI and/or the editor(s) disclaim responsibility for any injury to people or property resulting from any ideas, methods, instructions or products referred to in the content.

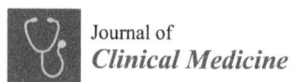

Article

Early Internal Fixation of Concomitant Clavicle Fractures in Severe Thoracic Trauma Prevents Posttraumatic Pneumonia

Julia Rehme-Röhrl [1], Korbinian Sicklinger [1,2], Andreas Brand [3,4], Julian Fürmetz [1,2], Carl Neuerburg [2], Fabian Stuby [1] and Christian von Rüden [3,5,*]

1. Department of Trauma Surgery, BG Unfallklinik Murnau, 82418 Murnau, Germany
2. Department of Orthopaedics and Trauma Surgery, Musculoskeletal University Center Munich, Ludwig-Maximilians University Munich, 81377 Munich, Germany
3. Institute for Biomechanics, Paracelsus Medical University, 5020 Salzburg, Austria
4. Institute for Biomechanics, BG Unfallklinik Murnau, 82418 Murnau, Germany
5. Department of Trauma Surgery, Orthopaedics and Hand Surgery, Weiden Medical Center, 92637 Weiden, Germany
* Correspondence: christian.vonrueden@kno.ag; Tel.: +49-961-30313041; Fax: +49-961-30313054

Abstract: Background: Severe thoracic trauma can lead to pulmonary restriction, loss of lung volume, and difficulty with ventilation. In recent years, there has been increasing evidence of better clinical outcomes following surgical stabilization of clavicle fractures in the setting of this combination of injuries. The aim of this study was to evaluate surgical versus non-surgical treatment of clavicle fractures in severe thoracic trauma in terms of clinical and radiological outcomes in order to make a generalized treatment recommendation based on the results of a large patient cohort. Patients and Methods: This retrospective study included 181 patients (42 women, 139 men) from a European level I trauma centre with a median of 49.3 years in between 2005 and 2021. In 116 cases, the clavicle fracture was stabilized with locking plate or hook plate fixation (group 1), and in 65 cases, it was treated non-surgically (group 2). Long-term functional outcomes at least one year postoperatively using the disabilities of the arm, shoulder and hand (DASH) questionnaire and the Nottingham Clavicle Score (NCS) as well as radiological outcomes were collected in addition to parameters such as hospital days, intensive care days, and complication rates. Results: The Injury Severity Score (ISS) was 17.8 ± 9.8 in group 1 and 19.9 ± 14.4 in group 2 (mean ± SEM; $p = 0.93$), the time in hospital was 21.5 ± 27.2 days in group 1 versus 16 ± 29.3 days in group 2 ($p = 0.04$). Forty-seven patients in group 1 and eleven patients in the group 2 were treated in the ICU. Regarding the duration of ventilation (group 1: 9.1 ± 8.9 days, group 2: 8.1 ± 7.7 days; $p = 0.64$), the functional outcome (DASH group 1: 11 ± 18 points, group 2: 13.7 ± 18. 4 points, $p = 0.51$; NCS group 1: 17.9 ± 8.1 points, group 2: 19.4 ± 10.3 points, $p = 0.79$) and the radiological results, no significant differences were found between the treatment groups. With an overall similar complication rate, pneumonia was found in 2% of patients in group 1 and in 14% of patients in group 2 ($p = 0.001$). Discussion: This study could demonstrate that surgical locking plate fixation of clavicle fractures in combination with CWI significantly reducing the development of posttraumatic pneumonia in a large patient collection and, therefore, can be recommended as standard therapeutic approach for severe thoracic trauma.

Keywords: clavicle fracture; chest wall injury (CWI); thoracic trauma; locking plate fixation; hook plate; disabilities of the arm; shoulder and hand (DASH); Nottingham Clavicle Score

Citation: Rehme-Röhrl, J.; Sicklinger, K.; Brand, A.; Fürmetz, J.; Neuerburg, C.; Stuby, F.; von Rüden, C. Early Internal Fixation of Concomitant Clavicle Fractures in Severe Thoracic Trauma Prevents Posttraumatic Pneumonia. *J. Clin. Med.* **2023**, *12*, 4878. https://doi.org/10.3390/jcm12154878

Academic Editors: Randall T. Loder and Shah-Hwa Chou

Received: 19 May 2023
Revised: 12 July 2023
Accepted: 19 July 2023
Published: 25 July 2023

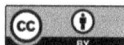

Copyright: © 2023 by the authors. Licensee MDPI, Basel, Switzerland. This article is an open access article distributed under the terms and conditions of the Creative Commons Attribution (CC BY) license (https://creativecommons.org/licenses/by/4.0/).

1. Introduction

Traditionally, displaced fractures of the clavicle have been treated non-operatively [1]. In recent years, a paradigm shift towards an increase in operative treatment occurred [2]. The benefits of surgical clavicle fracture management need to be weighed against the well-known risk of intraoperative or postoperative complications [3]. Although most of the clavicle fractures present as isolated injury, a part of the affected patients also sustains associated thoracic trauma. More than every second patient with an injury severity score (ISS) ≥16 suffers from thoracic trauma [4]. Particularly in polytraumatized patients, unstable chest wall injuries (CWI) are common [5]. Clavicle fractures are common in CWI with an incidence ranging up to 60% [6]. Even higher incidences have been described following open clavicle fractures [7]. Nevertheless, there is a wide range in the severity of the associated CWI. Concurrent rib fractures, for example, may negatively affect the stability of the clavicle fracture [8], since concomitant ipsilateral rib fractures have been reported to significantly increase the extent of displacement of unstable clavicle fractures [9]. While the clavicle is an important stabilizer of the upper quadrant of the chest, displacement and resulting pain can lead to a relevant loss of function of the shoulder girdle and a pronounced deformation of the ipsilateral chest wall [10]. In severe CWI, posttraumatic pneumonia delayed and retained hemothorax or empyema may result in permanent pulmonary restriction, loss of lung volume, and difficulty with ventilation and breathing. This clinical course might affect the treating surgeon's clavicle fracture management decision [11]. In contrast to the concomitant rib fracture, whose timely surgical stabilization is considered beneficial in preventing posttraumatic pneumonia [12], the effect of early clavicle fracture management in severe thoracic trauma of the seriously injured patient still remains unclear [13,14].

Therefore, the aim of this study was to evaluate clinical and radiological long-term outcomes following operative versus non-operative treatment of concomitant clavicle fractures in severe thoracic trauma to provide a sound general treatment recommendation based on the results of a large patient collection.

2. Patients and Methods

In this retrospective study, data from 181 consecutive patients with concomitant clavicle fractures combined with severe thoracic trauma (139 men, 42 women) with a median age of 49.3 (range 16 to 95) years in a European Level I Trauma Center between January 2005 and December 2021 were included. In all cases, patient management was conducted according to the ATLS® guidelines [15]. In group OP, operative management including open reduction and internal locking plate fixation within five days after trauma and in group NO non-operative treatment was performed. The following inclusion criteria were noted: age over 16 years, skeletal maturity, medial, lateral and midshaft fractures according to the Allman classification, combined with three or more unilateral segmental rib fractures or three or more bilateral rib fractures and/or sternal fracture and/or scapula fracture and/or pneumothorax/hemothorax [7,16]. According to Dehghan et al. [17], the exclusion criteria were as follows: Patients with upper airway injury requiring long-term intubation and mechanical ventilation (e.g., tracheal disruption), acute quadriparesis or tetraplegia, head and neck burn injuries, or inhalation burn injuries, dementia or other inability to complete follow-up questionnaires, cases with lack of informed consent from patient or substitute decision maker were excluded from the study. For the item ventilation time, both invasive and noninvasive ventilation were combined. The identical aftercare protocol was conducted with all patients [18]. In the group NO, non-operative treatment included immobilization in a shoulder sling providing patient comfort, especially in the initial phase after trauma [19]. After the symptoms subsided, early physiotherapy was started with passive–assistive exercises including humeral abduction and anteversion to 90° and without weight-bearing for six weeks.

2.1. Follow-Up

Follow-up studies were performed at regular intervals, including six weeks, 3, 12, and 24 months, as well as at the most recent visit to the outpatient department. Follow-up assessment included a thorough physical examination, functional evaluation, and diagnostic biplanar conventional radiological studies. The influence of the treatment outcome on patients' mental and physical health status was assessed using the disabilities of the arm, shoulder and hand (DASH) outcome measure [20] and the modified Nottingham Clavicle Score (NCS; modified version for German patients) [21]. For better understanding, both of the scores were analyzed in a similar way using five choices to answer ranging from "very good" to "very bad". For better comparability and understanding, the evaluation of the NCS was adapted exactly to the evaluation of the DASH outcome measure: best answer received 1 point and worst answer 5 points. Moreover, Visual Analogue Scale (VAS) was analyzed with a scale ranging from 1 (no pain) to 10 (strongest pain ever experienced). Radiological follow-up was assessed using anterior–posterior and lateral radiographs. According to Fisher et al., osseous healing was defined as formation of bridging callus at all four cortices, and absence of fracture lines [22]. Outcome measures were presented as mean and standard error of the mean (SEM).

2.2. Statistical Analysis

Statistical comparisons between groups were conducted using IBM SPSS® Statistics for Windows (IBM Corp., Armonk, NY, USA). Based on ordinal data scales, the Mann–Whitney U test was applied for comparisons of clinical scores (modified NCS, ISS, DASH) and for pain assessment (VAS). Additional clinical measures were compared using either the Mann–Whitney U test (time on ICU, ventilation time, time in hospital) or chi-squared test (Allman classification, polytrauma, pneumonia rate, gender, injury side). The two-sample t-test was used to compare age differences between groups. The level of significance was set at $p < 0.05$.

3. Results

An overview on patients' general data is displayed in Table 1. In 116 out of 181 patients, clavicle fractures were treated operatively using locking plate fixation (Figure 1a–c) with or without hook. In the remaining 65 cases, non-operative therapy was used. The mean ISS was 17.8 ± 9.8 in group 1 and 19.9 ± 14.4 in group NO ($p = 0.93$).

Table 1. Overview on patients' general data.

	Operative (Group OP)	Non-Operative (Group NO)	p-Value
Patients [number]	116	65	
Gender [male/female]	97/19	42/23	0.004
Age [years]	48 ± 14	53 ± 20	0.06
Injured side [right/left]	47/69	24/41	0.63
Allman classification [midshaft/lateral/medial]	88/25/3	35/29/1	<0.01
ISS (mean ± SD) [points]	17.8 ± 9.8	19.9 ± 14.4	0.93
Polytrauma [yes/no]	70/46	34/31	0.29

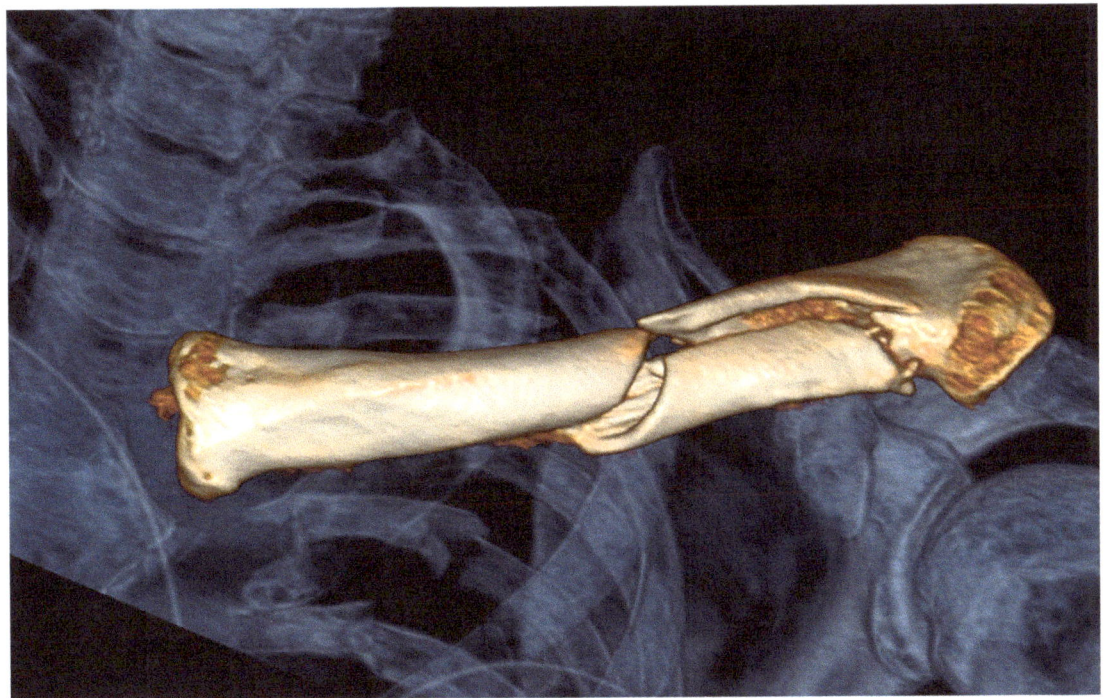

(a)

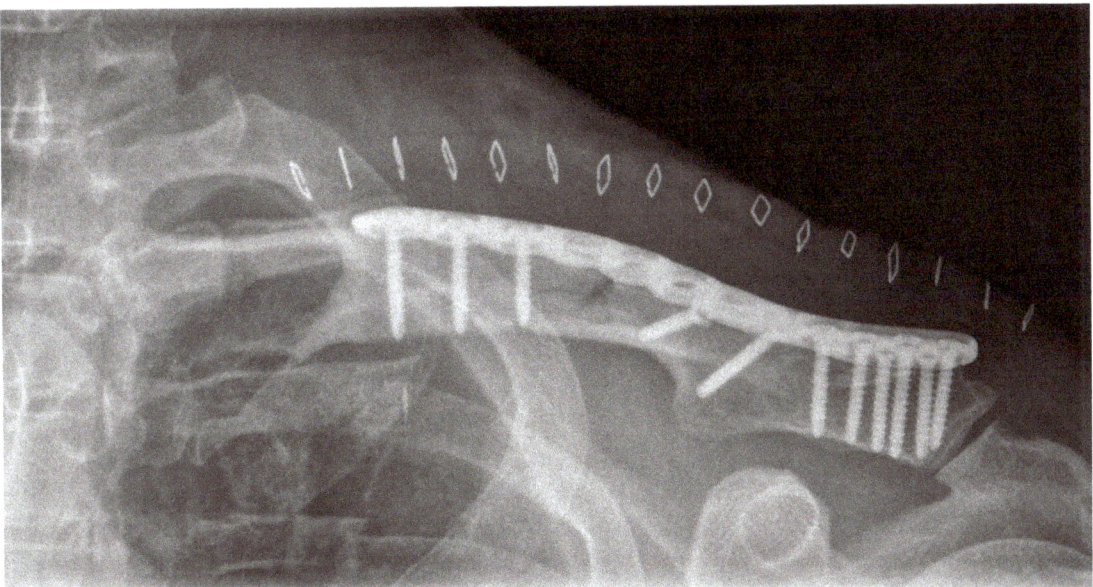

(b)

Figure 1. *Cont.*

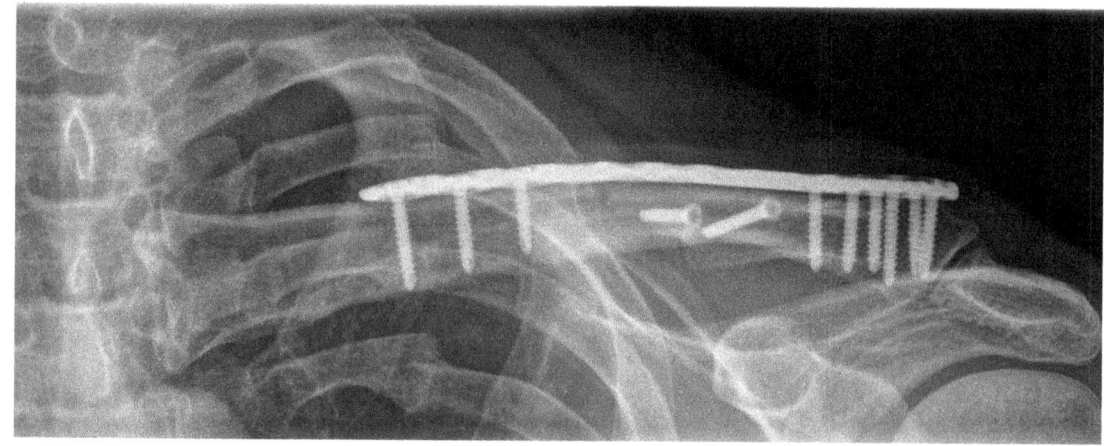

(c)

Figure 1. (a) Three-dimensional reconstructions of the polytrauma whole-body-computed tomography scan in a 51-year-old male patient after bicycle accident: Severe thoracic trauma including serial rib fractures and concomitant ipsilateral displaced multifragmentary clavicle fracture. (b) Postoperative anterior–posterior radiograph after internal precontoured locking plate fixation of the clavicle via longitudinal approach (skin clips). (c) Programmed radiological control demonstrated osseous healing one year after trauma. The serial rib fracture also healed after non-operative treatment.

One-hundred-and-four patients suffered from the clavicle fracture as part of polytraumatization. High-energy trauma was the cause of the thoracic trauma in 132 patients. Twenty-one patients had a car accident, thirty-eight patients had a motor bike accident, fifty-two patients had a bicycle accident, eight patients had a ski accident, five patients suffered a fall from horseback, and the remaining eight patients suffered a fall from a height over 3 m. Simple falls occurred in twenty-three patients and a blunt impact in five patients. Twenty-one patients could not be categorized clearly. According to the Allman classification, 123 fractures were located in the mid third, 54 fractures in the lateral third, and 4 fractures in the medial third. A significant difference was found between both groups regarding the midshaft location. In four patients, open clavicle fractures occurred. In about 60% of patients in both treatment groups, the left side of the thorax was affected.

There was no significant different concerning the range of time on ICU between the treatment groups, but operatively treated patients demonstrated significantly less ventilation time ($p = 0.04$) and significantly more days in hospital ($p = 0.04$) compared with non-operatively treated patients. Furthermore, the rate of posttraumatic pneumonia was significantly higher following non-operative treatment ($p < 0.001$) (Table 2). Since noninvasive ventilation was performed not only on ICU but also on the normal ward, a longer ventilation time was observed than time on ICU in the non-operative group.

Table 2. Parameters related to the hospital stay.

	Operative (Group OP)	Non-Operative (Group NO)	p-Value
Time on ICU [days]	9.1 ± 8.9	8.1 ± 7.7	0.25
Ventilation time [days]	7.5 ± 10	13.6 ± 9	0.04
Time in hospital [days]	21.5 ± 27.2	16 ± 29.3	0.04
Pneumonia [yes/no]	2/114	9/56	<0.001

Clinical long-term results using the DASH, modified NCS, and VAS are presented in Table 3. Median follow-up was 7 years (1–16 years) after trauma. Due to a loss of follow-up, data from 78 out of 181 patients (43%) could be included in the study (group OP: 56 patients; group NO: 22 patients). To ensure that potential posttraumatic pain was due to the trauma and not to other factors unrelated to the accident, the VAS was evaluated 12 months after the accident.

Table 3. Clinical long-term results.

	Operative (Group OP)	Non-Operative (Group NO)	p-Value
Follow-up period [years]	7 (1–15)	8 (1–16)	
DASH [points]	10 ± 17	13.7 ± 18.4	0.39
Modified NCS [points]	17.3 ± 7.5	19.4 ± 10.3	0.63
VAS [points]	1.9 ± 2.5	2.4 ± 2.3	0.29

Due to the above loss of a follow-up description, conventional radiographs were analyzed in 48 patients of group OP, in 6 patients of group NO after one year (Figure 1c), in 56 patients of group OP, respectively, and in 14 patients of group NO available for a final follow-up two years after trauma. Radiological results did not demonstrate any significant difference between the treatment groups ($p = 0.28$). Aseptic clavicle nonunion was observed in three patients of each treatment group one year after surgery and in one patient of each treatment group two years after surgery.

4. Discussion

The aim of this study was to evaluate if there is a significant difference between operative and non-operative treatment of clavicle fractures in combination with severe thoracic trauma. the lung function is especially known to have a decisive impact on the overall clinical outcome [17]. An isolated unstable clavicle fracture is known to be causative for an ineffective respiration and oxygenation [23–25]. Therefore, in combination with severe thoracic trauma, it may lead to increasing organ dysfunction and pulmonary failure [26]. Inadequate treatment of severe thoracic trauma might increase the risk of developing life-threatening complications, long-term morbidity, and elevated mortality rates [27–29]. In summary, the entire thoracic trauma in combination with the clavicle fracture represents the challenge for the treating surgeon. Operative treatment of CWI is known to be associated with advantages regarding the clinical course and long-term outcome following polytrauma [30,31]. The positive effects of rib fixation in preventing pneumonia following CWI have been well established [32]. In contrast, no studies have yet been performed on this topic for concomitant clavicle fractures, although surgical fixation of the clavicle fracture appears to be much easier and less likely to cause complications compared with osteosynthesis of rib fractures. To our knowledge, there was no information on the long-term effect following operative versus non-operative treatment of concomitant clavicle fractures associated with CWI in the literature yet. So far, the most interesting finding of the current study for daily clinical practice was the significantly lower pneumonia rate in the operative group compared to the non-operative group.

Nevertheless, no significant differences between the treatment groups concerning the remaining clinical and radiologic long-term results could be evaluated. Previous literature highlighted nonunion rates of up to 15% following non-surgical clavicle fracture management [33–35]. Interestingly, the current patient cohort demonstrated a nonunion rate of only 1% in the operative group versus 7% in the non-operative group.

Another important finding of the current study was the effect on clinically relevant outcome parameters during the initial stay in hospital and in the long-term clinical course. The ICU stay was comparable, but the ventilation time was prolonged compared to recently published data from polytrauma patients without thoracic trauma [36]. This was in line with a meta analysis provided by Leinicke et al., reporting that patients demonstrated shorter ventilation time following early internal clavicle fracture fixation than following non-operative treatment [30]. However, in the current study, the duration of treatment in hospital was significantly higher in the operative group. This was unexpected and in contrast to Leinicke et al. reporting that both the duration of treatment in the ICU and the total length of stay in the hospital were significantly decreased by operative treatment. One reason for this may be that these parameters might have been influenced by other injuries except the thoracic trauma or by certain comorbidities. On the other hand, in the current study, operative clavicle fracture treatment was only performed when the patients' overall clinical status was good enough for surgery. Furthermore, it was accepted as a relatively minor operative procedure compared to polytraumatization [37].

Generally, data of the current patient cohort corresponded with other studies reporting the epidemiology of concomitant clavicle fractures combined with severe thoracic trauma [17,23,38]. Mainly traffic accidents with high-energy trauma could be identified as cause of severe thoracic trauma [36,39,40].

According to the Allman classification, the study groups were statistically different regarding the midshaft location. Additionally, all open fractures were treated operatively and confirmed the current golden standard in open clavicle fracture management [41]. Furthermore, several authors recommended internal stabilization of clavicle fractures in thoracic trauma, particularly in the case of displaced fractures and associated serial rib fractures or flail chest injury [10]. Another subject was the heterogeneous patient collection regarding the decision for operative versus non-operative treatment. However, even upon reviewing the individual cases, the groups were comparable with respect to the ISS.

According to the results of this study, we recommend to include timely internal locked plating of concomitant clavicle fractures in the standard treatment regime after severe thoracic trauma aiming to prevent the development of pneumonia in the context of a severe posttraumatic course after severe CWI.

Study Limitations

The current study had limitations, such as its retrospective nature. First of all, the follow-up period of seven years after surgery was pleasingly relatively long and comparable with Nowak et al. [42], but unfortunately, it was also associated with a relatively high loss of follow-up. Furthermore, the number of patients treated non-operatively in the long-term follow-up was significantly lower than the number treated operatively, which complicated the comparability of the results. Accordingly, it was not possible to randomize age, gender, and indication for the treatment concepts. The advantages of the study were the exceedingly large cohort size and the fact that all patients were treated by the same team of surgeons in the same hospital according to the same treatment and aftercare protocol. Considering that the cases of clavicle fracture associated with CWI are relatively rare and difficult to collect and that only few cases are available in the literature, the results of this study with a long-term follow-up of consecutive patients may be highly relevant.

5. Conclusions

The clinical and radiologic long-term results of this study could demonstrate that timely open reduction and internal locking plate fixation of concomitant clavicle fractures associated with CWI significantly decreased the development of posttraumatic pneumonia in a large patient collection and, therefore, may be recommended as a standard surgical approach in cases of severe thoracic trauma with concurrent clavicle fracture.

Author Contributions: Study conception and design: C.v.R.; acquisition and/or interpretation of data: K.S., J.R.-R. and C.v.R.; statistical analysis: A.B.; drafting/revision of the work for intellectual content and context: C.v.R. and J.R.-R.; supervision and revision of the final draft: F.S., C.N. and J.F. All authors have read and agreed to the published version of the manuscript.

Funding: This research received no external funding.

Institutional Review Board Statement: All human examinations described in this study were carried out with the approval of the responsible institutional as well as the National Ethics Committee of the Bavarian State Medical Association (BLAEK; ID: 2021-1205), in accordance with national law and with the 1964 Helsinki Declaration and its later amendments. All information was completely anonymized. The study was conducted according to ICMJE guidelines. On 19 July 2022, it was retrospectively registered with the German Clinical Trials Registry (DRKS: 00029728).

Informed Consent Statement: All patients who may be identified by means of images or by other information within the manuscript gave their written consent for publication.

Data Availability Statement: The datasets analyzed during the current work are available from the corresponding author upon reasonable request.

Conflicts of Interest: All authors state that there are no conflict of interest within the meaning of the ICMJE requirements.

References

1. Huttunen, T.T.; Launonen, A.P.; Berg, H.E.; Lepola, V.; Fellander-Tsai, L.; Mattila, V.M. Trends in the incidence of clavicle fractures and surgical repair in Sweden: 2001–2012. *J. Bone Jt. Surg. Am.* **2016**, *98*, 1837–1842. [CrossRef]
2. Yan, M.Z.; Yuen, W.S.; Yeung, S.C.; Wing-Yin, C.W.; Wong, S.C.; Si-Qi, W.W.; Tian, E.; Rashed, S.; Yung, C.S.Y.; Fang, C.X. Operative management of midshaft clavicle fractures demonstrates better long-term outcomes: A systematic review and meta-analysis of randomised controlled trials. *PLoS ONE* **2022**, *17*, e0267861. [CrossRef] [PubMed]
3. Ronald, A.; Navarro, R.A.; Gelber, J.D.; Harrast, J.J.; Seiler, J.G.; Jackson, K.R.; Garcia, I.A. Frequency and complications after operative fixation of clavicular fractures. *J. Shoulder Elb. Surg.* **2016**, *25*, e125–e129. [CrossRef]
4. Vécsei, V.; Arbes, S.; Aldrian, S.; Nau, T. Chest Injuries in Polytrauma. *Eur. J. Trauma* **2005**, *31*, 239–243. [CrossRef]
5. Timm, A.; Maegele, M.; Lefering, R.; Wendt, K.; Wyen, H.; TraumaRegister DGU®. Pre-hospital rescue times and actions in severe trauma. A comparison between two trauma systems: Germany and the Netherlands. *Injury* **2014**, *45* (Suppl. S3), S43–S52. [CrossRef]
6. Robinson, C.M. Fractures of the clavicle in the adult. Epidemiology and classification. *J. Bone Jt. Surg. Br.* **1998**, *80*, 476–484. [CrossRef]
7. Kihlström, C.; Möller, M.; Lönn, K.; Wolf, O. Clavicle fractures: Epidemiology, classification and treatment of 2422 fractures in the Swedish Fracture Register; an observational study. *BMC Musculoskelet. Disord.* **2017**, *18*, 82. [CrossRef]
8. Sweet, A.A.R.; Beks, R.B.; IJpma, F.F.A.; de Jong, M.B.; Beeres, F.J.P.; Leenen, L.P.H.; Houwert, R.M.; van Baal, M.C.P.M. Epidemiology of combined clavicle and rib fractures: A systematic review. *Eur. J. Trauma Emerg. Surg.* **2022**, *48*, 3513–3520. [CrossRef]
9. Stahl, D.; Ellington, M.; Brennan, K.; Brennan, M. Association of Ipsilateral rib Fractures with Displacement of Midshaft clavicle fractures. *J. Orthop. Trauma* **2017**, *31*, 225–228. [CrossRef]
10. Langenbach, A.; Krinner, S.; Hennig, F.F.; Ekkernkamp, A.; Schulz-Drost, S. Injuries of the posterior and lateral chest wall-importance of an additional clavicular fracture. *Unfallchirurg* **2018**, *121*, 615–623. [CrossRef]
11. Majercik, S.; Pieracci, F.M. Chest Wall trauma. *Thorac. Surg. Clin.* **2017**, *27*, 113–121. [CrossRef] [PubMed]
12. Wang, Z.; Jia, Y.; Li, M. The effectiveness of early surgical stabilization for multiple rib fractures: A multicenter randomized controlled trial. *J. Cardiothorac. Surg.* **2023**, *18*, 118. [CrossRef] [PubMed]
13. Bakir, M.S.; Langenbach, A.; Pinther, M.; Lefering, R.; Krinner, S.; Grosso, M.; Ekkernkamp, A.; Schulz-Drost, S.; TraumaRegister, D.G.U. The significance of a concomitant clavicle fracture in flail chest patients: Incidence, concomitant injuries, and outcome of 12,348 polytraumata from the TraumaRegister DGU®. *Eur. J. Trauma Emerg. Surg.* **2022**, *48*, 3623–3634. [CrossRef] [PubMed]
14. Sawyer, E.; Wullschleger, M.; Muller, N.; Muller, M. Surgical Rib Fixation of Multiple Rib Fractures and Flail Chest: A Systematic Review and Meta-analysis. *J. Surg. Res.* **2022**, *276*, 221–234. [CrossRef]
15. von Rüden, C.; Bühren, V.; Perl, M. Polytrauma Management—Treatment of Severely Injured Patients in ER and OR. *Z. Orthop. Unfall.* **2017**, *155*, 603–622. [CrossRef] [PubMed]
16. Allman, F.L. Fractures and ligamentous injuries of the clavicle and its articulation. *J. Bone Jt. Surg. Am.* **1967**, *49*, 774–784. [CrossRef]
17. Dehghan, N.; Nauth, A.; Schemitsch, E.; Vicente, M.; Jenkinson, R.; Kreder, H.; McKee, M.; Canadian Orthopaedic Trauma Society and the Unstable Chest Wall RCT Study Investigators. Operative vs Nonoperative Treatment of Acute Unstable Chest Wall Injuries: A Randomized Clinical Trial. *JAMA Surg.* **2022**, *157*, 983–990. [CrossRef]
18. Caspari, R.B.; Beach, W.R. Arthroscopic anterior shoulder capsulorrhaphy. *Sports Med. Arthrosc.* **1993**, *1*, 237–241. [CrossRef]
19. Frima, H.; van Heijl, M.; Michelitsch, C.; van der Meijden, O.; Beeres, F.J.P.; Houwert, R.M.; Sommer, C. Clavicle fractures in adults; current concepts. *Eur. J. Trauma Emerg. Surg.* **2020**, *46*, 519–529. [CrossRef]
20. Hudak, P.L.; Amadio, P.C.; Bombardier, C. Development of an upper extremity outcome measure: The DASH (disabilities of the arm, shoulder and hand) [corrected]. The Upper Extremity Collaborative Group (UECG). *Am. J. Ind. Med.* **1996**, *29*, 602–608. [CrossRef]

21. Charles, E.R.; Kumar, V.; Blacknall, J.; Edwards, K.; Geoghegan, J.M.; Manning, P.A.; Wallace, W.A. A validation of the Nottingham Clavicle Score: A clavicle, acromioclavicular joint and sternoclavicular joint-specific patient-reported outcome measure. *J. Shoulder Elb. Surg.* **2017**, *26*, 1732–1739. [CrossRef]
22. Fisher, J.S.; Kazam, J.J.; Fufa, D.; Bartolotta, R.J. Radiologic evaluation of fracture healing. *Skelet. Radiol.* **2019**, *48*, 349–361. [CrossRef]
23. van Laarhoven, J.J.E.M.; Hietbrink, F.; Ferree, S.; Gunning, A.C.; Houwert, R.M.; Verleisdonk, E.M.M.; Leenen, L.P.H. Associated thoracic injury in patients with a clavicle fracture: A retrospective analysis of 1461 polytrauma patients. *Eur. J. Trauma Emerg. Surg.* **2019**, *45*, 59–63. [CrossRef] [PubMed]
24. Bonnevie, T.; Gravier, F.E.; Ducrocq, A.; Debeaumont, D.; Viacroze, C.; Cuvelier, A.; Muir, J.F.; Tardif, C. Exercise testing in patients with diaphragm paresis. *Respir. Physiol. Neurobiol.* **2018**, *248*, 31–35. [CrossRef]
25. Ramsook, A.H.; Molgat-Seon, Y.; Schaeffer, M.R.; Wilkie, S.S.; Camp, P.G.; Reid, W.D.; Romer, L.M.; Guenette, J.A. Effects of inspiratory muscle training on respiratory muscle electromyography and dyspnea during exercise in healthy men. *J. Appl. Physiol.* **2017**, *122*, 1267–1275. [CrossRef] [PubMed]
26. Ware, L.B.; Matthay, M.A. The acute respiratory distress syndrome. *N. Engl. J. Med.* **2000**, *342*, 1334–1349. [CrossRef] [PubMed]
27. Treggiari, M.M.; Hudson, L.D.; Martin, D.P.; Weiss, N.S.; Caldwell, E.; Rubenfeld, G. Effect of acute lung injury and acute respiratory distress syndrome on outcome in critically ill trauma patients. *Crit. Care Med.* **2004**, *32*, 327–331. [CrossRef]
28. Geiger, E.V.; Lustenberger, T.; Wutzler, S.; Lefering, R.; Lehnert, M.; Walcher, F.; Laurer, H.L.; Marzi, I.; TraumaRegister DGU®. Predictors of pulmonary failure following severe trauma: A trauma registry-based analysis. *Scand. J. Trauma Resusc. Emerg. Med.* **2013**, *21*, 34. [CrossRef]
29. Coppola, S.; Chiumello, D. Toracic trauma and acute respiratory distress syndrome: Mind the link! *Minerva Anestesiol.* **2017**, *83*, 83–1004. [CrossRef]
30. Leinicke, J.A.; Elmore, L.; Freeman, B.D.; Colditz, G.A. Operative management of rib fractures in the setting of fail chest. *Ann. Surg.* **2013**, *258*, 914–921. [CrossRef]
31. Schuurmans, J.; Goslings, J.C.; Schepers, T. Operative management versus non-operative management of rib fractures in fail chest injuries: A systematic review. *Eur. J. Trauma Emerg. Surg.* **2017**, *43*, 163–168. [CrossRef]
32. Liao, C.A.; Kuo, L.W.; Huang, J.F.; Fu, C.Y.; Chen, S.A.; Tee, Y.S.; Hsieh, C.H.; Liao, C.H.; Cheng, C.T.; Young, T.H.; et al. Timely surgical fixation confers beneficial outcomes in patients' concomitant flail chest with mild-to-moderate traumatic brain injury: A trauma quality improvement project analysis—A cohort study. *Int. J. Surg.* **2023**, *109*, 729–736. [CrossRef]
33. Neer CS 2nd. Nonunion of the clavicle. *J. Am. Med. Assoc.* **1960**, *172*, 1006–1011. [CrossRef] [PubMed]
34. Gossard, J.M. Closed treatment of displaced middle-third fractures of the clavicle gives poor results. *J. Bone Jt. Surg. Br.* **1998**, *80*, 558. [CrossRef]
35. Ahrens, P.M.; Garlick, N.I.; Barber, J.; Tims, E.M.; The Clavicle Trial Collaborative Group. The Clavicle Trial A Multicenter Randomized Controlled Trial Comparing Operative with Nonoperative Treatment of Displaced Midshaft Clavicle Fractures. *J. Bone Jt. Surg. Am.* **2017**, *99*, 1345–1354. [CrossRef] [PubMed]
36. Bayer, J.; Lefering, R.; Reinhardt, S.; Kühle, J.; Südkamp, N.P.; Hammer, T.; TraumaRegister, D.G.U. Severity-dependent diferences in early management of thoracic trauma in severely injured patients—Analysis based on the TraumaRegister DGU®. *Scand. J. Trauma Resusc. Emerg. Med.* **2017**, *25*, 10. [CrossRef]
37. von Rüden, C.; Rehme-Röhrl, J.; Augat, P.; Friederichs, J.; Hackl, S.; Stuby, F.; Trapp, O. Evidence on treatment of clavicle fractures. *Injury* **2023**, 110818, *Online ahead of print*. [CrossRef]
38. Eberbach, H.; Lefering, R.; Hager, S.; Schumm, K.; Bode, L.; Jaeger, M.; Maier, D.; Kalbhenn, J.; Hammer, T.; Schmal, H.; et al. Influence of surgical stabilization of clavicle fractures in multiply-injured patients with thoracic trauma. *Sci. Rep.* **2021**, *11*, 23263. [CrossRef] [PubMed]
39. Hill, A.B.; Fleiszer, D.M.; Brown, R.A. Chest trauma in a Canadian urban setting—Implications for trauma research in Canada. *J. Trauma* **1991**, *31*, 971–973. [CrossRef]
40. Grubmüller, M.; Kerschbaum, M.; Diepold, E.; Angerpointner, K.; Nerlich, M.; Ernstberger, A. Severe thoracic trauma—Still an independent predictor for death in multiple injured patients? *Scand. J. Trauma Resusc. Emerg. Med.* **2018**, *26*, 6. [CrossRef]
41. Biberthaler, P.; Schubert, E.C.; Kirchhoff, C.; Kanz, K.G. Current management of midshaft clavicle fractures. *MMW Fortschr. Med.* **2015**, *157*, 50–53. [CrossRef] [PubMed]
42. Nowak, J.; Holgersson, M.; Larsson, S. Can we predict long-term sequelae after fractures of the clavicle based on initial findings? A prospective study with nine to ten years of follow-up. *J. Shoulder Elb. Surg.* **2004**, *13*, 479–486. [CrossRef] [PubMed]

Disclaimer/Publisher's Note: The statements, opinions and data contained in all publications are solely those of the individual author(s) and contributor(s) and not of MDPI and/or the editor(s). MDPI and/or the editor(s) disclaim responsibility for any injury to people or property resulting from any ideas, methods, instructions or products referred to in the content.

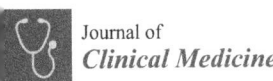

Brief Report

Prevalence and Characteristics of Patients Requiring Surgical Reinterventions for Ankle Fractures

Abraham Reyes-Valdés [1], Mirna Martínez-Ledezma [1], David Fernández-Quezada [2], José Guzmán-Esquivel [3] and Martha Irazema Cárdenas-Rojas [3,*]

1. Hospital General de Zona No. 1, Instituto Mexicano del Seguro Social, Av. Lapislázuli No. 250 Colonia La Haya, Villa de Álvarez, Colima 28984, Mexico; dr.reyes.abr@gmail.com (A.R.-V.); mirnamale21@gmail.com (M.M.-L.)
2. Centro Universitario de Ciencias de la Salud (CUCS), Laboratorio de Microscopía de Alta Resolución, Departamento de Neurociencias, Universidad de Guadalajara, Guadalajara 44340, Mexico; david.fernandez@academicos.udg.mx
3. Unidad de Investigación en Epidemiología Clínica, Instituto Mexicano del Seguro Social, Av. Lapislázuli No. 250 Colonia La Haya, Villa de Álvarez, Colima 28984, Mexico; pepeguzman_esquivel@outlook.com
* Correspondence: martha.cardenasr@imss.gob.mx or martha_irazema@hotmail.com

Abstract: (1) Background: Ankle fractures are common injuries that typically require surgical treatment. Complications may arise, leading to reinterventions with poor recovery and reduced quality of life for patients. The aim of this study was to determine the number of patients who underwent surgical reintervention for ankle fractures, characteristics, and associated factors. (2) Methods: A cross-sectional study was conducted to analyze the number of patients requiring surgical intervention for ankle fractures at General Hospital Zone No1 IMSS in Colima over a period of two years. The age, gender, comorbidities, laterality, cause of surgical reintervention, Weber classification, and elapsed time to reintervention were analyzed. (3) Results: A total of 33 patients were included in this study, of whom 63.3% were male, ranging in age from 18 to 51 years old. The predominant Danis–Weber classification for both sexes was suprasyndesmotic fracture (Type C). No established relationship was found between comorbidities and surgical reintervention; however, a significant relationship was observed between home accidents and the need for reintervention. (4) Conclusions: Reintervention in patients previously operated on for ankle fractures is more frequent in male patients and those who sustained the injury at home.

Keywords: ankle; bone fracture; surgical traumatology; Danis–Weber

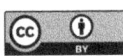

1. Introduction

Ankle fractures are a common type of injury, with an incidence of 187 per 100,000 adults per year. Women are more prone to suffer ankle fractures in advanced ages, while in men, they occur in youth [1]. However, they occur more frequently in patients with osteoporosis, peripheral arterial disease, and diabetes mellitus; the latter present three times more postoperative complications [2]. Among ankle injury cases treated in the emergency department, 15% present fractures. In Mexico, a total of 3755 ankle fracture surgeries were performed in one year [3].

The ankle is stabilized with three groups of ligaments: the lateral collateral ligament complex, the syndesmotic ligament complex, and the medial collateral ligament complex (deltoid) [4]. During trauma, the ankle can be in two different positions: pronation (eversion) and supination (inversion). Additionally, three deforming forces can occur, abduction, adduction, and external rotation, which determine the four mechanisms of injury: pronation-abduction, pronation-external rotation, supination-adduction, and supination-external rotation [5,6]. Ankle fractures are often the results of sustained torsion, typically due to low-energy injury. The position of the ankle at the time of injury and the posterior direction of force typically determines the fracture pattern [4,7,8].

The Lauge–Hansen classification describes the position of the foot at the time of injury and the deforming force on the ankle, providing additional information about stability and the necessary treatment [9,10]. The Danis–Weber classification system classifies ankle fractures based on the location of the distal fibular fracture in relation to the syndesmosis. This classification divides fractures into three groups: type A (below the level of the syndesmosis, type B (at the level of the syndesmosis, and type C (above the syndesmosis) [11]. Weber type A can be treated conservatively, while Weber B and C are usually treated with surgery [4]. Also, an additional classification based on fracture stability is employed, wherein a unimalleolar fracture is regarded as stable and amenable to conservative management, while bimalleolar and trimalleolar fractures are deemed unstable and require surgical intervention [12].

The purpose of surgery for an ankle fracture is to restore the anatomical congruence of the ankle joint. When achieving this anatomical relationship is not possible, altered loading occurs in the tibiotalar joint, leading to poor outcomes. The type of surgery to be performed for fracture reduction and fixation depends on the type of fracture and the characteristics of the patients [4]. In cases where the fracture is not reduced, there is a risk of vascular complications, ischemia, joint damage, and prolonged inflammation of the ankle's soft tissues, which could result in chronic pain. These unstable fractures are treated via open reduction and internal fixation in an operating room [7,8]. Despite the abundance of evidence to guide surgical management and achieve optimal outcomes in ankle fractures, results are often suboptimal [13]. The most frequent postoperative complications in the short term include wound hematoma and wound-edge necrosis, compartment syndrome, compromised wound healing, infection (reported in 2% of the patients), dislocation, malpositioned screw, inadequate reduction, and Complex Regional Pain Syndrome. In the mid to long term, patients may experience non-union, malposition, impingement syndrome, a restricted range of motion, and, in 10% of the cases, ankle arthrosis, with many necessitating reoperation [4].

Reported indications for performing surgical reintervention include problems with syndesmosis reduction and fibular shortening [14].

Although there are reports of complications following ankle fracture surgery, the frequency of this requirement is poorly documented. Based on previous reports, we anticipate that less than 29% of the patients will necessitate reintervention [15].

The aim of this study was to determine the number of patients requiring reintervention after open reduction with internal fixation of the ankle, as well as their characteristics and associated factors.

2. Materials and Methods

A cross-sectional retrospective study was conducted at General Hospital Zone No. 1, located in the western region of México, from 1 March 2018 to 31 December 2020. A comprehensive search was conducted in the INTQX database to identify all patients who underwent ankle fracture surgery. The patients undergoing ankle surgery presented a fracture displacement greater than 2 mm. The performed surgery was an open reduction with internal fixation using a plate for fractures with long lines or with multifragmentation, and screws were used for fractures with simple lines. After surgery, wound care was performed on patients, and they were administered antibiotics, analgesics, and anti-inflammatory drugs. The following day joint mobilization without weight-bearing was initiated. The patients had their sutures removed 15 days post-surgery, followed by radiographic assessment. Subsequently, they were examined every month for three months, then at sixth month, and went through a final review one year after the surgery. The criteria for discharging a patient following ankle fracture surgery are that they exhibit ranges of motion greater than 80% and do not experience incapacitating pain.

We enrolled all eligible patients meeting the predefined inclusion criteria, which encompassed individuals who underwent a surgical reintervention, defined by the necessity for additional surgical procedures for the ankle fracture. This study encompassed both sexes, individuals aged 18 years or older, and those fulfilling the Danis–Weber classification for ankle fracture diagnosis. Patients who underwent surgical reintervention to remove osteosynthesis material in cases of consolidated ankle fracture were excluded, as well as those in whom an osteosynthesis screw was removed under appropriate conditions. Additionally, patients whose initial surgery was performed at another medical facility were excluded. Patients with incomplete medical records were also eliminated from the analysis. Figure 1 shows the flowchart for patient inclusion.

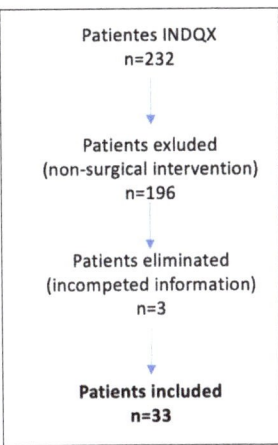

Figure 1. Flowchart for patients' inclusion.

All patients who met the inclusion criteria were selected by sampling for convenience.

Information on age, gender, comorbidities (diabetes mellitus, high blood pressure, hyperuricemia, and chronic renal disease), laterality, cause of surgical intervention, Weber classification, and time elapsed until reintervention was obtained using the Electronic Medical Record and the Official Bed Information System, which are the electronic platforms used to store all patient's information for outpatient consultation and hospitalizations, respectively.

Descriptive statistical analysis was performed using measures of central tendency, standard deviation, frequencies, and percentages for categorical variables, while the chi-square test was used for inferential analysis, considering statistical significance at a p-value < 0.05. The software used for the analysis was SPSS V.25

This study was approved by de Local Research Committee-601, with registration number R-2021-601-041.

3. Results

3.1. Characteristics of the Population

A total of 232 patients with ankle fractures underwent surgical intervention, among whom 33 individuals (14%) necessitated surgical reintervention and met the inclusion criteria. Table 1 presents the characteristics of the study population.

3.2. Diagnosis and Treatment of Ankle Fracture

According to the Weber classification, the majority of patients requiring surgical reintervention had a higher frequency of Weber C classification at 81.8% (n = 27), followed by Weber B classification at 18.2% (n = 6). 1. Additionally, among the patients who required surgical reintervention, 16 (48.3%) presented with unimalleolar fractures, 7 (21.1%) had bimalleolar fractures, 9 (27.3%) had trimalleolar fractures, and 1 (3%) exhibited pseudoarthrosis.

Table 1. Characteristics of the study population.

	n = 33 Patients	Measure
Age (years)		
18–35	11	33.3 *
36–51	11	33.33 *
52–68	9	27.3 *
69–85	2	6.1 *
Gender		
Male	21	63.6 *
Female	12	36.4 *
Weight (years)		
18–35	11	74.6 +
36–51	11	71.13 +
52–68	9	74.0 +
69–85	2	62.0 +
Side of injury		
Left	11	33.3 *
Right	22	66.7 *
Injury cause		
Activities at home (fall or blow)	15	45.5 *
Sport	4	12.1 *
Traffic accidents	10	30.3 *
Activities at work	4	12.1 *
Comorbidity		
Hyperuricemia	1	3 *
Type 2 diabetes mellitus	5	15.2 *
High blood pressure	2	6.1 *
Chronic kidney disease	1	3 *
None	24	73.7 *

* Percentage. + Kilograms.

A total of 27 patients (82%) exhibited syndesmosis instability and were subject to positioning screw and plate placement. One patient (3%) received a plate and suture on the medial malleolus, two patients (6%) underwent sole plate fixation, and three patients (9%) received medial malleolar screw placement.

When analyzing the time interval between the first open reduction with internal fixation and the surgical reintervention for ankle fracture, a wide variation was observed, ranging from 1 to 1095 days. The mode was 3 days, corresponding to 12 cases (36.4%). Table 2 presents all the causes that required surgical reintervention for ankle fractures.

Table 2. Causes of surgical reintervention in patients with ankle fractures.

	Frequency (n)	Percentage (%)
Osteoarthritis and residual ankle deformity	1	3
Osteoarthritis and ankle pain + talar necrosis	1	3
Displaced fragments/ankle instability	4	12.1
Inadequate closure of the syndesmosis	7	21.2
Inadequate closure of the medial clear space	1	3
Dislocated medial clear space	1	3
Ankle pain/wound exudate	1	3
Pain/exposure to osteosynthesis material	1	3
Lack of mobility due to inadequate rehabilitation	1	3
Osteosynthesis material fatigue	1	3
Fistula + exposure to osteosynthesis material	2	6.1
Surgical wound infection	1	3
Intolerance to osteosynthesis material	1	3
Intolerance to osteosynthesis material + fistula	1	3

Table 2. Cont.

	Frequency (n)	Percentage (%)
Insufficient material, displacement of fracture fragments	2	6.1
Osteomyelitis + rejection of osteosynthesis material	1	3
Left ankle osteomyelitis	1	3
Ankle nonunion fracture	1	3
Inadequate reduction in lateral malleolus	1	3
Displaced fracture line	3	9.1

3.3. Factors Associated with Surgical Reintervention

It was determined that age is not associated with the type of fracture and the need for surgical reintervention, as shown in Table 3.

Table 3. Analysis of the association between age and fracture type in patients undergoing surgical reintervention.

Age (Years)	Unimalleolar Fracture (n)	Bimalleolar Fracture (n)	Trimalleolar Fracture (n)	Non-Union (n)	*p* Value *
18–35	4	4	2	1	
36–51	7	0	4	0	
52–68	3	3	3	0	0.328
69–85	2	0	0	0	
Total	16	7	9	1	

* Chi-square.

The association between gender and ankle fracture type in patients undergoing surgical reintervention is shown in Table 4. Despite the fact that gender is not associated with surgical reintervention, a higher frequency is observed among male individuals.

Table 4. Association between gender and fracture type in patients undergoing surgical reintervention for ankle fracture.

Gender	Unimalleolar Fracture (n)	Bimalleolar Fracture (n)	Trimalleolar Fracture (n)	Non-Union (n)	*p* Value *
Female	5	4	3	0	
Male	11	3	6	1	0.553
Total	16	7	9	1	

*Chi-square.

No association was observed between fracture type and comorbidities in patients undergoing surgical reintervention, as shown in Table 5.

Table 5. Association between comorbidities and fracture type.

Comorbidities	Unimalleolar Fracture (n)	Bimalleolar Fracture (n)	Trimalleolar Fracture (n)	Non-Union (n)	*p* Value *
Hyperuricemia	1	0	0	0	
Type 2 diabetes mellitus	2	1	2	0	
High blood pressure	0	2	0	0	0.428
Chronic kidney disease	0	0	1	0	
None	13	4	6	1	

* Chi-square.

A statistically significant association was found between the type of accident and ankle fracture, with a *p*-value of 0.014. Home accidents showed an association with the need for surgical interventions in patients who had unimalleolar fractures. The details of this association are presented in Table 6.

Table 6. Association between the type of accident and fracture type in patients undergoing surgical reintervention.

Accident	Unimalleolar Fracture (n)	Bimalleolar Fracture (n)	Trimalleolar Fracture (n)	Non-Union (n)	p Value *
Sport	4	0	0	0	
Home	9	3	3	0	0.014
Work	0	0	3	1	
Traffic	3	4	3	0	

* Chi-square.

4. Discussion

A surgical reintervention was required in 14% of the patients, which is slightly lower than the previously reported [15]. This discrepancy could be attributed to differences in study design and the inclusion criteria utilized. It was observed that the most frequent group of patients undergoing reintervention comprised individuals aged between 18 and 51 years [13], with males being the most common [16]. This coincides with previous findings that also reported a higher frequency of ankle fractures in this age group, possibly due to the occupational and sports activities they engage in. The fact that this group is more prone to ankle fractures also predisposes them to require more surgical reinterventions.

Regarding weight, an average of 70 kg was found, considered within the normal range, and no association was found between weight and the need for surgical reintervention in our study, as previously reported [17].

However, other reports indicate that diabetes mellitus and the high body mass index are risk factors for open reduction with internal fixation of the syndesmosis in ankle malleolar fractures, as well as worse outcomes and poor functional results [2,18,19]. These differences could be due to variations in study design and sample size, which are larger than in previous studies. Similar to this study, it has been previously reported that 64% of ankle fractures occur due to accidents during domestic or everyday activities, so this cause should not be underestimated [20]. Regarding laterality, a higher frequency of fracture was observed on the right side, in line with previous findings that investigated postoperative complications and reoperation rates in ankle fractures. In their results, they found that 51.2% of the reinterventions were classified as Danis–Weber C [21]. When analyzing comorbidities, it was found that type 2 diabetes mellitus is the most common disease among patients undergoing reintervention for ankle fracture, although this association was not statistically significant. However, diabetes mellitus has effects on fracture risk and is associated with higher morbidity compared to the general population. A higher risk of fractures has been reported in patients with diabetes mellitus, including an increased risk of lower extremity fractures and other fractures [22]. The presence of diabetes mellitus in patients with ankle fractures can complicate surgery and postoperative recovery, even with the care of an experienced surgeon. Although evidence on surgical management and decision-making in ankle fractures in diabetic patients is limited, it has been shown that immediate surgical intervention is appropriate in closed ankle fractures in patients with decompensated diabetes mellitus type 2 prior to operation [23,24].

Regarding the time interval between open reduction and internal fixation and surgical reintervention in ankle fracture patients, it was found to be 3 days. This result differs from a previous study where most intervened patients returned to the hospital eight weeks or later after the initial surgery, which was one of the inclusion criteria [25,26].

Regarding the causes of surgical reintervention, inadequate syndesmosis closure was found to be the most frequent cause. The authors agree that syndesmosis injuries require surgical treatment, as their integrity is essential for maintaining normal movement. An unresolved injury to this structure can lead to various complications, including arthritis.

The limitations of this study include its retrospective design and relatively small sample size, which restricted the analysis to a specific population without considering the entire cohort of patients who underwent ankle surgery.

5. Conclusions

Reintervention in patients previously operated for ankle fractures is more frequent in male patients and those who sustained the injury at home.

Author Contributions: Methodology, D.F.-Q.; Formal analysis, J.G.-E.; Investigation, A.R.-V. and M.M.-L.; Writing—review & editing, M.I.C.-R. All authors have read and agreed to the published version of the manuscript.

Funding: This research received no external funding.

Institutional Review Board Statement: This study was conducted in accordance with the Declaration of Helsinki and approved by the Institutional Review Board (or Ethics Committee) of Local Research Committee-601, with registration number R-2021-601-041 for studies involving humans of the Mexican Institute of Social Security.

Informed Consent Statement: Informed consent was obtained from all subjects involved in this study.

Data Availability Statement: No new data were created or analyzed in this study. Data sharing is not applicable to this article.

Conflicts of Interest: The authors declare no conflict of interest.

References

1. Wire, J.; Hermena, S.; Slane, V.H. Ankle Fractures. In *StatPearls*; StatPearls Publishing: Treasure Island, FL, USA, 2023.
2. Ziegler, P.; Schlemer, D.; Flesch, I.; Bahrs, S.; Stoeckle, U.; Werner, S.; Bahrs, C. Quality of life and clinical-radiological long-term results after implant-associated infections in patients with ankle fracture: A retrospective matched-pair study. *J. Orthop. Surg. Res.* **2017**, *12*, 114. [CrossRef] [PubMed]
3. Dominguez Gasca, L.G.; Orozco Villasenor, S.L. Frecuencia y tipos de fracturas clasificadas por la Asociación para el Estudio de la Osteosíntesis en el Hospital General de León durante un año. *Acta Méd. Grupo Ángeles México* **2017**, *15*, 275–286. Available online: http://www.scielo.org.mx/scielo.php?script=sci_arttext&pid=S1870-72032017000400275&lng=es&nrm=iso (accessed on 12 June 2023).
4. Goost, H.; Wimmer, M.D.; Barg, A.; Kabir, K.; Valderrabano, V.; Burger, C. Fractures of the ankle joint: Investigation and treatment options. *Dtsch. Arztebl. Int.* **2014**, *111*, 377–388. [CrossRef] [PubMed]
5. Lubrano, E.; Marchesoni, A.; Olivieri, I.; D'angelo, S.; Palazzi, C.; Scarpa, R.; Ferrara, N.; Parsons, W.J.; Brunese, L.; Helliwell, P.S.; et al. The Radiological Assessment of Axial Involvement in Psoriatic Arthritis. *J. Rheumatol.* **2012**, *89*, 54–56. [CrossRef] [PubMed]
6. Bruno, F.; Arrigoni, F.; Splendiani, A.; Di Cesare, E.; Zappia, M.; Guglielmi, G.; Masciocchi, C.; Barile, A. Emergency and Trauma of the Ankle. *Semin. Musculoskelet. Radiol.* **2017**, *21*, 282–289. [CrossRef]
7. Strudwick, K.; McPhee, M.; Bell, A.; Martin-Khan, M.; Russell, T. Review article: Best practice management of common ankle and foot injuries in the emergency department (part 2 of the musculoskeletal injuries rapid review series). *Emerg. Med. Australas.* **2018**, *30*, 152–180. [CrossRef]
8. Bachmann, L.M.; Kolb, E.; Koller, M.T.; Steurer, J.; ter Riet, G. Accuracy of Ottawa ankle rules to exclude fractures of the ankle and mid-foot: Systematic review. *BMJ* **2003**, *326*, 417. [CrossRef]
9. Bekerom, M.P.J.v.D.; Mutsaerts, E.L.A.R.; van Dijk, C.N. Evaluation of the integrity of the deltoid ligament in supination external rotation ankle fractures: A systematic review of the literature. *Arch. Orthop. Trauma Surg.* **2009**, *129*, 227–235. [CrossRef]
10. Gardner, M.J.; Demetrakopoulos, D.; Briggs, S.M.; Helfet, D.L.; Lorich, D.G. The Ability of the Lauge-Hansen Classification to Predict Ligament Injury and Mechanism in Ankle Fractures: An MRI Study. *J. Orthop. Trauma* **2006**, *20*, 267–272. [CrossRef]
11. Mandi, D.M. Ankle Fractures. *Clin. Podiatr. Med. Surg.* **2012**, *29*, 155–186. [CrossRef]
12. Ovaska, M.; Madanat, R.; Mäkinen, T.; Lindahl, J. Complications in ankle fracture surgery. *Duodecim* **2015**, *131*, 1451–1459. (In Finnish) [CrossRef] [PubMed]
13. Whitehouse, S.; Mason, L.; Jayatilaka, L.; Molloy, A. Fixation of ankle fractures—A major trauma centre's experience in improving quality. *Ann. R. Coll. Surg. Engl.* **2019**, *101*, 387–390. [CrossRef] [PubMed]
14. Ovaska, M.T.; Mäkinen, T.J.; Madanat, R.; Kiljunen, V.; Lindahl, J. A comprehensive analysis of patients with malreduced ankle fractures undergoing re-operation. *Int. Orthop.* **2014**, *38*, 83–88. [CrossRef] [PubMed]

15. White, T.O.; Bugler, K.E.; Olsen, L.M.; Lundholm, L.H.; Holck, K.; Madsen, B.L.; Duckworth, A.D. A Prospective, Randomized, Controlled, Two-Center, International Trial Comparing the Fibular Nail With Open Reduction and Internal Fixation for Unstable Ankle Fractures in Younger Patients. *J. Orthop. Trauma* **2022**, *36*, 36–42. [CrossRef]
16. Ng, R.; Broughton, N.; Williams, C. Measuring Recovery After Ankle Fractures: A Systematic Review of the Psychometric Properties of Scoring Systems. *J. Foot Ankle Surg.* **2018**, *57*, 149–154. [CrossRef]
17. López Contreras, K.O. Tesis. 2016. Available online: http://repositorio.ug.edu.ec/handle/redug/24340 (accessed on 12 April 2021).
18. Goodloe, J.B.; Caughman, A.A.; Traven, S.A.; Gross, C.E.; Slone, H.S. Obesity and risk for open reduction and internal fixation of syndesmotic injuries in the setting of concomitant ankle fractures. *J. Orthop.* **2020**, *23*, 83–87. [CrossRef]
19. Audet, M.A.; Benedick, A.; Breslin, M.A.; Schmidt, T.; Vallier, H.A. Determinants of functional outcome following ankle fracture. *OTA Int. Open Access J. Orthop. Trauma* **2021**, *4*, e139. [CrossRef]
20. Cardoso, D.V.; Dubois-Ferrière, V.; Gamulin, A.; Baréa, C.; Rodriguez, P.; Hannouche, D.; Lübbeke, A. Operatively treated ankle fractures in Switzerland, 2002–2012: Epidemiology and associations between baseline characteristics and fracture types. *BMC Musculoskelet. Disord.* **2021**, *22*, 266. [CrossRef]
21. Macera, A.; Carulli, C.; Sirleo, L.; Innocenti, M. Postoperative Complications and Reoperation Rates Following Open Reduction and Internal Fixation of Ankle Fracture. *Joints* **2018**, *6*, 110–115. [CrossRef]
22. Walsh, J.S.; Vilaca, T. Obesity, Type 2 Diabetes and Bone in Adults. *Calcif. Tissue Int.* **2017**, *100*, 528–535. [CrossRef]
23. Manway, J.M.; Blazek, C.D.; Burns, P.R. Special Considerations in the Management of Diabetic Ankle Fractures. *Curr. Rev. Musculoskelet. Med.* **2018**, *11*, 445–455. [CrossRef] [PubMed]
24. Guo, J.J.; Yang, H.; Xu, Y.; Wang, G.; Huang, L.; Tang, T. Results after immediate operations of closed ankle fractures in patients with preoperatively neglected type 2 diabetes. *Injury* **2009**, *40*, 894–896. [CrossRef] [PubMed]
25. Walsh, A.S.; Sinclair, V.; Watmough, P.; Henderson, A.A. Ankle fractures: Getting it right first time. *Foot* **2018**, *34*, 48–52. [CrossRef] [PubMed]
26. Pogliacomi, F.; De Filippo, M.; Casalini, D.; Longhi, A.; Tacci, F.; Perotta, R.; Pagnini, F.; Tocco, S.; Ceccarelli, F. Acute syndesmotic injuries in ankle fractures: From diagnosis to treatment and current concepts. *World J. Orthop.* **2021**, *12*, 270–291. [CrossRef]

Disclaimer/Publisher's Note: The statements, opinions and data contained in all publications are solely those of the individual author(s) and contributor(s) and not of MDPI and/or the editor(s). MDPI and/or the editor(s) disclaim responsibility for any injury to people or property resulting from any ideas, methods, instructions or products referred to in the content.

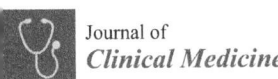

Review

Current Management of Diaphyseal Long Bone Defects—A Multidisciplinary and International Perspective

Steffen Bernd Rosslenbroich [1,*], Chang-Wug Oh [2], Thomas Kern [3], John Mukhopadhaya [4], Michael Johannes Raschke [1], Ulrich Kneser [5] and Christian Krettek [6]

1. Department of Trauma, Hand and Reconstructive Surgery, University Hospital Muenster, 48149 Münster, Germany; michael.raschke@ukmuenster.de
2. Department of Orthopedic Surgery, School of Medicine, Kyungpook National University, Kyungpook National University Hospital, Jung-gu, Daegu 41944, Republic of Korea; cwoh@knu.ac.kr
3. Department of Trauma Surgery/Murnau, BG Unfallklinik Murnau, 82418 Murnau am Staffelsee, Germany; thomas.kern@bgu-murnau.de
4. Orthopedic and Trauma Department, Paras HMRI Hospital, Patna 800014, Bihar, India; mukhoj@gmail.com
5. BG Trauma Center Ludwigshafen, Department of Plastic Surgery, University of Heidelberg/Ludwigshafen, 67059 Heidelberg, Germany; ulrich.kneser@bgu-ludwigshafen.de
6. Trauma Department/Hannover, Hannover Medical School, 30625 Hannover, Germany; krettek.christian@mh-hannover.de
* Correspondence: steffen.rosslenbroich@ukmuenster.de

Abstract: The treatment of defects of the long bones remains one of the biggest challenges in trauma and orthopedic surgery. The treatment path is usually very wearing for the patient, the patient's environment and the treating physician. The clinical or regional circumstances, the defect etiology and the patient´s condition and mental status define the treatment path chosen by the treating surgeon. Depending on the patient´s demands, the bony reconstruction has to be taken into consideration at a defect size of 2–3 cm, especially in the lower limbs. Below this defect size, acute shortening or bone grafting is usually preferred. A thorough assessment of the patient´s condition including comorbidities in a multidisciplinary manner and her or his personal demands must be taken into consideration. Several techniques are available to restore continuity of the long bone. In general, these techniques can be divided into repair techniques and reconstructive techniques. The aim of the repair techniques is anatomical restoration of the bone with differentiation of the cortex and marrow. Currently, classic, hybrid or all-internal distraction devices are technical options. However, they are all based on distraction osteogenesis. Reconstructive techniques restore long-bone continuity by replacing the defect zone with autologous bone, e.g., with a vascularized bone graft or with the technique described by Masquelet. Allografts for defect reconstruction in long bones might also be described as possible options. Due to limited access to allografts in many countries and the authors' opinion that allografts result in poorer outcomes, this review focuses on autologous techniques and gives an internationally aligned overview of the current concepts in repair or reconstruction techniques of segmental long-bone defects.

Keywords: bone defect; callus distraction; all-internal distraction; Ilizarov

1. Introduction

Defects of the long bones are challenging for the patient, the patient´s environment and the treating physician. Depending on the clinical or regional circumstances, the distribution of the defect etiology differs. The main reasons for defects of the long bones are the following:

- traumatic substance loss due to open fracture or debridement
- fracture-associated infection or osteomyelitis
- nonunion

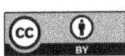

- tumor

Defects with a defect size of up to 2–3 cm are usually treated with grafting or acute shortening. Defects larger than 3 cm, especially in the lower limbs, are frequently restored to normal to avoid further functional impairment. A thorough assessment of the patient´s condition including comorbidities in a multidisciplinary manner and her or his personal demands must be taken into consideration. The mental stability and the strength of the patient to collaborate in these often very exhausting treatments are frequently underestimated. These considerations, the experience of the treating surgeon and the healthcare circumstances define the treatment path. Several techniques are available to restore continuity of the long bone. These techniques can be used alternatively or subsequently. Knowledge of all options and their individual pros and cons might be helpful for the physician to avoid problems and obstacles in these lengthy limb-saving procedures. In general, these techniques can be divided into *repair* techniques and *reconstructive* techniques.

The aim of the repair techniques is anatomical restoration of the bone with differentiation of the cortex and marrow. The basis for these techniques is distraction osteogenesis, which was influenced by names such as Langenbeck, Codovilla, Bier and Magnussen. The milestone work by Ilizarov in terms of instrument development and scientific research made distraction osteogenesis available for modern medicine. The term mechanotransduction was defined by his work that described the cellular mechanism for bone adaptation to mechanical loading, resembling the foundation for distraction osteogenesis.

Currently, classic, hybrid or all-internal distraction devices are technical options. However, they are all based on gradual distraction and consecutive bone transport or limb lengthening in osseous defect situations.

Reconstructive techniques restore long-bone continuity by replacing the defect zone with autologous bone, e.g., with a vascularized bone graft or with the technique described by Masquelet. Allografts for defect reconstruction in long bones might also be described as possible options. Due to the limited access to allografts in many countries and the authors' opinion that allografts result in poorer outcomes, this review focuses on autologous techniques and gives an internationally aligned overview of the current concepts in repair or reconstruction techniques of segmental long-bone defects.

1.1. Classic Bone Transport

Bone transport is defined as the gradual relocation of a bone segment from a healthy area to a region of bone loss and regeneration by distraction osteogenesis (Figure 1). Many small steps were necessary before the classical bone-transport method was developed. As early as the mid-19th century, Bernhard von Langenbeck described that the longitudinal growth of bones could be increased by distraction [1].

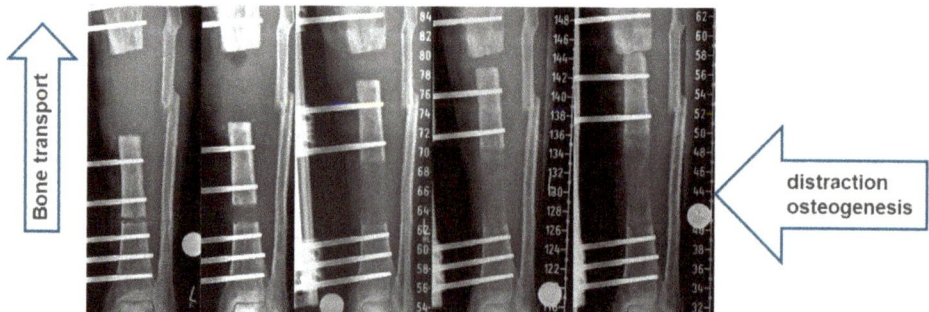

Figure 1. Distraction osteogenesis as classic segmental bone transport in the left tibia.

Léopold Ollier recognized the importance of the periosteum for bone growth [2]. Even though Alesandro Codivilla had already gained experience with limb lengthening in 1905, those attempts were usually associated with very high complication rates [3]. Louis Ombrédanne was the first to use slow–gradual lengthening for the first time [4], and Vittorio Putti improved the fixator technique [5]. August Bier recognized the importance of hematoma for bone healing [6]. The latency period after osteotomy to start lengthening was pioneered by Leroy Abbott [7]. Drilling osteoclasis was first described by Max Brandes [8], and Bosworth named the procedure bone distraction [9].

Raimund Wittmoser devised a ring fixator in 1944, but Lorenz Boehler did not recognize the brilliance and forbade him from publishing those ideas [10]. In 1951, Pierre Bertrand first used intramedullary nails for stabilization for femoral distraction [11]. Heinz Wagner recognized the importance of early mobilization and, therefore, developed a more stable fixator system [12]. After isolation by the Iron Curtain, Gavriil Ilizarov developed the method of bone transport. In 1952, he received a Russian patent for his ring fixator and then published "Compression osteosynthesis with the author's device" in 1968. He performed many experimental studies on the biology of bone formation and developed a method for bone transport by callus distraction [13–16].

The Ilizarov ring fixator has been available in the West only since 1981.

The foundation for all repair techniques is the technique of distraction osteogenesis, a low-energy osteotomy is performed with gentle drilling (osteoclasia without heat) or a gigli saw, preferably at the proximal or distal part of the affected bone at the metaphyseal area. The focus should be on minimal soft-tissue and periosteal compromise to preserve blood supply. At the osteotomy site, the hematoma changes to a viscous callus that can be distracted after a latency period of 3–7 days. Ilizarov described the optimal speed of distraction as 1 mm/day in four steps. Depending on the patient's condition and the soft-tissue situation and radiographic callus formation, the speed of distraction is individually modified. Raschke described intramedullary bone transport combined with a monolateral fixation system 30 years ago [17]. Since then there was a strong development of new instruments external and internal which are discussed throughout this review.

Segmental transport can be performed with various devices, such as ring/circular fixators, monolateral fixators and intramedullary nail systems, or by combinations of more than one device. Each device or technique has its own advantages and disadvantages. For bone transport, a stabilization system and a motor are needed.

We define "classic bone transport" as procedures in which only external devices are used. On the femur, problems arise because of the large soft tissue cover; monolateral systems become unstable, and ring fixators become uncomfortable. That is why we only use classic bone transport on the femur in special cases.

We observe an indication for classic bone transport, especially at the tibia, radius and ulna (Figure 2).

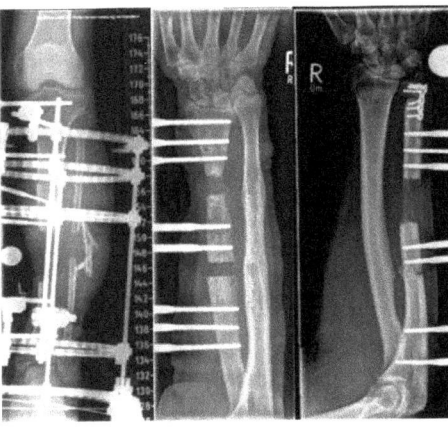

Figure 2. Classic segmental bone transport in the left tibia, right radius and right ulna.

To use a monolateral fixator, sufficiently long bone fragments are needed. This usually works for diaphyseal defects. If we have short bone ends, a classic Ilizarov ring fixator must be used.

If the joint line at one end of the bone is completely missing, and docking arthrodesis is required, the ring fixator is a possible way to solve the problem.

In the case of plastic reconstruction, cable systems can be used when a flap forbids us from pulling wires through it. Cable systems are also suitable for long transport distances, as the transport fragment then arrives at the docking point without translation (Figure 3).

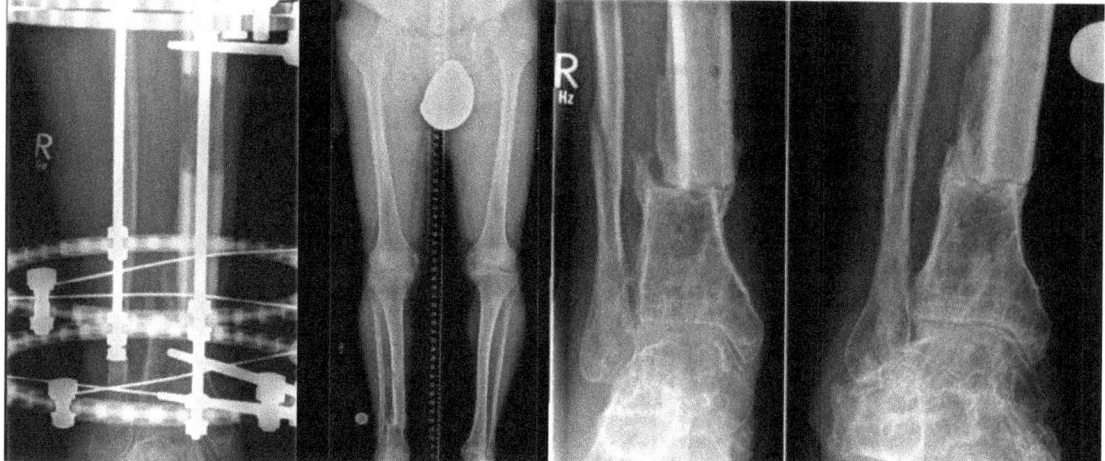

Figure 3. Translation with remodeling after docking in the course of consolidation.

Although patients rarely ask for an external fixator, we still observe classic bone transport as an indispensable method for many cases. Despite the risks associated with the long time that an external fixator has to be in place, it is a safe procedure with reproducibly good results.

Figure 4A–E show a case that could hardly be solved in a joint-preserving manner without classical bone transport in a ring fixator.

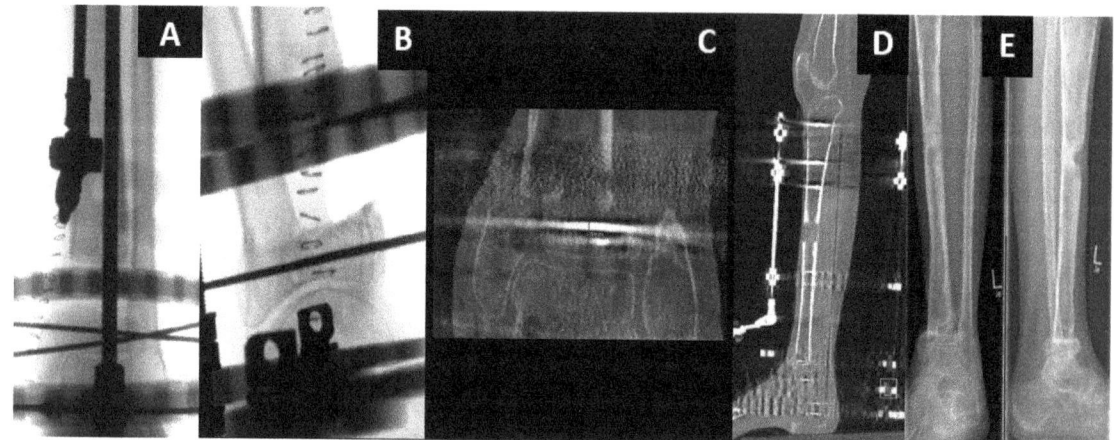

Figure 4. Example of classic bone transport.

After a pilon tibial fracture, the joint section had healed, but osteomyelitis developed directly above it. After definitive treatment of the infection, only an 8 mm thin slice of distal tibia remained. We built up a ring fixator across the ankle joint and fixed the pilon fragment with two wires (Figure 4A,B). A gentle drilling osteoclasia (without heat) produced a transport segment in the proximal part. Six to nine days after surgery, transport began three times 0.25 mm per day. In the subsequent process, the distraction speed can be adjusted depending on the radiographic callus formation. When the transport segment arrives (Figure 4C,D), surgical docking with autologous bone grafting and compression can reduce the time to fixator removal. When the docking zone has healed and the regenerate has hardened, the fixator can be removed (Figure 4E). During the entire process, the leg axis, length and torsion must be controlled.

1.2. Hybrid Techniques of Segmental Bone Transport

Classic bone transport using an external fixator (EF) has many advantages, including an unlimited amount of bone regeneration, the capacity to correct the deformity and early weight bearing. However, it requires a long period of external fixation, including the distraction period, healing at the docking site and consolidation of the distraction callus. Therefore, avoiding complications, such as pin-related problems and joint contractures, is difficult and can result in poor outcomes [18]. Although multifocal bone transport techniques (Figure 5) have reduced the distraction period, consolidation of the distraction callus may still require a long period until it is safe to remove the EF. Therefore, secondary nailing that follows the distraction phase might be an option.

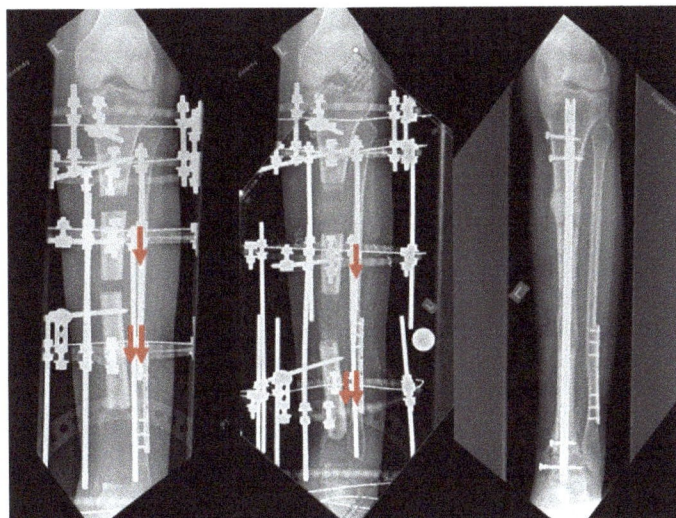

Figure 5. A thirty-year-old female patient after post-traumatic osteomyelitis and resection of the distal tibia received multifocal bone transport (tandem-technique), doubling distraction speed of the distal fragment. After docking, the approach was changed to an antibiotic-coated nail for consolidation and partial weight bearing. Red arrows show the distraction direction—the segment with the double arrows is transported with twice the speed.

Unless the distraction callus is sufficiently hard, EF removal may result in a fractured callus, nonunion of the docking site, malunion or even ultimate failure of bone transport. To reduce the external fixation time (EFT) as well as its resultant complications, hybrid bone-transport techniques have been developed. A combination of an EF and an internal implant (either a nail or a plate) can be performed simultaneously, while the EF can be removed early before completion of the consolidation. With its mechanical advantage to support the distraction callus and protect it against refracture, it may help the patient´s comfort and convenience.

Bone transport over a nail (BTON) is a commonly used hybrid technique that eliminates the consolidation period of the distraction callus with the stabilization provided by the intramedullary (IM) nail. BTON remarkably reduced EFT, which was associated with increased patient comfort, a decreased complication rate and convenient and rapid rehabilitation [19]. However, the conventional BTON technique should maintain EF until docking-site consolidation is completed. Therefore, modifications of BTON have been attempted to achieve stability and compression at the docking site by performing additional plate fixation or by locking the transported segment to the predrilled, custom-made, intramedullary nail via the extra locking holes [20]. BTON has a potential risk of developing a deep infection in the medullary canal. As close proximity is inevitable between the nail and EF pins, cross-contamination from the infected pin track may lead to bone reconstruction failure [21].

Bone transport over a plate (BTOP) combines plate fixation with EF. Compared with BTON, BTOP may decrease the risk of deep infection because it can minimize possible contact between the plate and EF pins [22]. Since the transported fragment is fixed to the plate with screws at the time of docking, BTOP requires the external fixator only during the distraction period, eliminating both the consolidation periods of the docking site and the distraction callus. A recent comparative study proved that BTOP had a significantly shorter EFT than BTON, while the final outcomes were similar in segmental tibial bone defects [23]. Nail fixation is also difficult when the defect is too close to the joint line and when the proximal or distal segment is too short for nail locking. BTON may be difficult to perform in forearm bones because of a very limited intramedullary space between the nail and EF. Under these conditions, BTOP is an ideal alternative since plate fixation is relatively free without anatomical restrictions. In summary, both hybrid bone-transport techniques are safe and achieve satisfactory outcomes for treating segmental defects of the long bone. The BTOP technique shows benefits over the BTON technique because of the shorter EFT and wider indications; however, in the lower leg, more stability is achieved with BTON.

A 15-year-old girl suffered reaming necrosis of the tibial shaft after tibial nailing (Figure 6A). A complete resection of necrotic bone resulted in a 3.5 cm segmental defect (Figure 6B). The BTOP procedure was performed. Figure 6C shows the lateral radiograph immediately after locked plate insertion on the medial aspect, corticotomy and application of an EF on the anterior aspect. Figure 6D shows the lateral radiograph after the completion of bone transport. Figure 6E shows the AP radiograph after screw fixation at the transported segment, autogenous iliac bone grafting at the docking site and removal of EF. Figure 6F shows the AP and lateral radiograph of the tibia showing bony healing of the docking site and distraction site 1 year after transport.

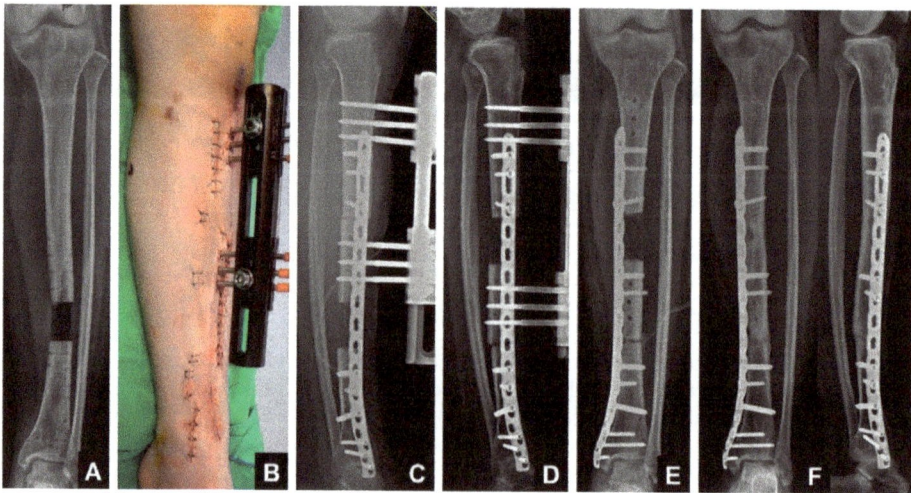

Figure 6. Example of hybrid bone transport.

1.3. Induced Membrane Technique—Masquelet

Membrane-induced osteogenesis, first reported by Masquelet in 2000, is a popular technique for the reconstruction of bone defects [24]. Among thirty-five patients with defects from 4 cm to 25 cm, union rates of 100% were reported. It has revolutionized our understanding of bone healing and has become a popular method of treating bone defects. Subsequently, many authors have reported on the success of this technique [25–29].

1.4. Principle

The bone defect is filled with cement (polymethylmethacrylate), which provokes a foreign-body reaction that results in the formation of a strongly vascularized membrane. This later functions as a biological chamber that can be filled with autologous bone grafts, resulting in solid cylindrical bone formation. The membrane prevents graft absorption and promotes bone healing via several vascular and growth factors.

1.5. Technique

The technique is a two-stage procedure. In the first stage, all nonviable bone and soft tissues are debrided. This is possibly the most important stage in the procedure. The limb needs to be stabilized, and the defect is filled with bone cement mixed with antibiotics, overlapping the cortices at the two ends. Good soft tissue cover is essential.

In the second stage, the membrane is incised, and the cement is removed. The medullary canals at the two ends are opened, the defect is filled with cancellous bone graft, and the membrane closes over it along with the soft tissue.

Masquelet in his series used external fixation for stabilization and cancellous autografts. However, other implants, such as interlocking nails [29,30], may be used. Similarly, authors have combined autologous bone grafts with bone substitutes, such as demineralized bone matrix or BMP [31], or used reamer-irrigation-aspirator (RIA) bone grafts [30,32].

Many articles have been written on the details of the technique using minor modifications [33–38].

2. Membrane Characteristics

The biologic activity of the induced membrane has been studied extensively. Pellesier et al. [37] showed that the induced membrane secreted growth factors, including vascular and osteoinductive factors, which could stimulate bone regeneration. Authors have studied the histologic and biochemical properties of the membrane in animal studies and have shown that, within two weeks, the membrane forms two distinct layers. Most studies have shown a significant increase in various factors that promote osteogenesis [37,39–41].

The vascularity of the outer part is more than that of the part in contact with the cement spacer and progressively increases from 2 to 4 weeks and decreases after 4–6 weeks.

Aho et al. [39] have shown that the membrane from human femur or tibia defects is significantly less vascular at 3 months than at 1 month.

Spacer Material

Masquelet used PMMA to fill the defect after debridement. The addition of antibiotics should help to combat infection due to the elution of high concentrations of local antibiotics [42–45].

Nau et al. [40] showed that different antibiotics may affect the membrane characteristics and that clindamycin produced a thinner membrane than vancomycin or gentamycin.

PMMA is conveniently available and most commonly used in clinical practice [46]. Alternative spacers, such as silicone epoxies and biosynthetic materials, may have a role in the future [47].

Bone graft materials

Autogenous cancellous bone grafting is still the gold standard. RIA has become popular more recently because of the large volume of grafts with reduced complications Bone substitutes, such as hydroxyapatite, may have benefits in increasing graft volume but not osteogenesis. BMP may help increase osteogenic properties, but clinical trials are still equivocal [31].

In conclusion, this method is very popular due to the excellent reports in complex situations. The renerate however, has a column-like structure, which might require further protection with an implant (e.g., plate or nail) until full weight bearing can be permitted.

Figures 7 and 8 show an example of the induced membrane technique—Masquelet.

Stage One:

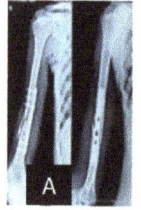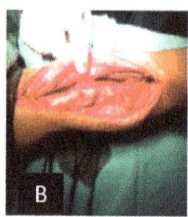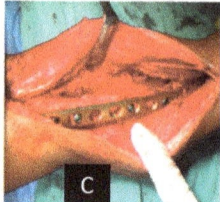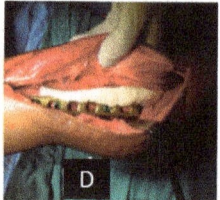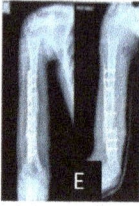

Figure 7. A 19-year-old patient was referred with swelling induration and sinus discharge 6 months after operative management of a humerus shaft fracture. (**A**) Preoperative X-ray: AP and lateral view. (**B**) Intraoperative photographs showing purulent discharge. (**C**) Through debridement excision of sequestrated bone stabilization with a locking compression plate (LCP) using locking screws only. (**D**) Filling of the bone defect with antibiotic-impregnated bone cement. (**E**) AP and lateral views after stage one.

Stage Two:

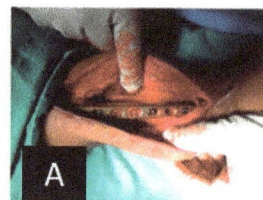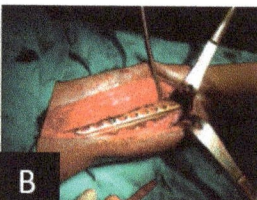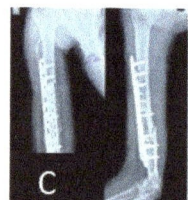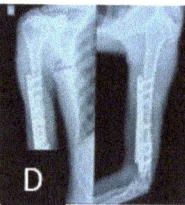

Figure 8. After six weeks, membrane formation was induced after removal of the cement spacer in stage two. (**A,B**) The defect was filled with a bone graft and an additional orthogonal plate for enhanced rotational stability. (**C**) Subsequent postoperative X-ray, AP and lateral views. (**D**) AP and lateral radiographs at the one-year follow-up showed successful healing.

2.1. Reconstruction with Vascularized Bone Graft

Vascularized bone grafts are an additional option for extensive bone defects or bone defects with impaired regenerative potential that require simultaneous structural support, bone regeneration and vascularization. In contrast to conventional bone grafts, vascularized bone grafts allow for direct healing and bridging of bony defects and do not require a process of partial necrosis or regeneration (creeping substitution) [48]. Over the last 40 years, a plethora of different vascularized bone grafts have been described for the reconstruction of bone defects in any region of the human body, including the extremities, trunk and head and neck [49]. Since its first description in 1975 by Taylor et al. [50], the free fibula graft has become the working horse flap for the reconstruction of large segmental bone defects. It is a long and straight graft and can be raised with a skin island that allows for the repair of concomitant soft-tissue defects. Donor-site morbidity is tolerable if 6–7 cm of the distal and proximal fibula is preserved [51]. Stress fractures are not uncommon after reconstruction of lower extremity bone defects with the free fibula graft, and it can sometimes take more than one year for graft hypertrophy to allow for full weight-bearing mobility [52]. At the lower extremities, the combination of free vascularized fibula grafts and allogenic bone grafts combines high mechanical stability and osteogenic potential and provides safe and stable healing in aseptic bone defects [53]. Shorter bone defects can also be addressed with a "double barrel" fibula graft for increased stability [54]. Free iliac crest [55] and scapula grafts [56] represent alternative options that are applicable in shorter defects or if the fibula graft is not available. While bone transport and membrane-guided bone regeneration are alternatives to free vascularized bone grafts at the lower extremities, free vascularized bone grafts represent the gold standard for segmental bone defects at the upper extremities due to their healing potential, mechanical properties and single-stage surgery that allow for early mobilization and physical therapy.

A 50-year-old female patient with a 3rd degree open radius and ulna fracture, showing ORIF radius and ulna at day 0; revision and cancellous bone grafting at days 24 and 63; severe bone and soft tissue infection, wound revision and sequestrectomy at day 75; and radius segment resection, spacer and external fixator at day 94 (Figure 9A–C). Reconstruction of an 8 cm segmental radius defect with free vascularized osteocutaneous fibula graft (Figure 9D). and ORIF (2 LCP plates) was performed at day 116 (Figure 9E–G). At day 120, the venous anastomosis was revised, and the flap was salvaged. The further course was uneventful, and bone healing was completed after 4 months.

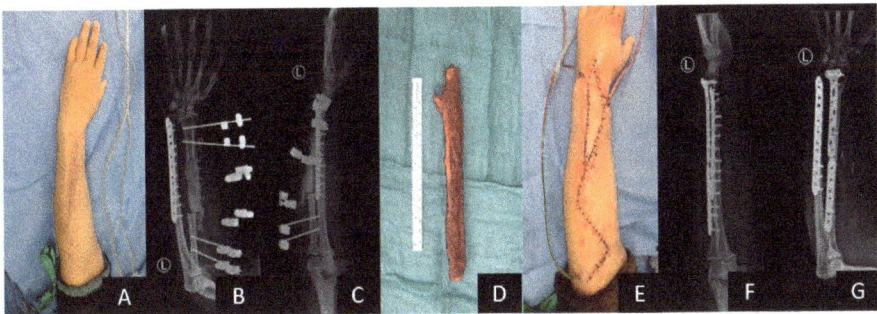

Figure 9. Example of vascularized bone graft. (**A–C**) Local wound situation and X-ray before reconstruction. Segmental bone defect is filled with a gentamycin spacer and stabilized with external fixation. (**D**) Free fibula graft prior to inset. (**E**) Primary closure with the skin island of the osteocutaneous fibula flap. (**F,G**) Stabile bony union at 12 months after reconstruction.

2.2. All-Internal Segmental Bone Transport with Motorized Nails

External fixation has been a great addition to the treatment of musculoskeletal bone defects, but external fixators are related to a variety of problems and complications, including pain, pin tract infection, joint stiffness, interference with gait, discomfort and a host of aesthetic and psychological problems (Video S1).

Motorized nails have been described for limb lengthening [57–59] (Video S2). The motor of the nail can be activated with mechanical energy by gait or, in more recent developments, with electrical energy either from a battery or magnetically induced with an actuating device. These devices have been adapted to bone defect situations where the lengthening nail functions as the driving motor for the bone segment for an 'all-internal' segmental bone transport. This can be reached with three different configurations (Figure 10, Table 1).

Table 1. Different options for all-internal distraction.

	Plate-Assisted Bone Segment Transport (PABST) [60,61]	Segment Transport Nails(STN) [62–65]	Nail-in-Nail System(MagicTube) [66,67]
Concept	• Defect is bridged with a plate. • Conventional motorized lengthening nail transports the osteotomized bone	• These nails consist of a proximal and distal locked and centrally slotted bridging element. • central motorized piston is connected to the transport segment	• Bridging the proximal to the distal main segment is performed with a simple slotted tube with several locking holes

Table 1. Cont.

	Plate-Assisted Bone Segment Transport (PABST) [60,61]	Segment Transport Nails(STN) [62–65]	Nail-in-Nail System(MagicTube) [66,67]
Advantage	• Flexible use of commercially available standard implants (locking plate, lengthening nail). Allows for short proximal and distal main segments.	• Consists of the one nail component only. No need for an additional plate.	• Does not require an additional plate to bridge proximal and distal main segment • No special segment transport nail needed • Applicable to any lengthening nail • Fragment size opposite the motor side can be as short as 3 cm • Optional additional lengthening
Disadvantage	• Difficulty achieving fixation in short metaphyseal segments • Locking plate might interfere with soft tissues and/or nail • Position of the piston locking holes might not be at the level of the transport segment, requiring a pulley system. • Flexible pulley systems only allow pull, not push mode. • Does not allow for sequential lengthening. • Maximum transport length only limited by nail stroke	• Difficulty maintaining alignment in short metaphyseal segments • Less forgiveness in execution and very little chance of correcting as the transport is underway • Does not allow for sequential lengthening • Additional surgical procedure required when transport length exceeds 70 mm	• Difficulty maintaining alignment in short metaphyseal segments • Adds to the thickness of the lengthening nail • Not FDA approved or CE marked • Maximum transport length only limited by nail stroke

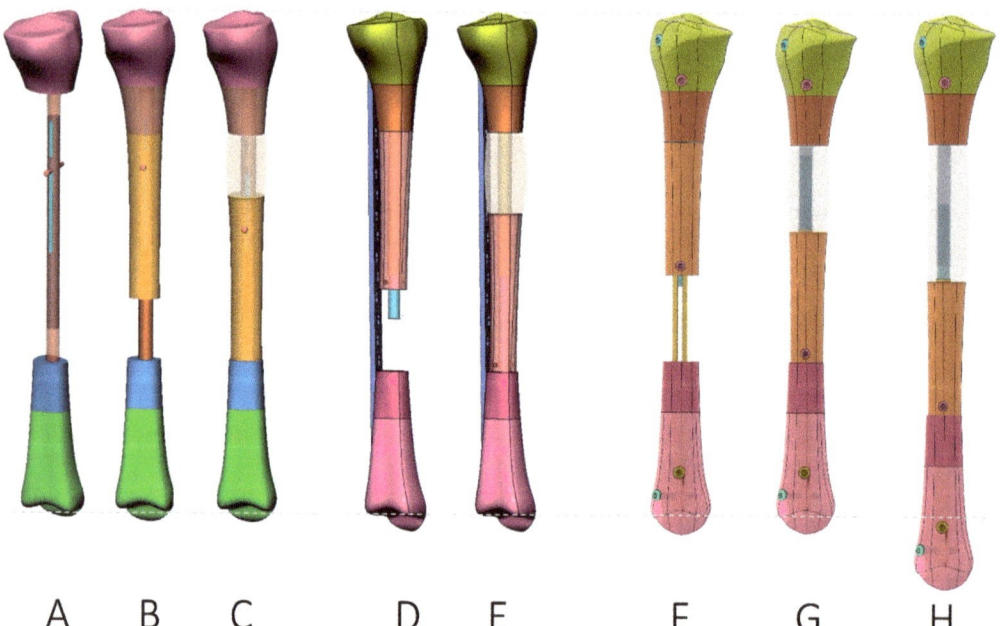

Figure 10. Different options for segmental bone transport with motorized nails. (**A–C**) Bone segment transport nail. (**D,E**) Plate-assisted bone segment transport (PABST). (**F–H**) MagicTube.

2.3. Bone Segment Transport Nails (STN)

These nails consist of a proximal and distal lock and a slotted bridging element. A central motorized piston is connected to the transport segment through the slot. With the movement of the piston, the connecting locking bolts glide in the slots of the central nail part and drive the bone segment [60,61] (Video S3).

2.4. Plate-Assisted Bone Segment Transport (PABST)

Here, a locking plate bridges the bone defect, and a conventional motorized lengthening nail transports the osteotomized bone segment into the defect [62,63] (Video S4).

2.5. MagicTube

The magic tube consists of a simple slotted tube that is slid over a motorized nail. The far end of the tube contains screw holes. This concept does not require an additional plate construct to bridge the proximal and distal main segments nor does it need a special segment transport nail since it is applicable to any lengthening nail (Videos S5 and S6). It also allows for additional lengthening if needed [64,65] (Videos S5 and S7).

3. Discussion

There are several techniques to choose from in the treatment of long-bone defects, as demonstrated above. The most significant difference is whether anatomical repair or reconstruction for continuity of the bone should be performed. The physical demand of the upper or lower limb must be taken into consideration, similar to the physical demand of the patient. Since the biomechanical characteristics of reconstruction techniques, such as fibula grafts of Masquelet, are generally inferior compared to anatomical repair, these techniques are more often used in the upper limbs. Because of the soft-tissue situation and the nearby anatomical structures in the upper limbs, which are potentially more at risk with distraction techniques with reduced time wearing an external fixator, this recommendation is supported from a safety and comfort perspective.

For lower-limb defects, restoration of the anatomical situation and biomechanical weight-bearing capacity seem essential, especially in younger patients. The Masquelet technique allows for quick reconstruction of bone continuity by missing cortex marrow differentiation. Fibula graft techniques have to double-fold the graft to gain a sufficient diameter if reconstruction, e.g., in the femur, is performed. This limits the length of the possible defects that can be reconstructed. Donor-site morbidity is also a relevant aspect to take into consideration when choosing the proper technique. Therefore, distraction osteogenesis in a classic, hybrid or all-internal manner shows advantages in the lower limbs. Classic and hybrid distraction devices are available around the globe and allow for the treatment of a great variety of defect morphologies and localizations in a cost-effective manner.

Nevertheless, external fixation is related to relative discomfort for the patient and a variety of possible complications, e.g., pin tract infections. To rule out these disadvantages, all-internal devices were developed that differ in the manner of activating the distraction device. Recently developed magnetically activated nails [66–68] have advantages over gait-activated systems [57], which are difficult to control (speed, stop) and cannot reverse direction. Magnetically or electrically activated motorized nails overcome these disadvantages. They allow for reliable control of the start and stop as well as the direction and speed.

All motorized segment transport nail systems benefit from internal components. All three technologies allow for the control of transport speed and direction. However, motorized nail systems have the disadvantage that they require a certain minimum length of the nail, which can be problematic in short proximal or distal fragments. In these circumstances, direct locking of the transport fragment may not be possible, and pulley systems (wire, plate) may need to be considered. Another disadvantage of magnetically motorized nails is the fact that the induction of energy is related to the distance between the external actuator and the internal receiver in the nail. In obese patients and limbs with a large soft-tissue envelope, the amount of energy transferred is less compared to normal-weight patients and slim limbs. Most of these patients with segmental defects also have some shortening. Additionally, there is frequently some shortening associated with debridement at the docking site. The MagicTube is the only device that allows for additional lengthening without further surgery just by continuing the segment transport. When STM was compared with PABST, it was shown that there are difficulties in maintaining alignment in short metaphyseal segments and fewer options to manage this when compared with the PABST procedure [61].

Due to the high costs of these devices, the availability and utilization of all-internal distraction devices are limited in health care systems worldwide.

4. Conclusions

The treatment of long-bone defects is challenging for the treating surgeon and the patient and his or her environment. In every case, the underlying pathology must be managed, such as infection eradication or resection of the tumor, before restoration of the defect can begin.

The physical demand of the patient and the localization of the defect influence whether repair or reconstruction techniques are used. Reconstruction techniques, such as Masquelet and vascularized fibula grafts, show good results and reduce the time of external fixation. Biomechanical disadvantages focus these techniques on the upper limbs. Repair techniques are mainly based on the work by Ilizarov [13–16], which can be performed in a classic all-external manner. Hybrid techniques reduce the time of the external fixator and show benefits at the time-point of docking. All-internal devices limit the complications of the external fixators but are limited in use because of the high cost.

Since the long process of restoration of a bone defect is demanding for the patient and the surgeon, the faith of the patient in the treating surgeon and the trustful cooperation of the patient and surgeon are as important for treatment success as the technique used.

Supplementary Materials: The following supporting information can be downloaded at: https://www.mdpi.com/article/10.3390/jcm12196283/s1, Video S1: EF. Video S2: motorized nails for limb lengthenig, Video S3: Bone segment transport, Video S4: plate assisted bone segment transport, Video S5: Magic tube, Video S6: Magic tube.

Author Contributions: All authors had significant impact in Conceptualization, writing—original draft preparation, writing—review and editing of this review. All authors have read and agreed to the published version of the manuscript.

Funding: This research received no external funding.

Conflicts of Interest: The authors declare no conflict of interest.

References

1. Langenbeck, B. Über krankhaftes Längenwachstum der Röhrenknochen und seine Verwertung für die chirurgische Praxis. *Berl. Klin. Wochenschr.* **1869**, *6*, 265–270.
2. Ollier, L. *Traité Expérimental et Clinique de la Régénération des os et de la Production Artificielle du Tissu Osseux*; Victor Masson Et Fils: Paris, France, 1867; Volume 2.
3. Codivilla, A. On the Means of Lengthening in the Lower Limbs, the Muscles and the Tissues which are Shortened through Deformity. *Am. J. Orthop. Surg.* **1905**, *2*, 353. [CrossRef]
4. Ombredanne, L. Allongement d'un fémur sur un membre trop court. *Bull. Mem. Soc. Chir.* **1913**, *39*, 1177.
5. Putti, V.; Peltier, L.F. The operative lengthening of the femur. *JAMA* **1921**, *77*, 934–935. [CrossRef]
6. Bier, A. Die Bedeutung des Blutergusses für die Heilung des Knochenbruches. Heilung von Pseudarthrosen und von verspäteter Callusbildung durch Bluteinspritzung Med Klinik. Urban&Schwarzenberg Berlin. *Med. Klinik* **1905**, 6–7.
7. Abbott, L.C.; Crego, C.H.; Adams, A.O. The operative lengthening of the lower extremity. *Int. J. Orthod. Oral Surg. Radiogr.* **1929**, *15*, 110–124. [CrossRef]
8. Brandes, M. Über Störungen der Konsolidation nach orthopädischen Osteotomien langer Röhrenknochen. *Verh. Deut. Orthop. Ges.* **1928**, *2*, 775.

9. Bosworth, D.M. Skeletal distraction of the tibia. *Surg. Gynaecol.* **1938**, *66*, 912–924.
10. Wittmoser, R. Pressure osteosynthesis. *Langenbeck's Arch. Klin. Chir. Ver. Dtsch. Z. Chir.* **1953**, *276*, 229–231.
11. Bertrand, P. Technic of lengthening of the femur in extreme shortness. *Rev. Chir. Orthop. Reparatrice Appar. Mot.* **1951**, *37*, 530–533.
12. Wagner, H. Surgical leg prolongation. *Chirurgei* **1971**, *42*, 260–266.
13. Ilizarov, G.A.; Lediaev, V.I.; Shitin, V.P. The course of compact bone reparative regeneration in distraction osteosynthesis under different conditions of bone fragment fixation (experimental study). *Eksp. Khir. Anesteziol.* **1969**, *14*, 3–12. [PubMed]
14. Ilizarov, G.A. *Transosseous Osteosynthesis: Theoretical and Clinical Aspects of the Regeneration and Growth of Tissue*; Springer: New York, NY, USA; Berlin/Heidelberg, Germany, 1992.
15. Ilizarov, G.A. The tension-stress effect on the genesis and growth of tissues. Part I. The influence of stability of fixation and soft-tissue preservation. *Clin. Orthop. Relat. Res.* **1989**, *238*, 249–281. [CrossRef]
16. Ilizarov, G.A. The tension-stress effect on the genesis and growth of tissues: Part II. The influence of the rate and frequency of distraction. *Clin. Orthop. Relat. Res.* **1989**, *239*, 263–285. [CrossRef]
17. Raschke, M.J.; Mann, J.W.; Oedekoven, G.; Claudi, B.F. Segmental transport after unreamed intramedullary nailing. Preliminary report of a "Monorail" system. *Clin. Orthop. Relat. Res.* **1992**, *282*, 233–240.
18. Kocaoglu, M.; Eralp, L.; Rashid, H.U.; Sen, C.; Bilsel, K. Reconstruction of segmental bone defects due to chronic osteomyelitis with use of an external fixator and an intramedullary nail. *J. Bone Jt. Surg.* **2006**, *88*, 2137–2145.
19. Oh, C.W.; Song, H.R.; Roh, J.Y.; Oh, J.K.; Min, W.K.; Kyung, H.S.; Kim, J.W.; Kim, P.T.; Ihn, J.C. Bone transport over an intramedullary nail for reconstruction of long bone defects in tibia. *Arch. Orthop. Trauma Surg.* **2008**, *128*, 801–808. [CrossRef]
20. Bas, A.; Daldal, F.; Eralp, L.; Kocaoglu, M.; Uludag, S.; Sari, S. Treatment of Tibial and Femoral Bone Defects With Bone Transport Over an Intramedullary Nail. *J. Orthop. Trauma* **2020**, *34*, e353–e359. [CrossRef]
21. Kim, S.J.; Mandar, A.; Song, S.H.; Song, H.R. Pitfalls of lengthening over an intramedullary nail in tibia: A consecutive case series. *Arch. Orthop. Trauma Surg.* **2012**, *132*, 185–191. [CrossRef]
22. Oh, C.W.; Apivatthakakul, T.; Oh, J.K.; Kim, J.W.; Lee, H.J.; Kyung, H.S.; Baek, S.G.; Jung, G.H. Bone transport with an external fixator and a locking plate for segmental tibial defects. *Bone Jt. J.* **2013**, *95*, 1667–1672. [CrossRef]
23. Park, K.H.; Oh, C.W.; Kim, J.W.; Oh, J.K.; Yoon, Y.C.; Seo, I.; Ha, S.S.; Chung, S.H. Matched Comparison of Bone Transport Using External Fixator Over a Nail Versus External Fixator Over a Plate for Segmental Tibial Bone Defects. *J. Orthop. Trauma* **2021**, *35*, e397–e404. [CrossRef] [PubMed]
24. Masquelet, A.C.; Fitoussi, F.; Begue, T.; Muller, G.P. Reconstruction of the long bones by the induced membrane and spongy autograft. *Ann. Chir. Plast. Esthet.* **2000**, *45*, 346–353. [PubMed]
25. Cuthbert, R.J.; Churchman, S.M.; Tan, H.B.; McGonagle, D.; Jones, E.; Giannoudis, P.V. Induced periosteum a complex cellular scaffold for the treatment of large bone defects. *Bone* **2013**, *57*, 484–492. [CrossRef] [PubMed]
26. Karger, C.; Kishi, T.; Schneider, L.; Fitoussi, F.; Masquelet, A.C. Treatment of posttraumatic bone defects by the induced membrane technique. *Orthop. Traumatol. Surg. Res.* **2012**, *98*, 97–102. [CrossRef]
27. Taylor, B.C.; Hancock, J.; Zitzke, R.; Castaneda, J. Treatment of Bone Loss with the Induced Membrane Technique: Techniques and Outcomes. *J. Orthop. Trauma* **2015**, *29*, 554–557. [CrossRef]
28. Zappaterra, T.; Ghislandi, X.; Adam, A.; Huard, S.; Gindraux, F.; Gallinet, D.; Lepage, D.; Garbuio, P.; Tropet, Y.; Obert, L. Induced membrane technique for the reconstruction for the reconstruction of bone defects in upper limb. A prospective single center study of nine cases. *Chir. Main* **2011**, *30*, 255–263. [CrossRef]
29. Mauffrey, C.; Barlow, B.T.; Smith, W. Management of segmental bone defects. *J. Am. Acad. Orthop. Surg.* **2015**, *23*, 143–153.
30. Giannoudis, P.V.; Faour, O.; Goff, T.; Kanakaris, N.; Dimitriou, R. Masquelet technique for the treatment of bone defects: Tips-tricks and future directions. *Injury* **2011**, *42*, 591–598. [CrossRef]
31. Masquelet, A.C.; Begue, T. The concept of induced membrane for reconstruction of long bone defects. *Orthop. Clin. N. Am.* **2010**, *41*, 27–37. [CrossRef]
32. Donegan, D.J.; Scolaro, J.; Matuszewski, P.E.; Mehta, S. Staged bone grafting following placement of an antibiotic spacer block for the management of segmental long bone defects. *Orthopedics* **2011**, *34*, e730–e735. [CrossRef]
33. Taylor, B.C.; French, B.G.; Fowler, T.T.; Russell, J.; Poka, A. Induced membrane technique for reconstruction to manage bone loss. *J. Am. Acad. Orthop. Surg.* **2012**, *20*, 142–150. [CrossRef] [PubMed]
34. Hak, D.J.; Pittman, J.L. Biological rationale for the intramedullary canal as a source of autograft material. *Orthop. Clin. N. Am.* **2010**, *41*, 57–61. [CrossRef] [PubMed]
35. Schmidmaier, G.; Herrmann, S.; Green, J.; Weber, T.; Scharfenberger, A.; Haas, N.P.; Wildemann, B. Quantitative assessment of growth factors in reaming aspirate, iliac crest, and platelet preparation. *Bone* **2006**, *39*, 1156–1163. [CrossRef] [PubMed]
36. Porter, R.M.; Liu, F.; Pilapil, C.; Betz, O.B.; Vrahas, M.S.; Harris, M.B.; Evans, C.H. Osteogenic potential of reamer irrigator aspirator (RIA) aspirate collected from patients undergoing hip arthroplasty. *J. Orthop. Res.* **2009**, *27*, 42–49. [CrossRef] [PubMed]
37. Pelissier, P.; Masquelet, A.C.; Bareille, R.; Pelissier, S.M.; Amedee, J. Induced membranes secrete growth factors including vascular and osteoinductive factors and could stimulate bone regeneration. *J. Orthop. Res.* **2004**, *22*, 73–79. [CrossRef]
38. Sagi, H.C.; Young, M.L.; Gerstenfeld, L.; Einhorn, T.A.; Tornetta, P. Qualitative and quantitative differences between bone graft obtained from the medullary canal (with a Reamer/Irrigator/Aspirator) and the iliac crest of the same patient. *J. Bone Jt. Surg. Am.* **2012**, *94*, 2128–2135. [CrossRef]

39. Aho, O.M.; Lehenkari, P.; Ristiniemi, J.; Lehtonen, S.; Risteli, J.; Leskela, H.V. The mechanism of action of induced membranes in bone repair. *J. Bone Jt. Surg. Am.* **2013**, *95*, 597–604. [CrossRef]
40. Nau, C.; Seebach, C.; Trumm, A.; Schaible, A.; Kontradowitz, K.; Meier, S.; Buechner, H.; Marzi, I.; Henrich, D. Alteration of Masquelet's induced membrane characteristics by different kinds of antibiotic enriched bone cement in a critical size defect model in the rat's femur. *Injury* **2016**, *47*, 325–334. [CrossRef]
41. Liu, H.; Hu, G.; Shang, P.; Shen, Y.; Nie, P.; Peng, L.; Xu, H. Histological characteristics of induced membranes in subcutaneous, intramuscular sites and bone defect. *Orthop. Traumatol. Surg. Res.* **2013**, *99*, 959–964. [CrossRef]
42. Viateau, V.; Guillemin, G.; Calando, Y.; Logeart, D.; Oudina, K.; Sedel, L.; Hannouche, D.; Bousson, V.; Petite, H. Induction of a barrier membrane to facilitate reconstruction of massive segmental diaphyseal bone defects: An ovine model. *Vet. Surg.* **2006**, *35*, 445–452. [CrossRef]
43. Wang, X.; Luo, F.; Huang, K.; Xie, Z. Induced membrane technique for the treatment of bone defects due to post-traumatic osteomyelitis. *Bone Jt. Res.* **2016**, *5*, 101–105. [CrossRef]
44. Apard, T.; Bigorre, N.; Cronier, P.; Duteille, F.; Bizot, P.; Massin, P. Two-stage reconstruction of post-traumatic segmental tibia bone loss with nailing. *Orthop. Traumatol. Surg. Res.* **2010**, *96*, 549–553. [CrossRef] [PubMed]
45. Scholz, A.O.; Gehrmann, S.; Glombitza, M.; Kaufmann, R.A.; Bostelmann, R.; Flohe, S.; Windolf, J. Reconstruction of septic diaphyseal bone defects with the induced membrane technique. *Injury* **2015**, *46* (Suppl. 4), S121–S124. [CrossRef] [PubMed]
46. Chan, Y.S.; Ueng, S.W.; Wang, C.J.; Lee, S.S.; Chen, C.Y.; Shin, C.H. Antibiotic-impregnated autogenic cancellous bone grafting is an effective and safe method for the management of small infected tibial defects: A comparison study. *J. Trauma* **2000**, *48*, 246–255. [CrossRef]
47. Tarchala, M.; Engel, V.; Barralet, J.; Harvey, E.J. A pilot study: Alternative biomaterials in critical sized bone defect treatment. *Injury* **2018**, *49*, 523–531. [CrossRef]
48. Cavadas, P.C.; Landin, L.; Ibanez, J.; Nthumba, P. Reconstruction of major traumatic segmental bone defects of the tibia with vascularized bone transfers. *Plast. Reconstr. Surg.* **2010**, *125*, 215–223. [CrossRef]
49. Yazar, S.; Lin, C.H.; Wei, F.C. One-stage reconstruction of composite bone and soft-tissue defects in traumatic lower extremities. *Plast. Reconstr. Surg.* **2004**, *114*, 1457–1466. [CrossRef]
50. Taylor, G.I.; Miller, G.D.; Ham, F.J. The free vascularized bone graft. A clinical extension of microvascular techniques. *Plast. Reconstr. Surg.* **1975**, *55*, 533–544. [CrossRef]
51. Attia, S.; Diefenbach, J.; Schmermund, D.; Böttger, S.; Pons-Kühnemann, J.; Scheibelhut, C.; Heiss, C.; Howaldt, H.P. Donor-Site Morbidity after Fibula Transplantation in Head and Neck Tumor Patients: A Split-Leg Retrospective Study with Focus on Leg Stability and Quality of Life. *Cancers* **2020**, *12*, 2217. [CrossRef]
52. Taylor, G.I. The current status of free vascularized bone grafts. *Clin. Plast. Surg.* **1983**, *10*, 185–209. [CrossRef]
53. Donati, D.; Di Liddo, M.; Zavatta, M.; Manfrini, M.; Bacci, G.; Picci, P.; Capanna, R.; Mercuri, M. Massive bone allograft reconstruction in high-grade osteosarcoma. *Clin. Orthop. Relat. Res.* **2000**, *377*, 186–194. [CrossRef]
54. Banic, A.; Hertel, R. Double vascularized fibulas for reconstruction of large tibial defects. *J. Reconstr. Microsurg.* **1993**, *9*, 421–428. [CrossRef]
55. Taylor, G.I.; Watson, N. One-stage repair of compound leg defects with free, revascularized flaps of groin skin and iliac bone. *Plast. Reconstr. Surg.* **1978**, *61*, 494–506. [CrossRef]
56. Sekiguchi, J.; Kobayashi, S.; Ohmori, K. Use of the osteocutaneous free scapular flap on the lower extremities. *Plast. Reconstr. Surg.* **1993**, *91*, 103–112. [CrossRef]
57. Cole, J.D.; Justin, D.; Kasparis, T.; DeVlught, D.; Knobloch, C. The intramedullary skeletal kinetic distractor (ISKD): First clinical results of a new intramedullary nail for lengthening of the femur and tibia. *Injury* **2001**, *32* (Suppl. 4), SD129–SD139. [CrossRef]
58. Laubscher, M.; Mitchell, C.; Timms, A.; Goodier, D.; Calder, P. Outcomes following femoral lengthening: An initial comparison of the Precice intramedullary lengthening nail and the LRS external fixator monorail system. *Bone Jt. J.* **2016**, *98*, 1382–1388. [CrossRef]
59. Liodakis, E.; Kenawey, M.; Krettek, C.; Ettinger, M.; Jagodzinski, M.; Hankemeier, S. Segmental transports for posttraumatic lower extremity bone defects: Are femoral bone transports safer than tibial? *Arch. Orthop. Trauma Surg.* **2011**, *131*, 229–234. [CrossRef]
60. Baumgart, R.; Betz, A.; Schweiberer, L. A fully implantable motorized intramedullary nail for limb lengthening and bone transport. *Clin. Orthop. Relat. Res.* **1997**, *343*, 135–143. [CrossRef]
61. Gardner, M.P.; Beason, A.M. Plate-Assisted Bone Segment Transport Versus Precice Bone Transport Nail. *J. Orthop. Trauma* **2021**, *35* (Suppl. 4), S19–S24. [CrossRef]
62. Kahler, O.U. Plate-assisted segmental bone transport with a lengthening nail and a plate: A new technique for treatment of tibial and femoral bone defects. *Unfallchirurg* **2018**, *121*, 874–883. [CrossRef]
63. Barinaga, G.; Beason, A.M.; Gardner, M.P. Novel Surgical Approach to Segmental Bone Transport Using a Magnetic Intramedullary Limb Lengthening System. *J. Am. Acad. Orthop. Surg.* **2018**, *26*, e477–e482. [CrossRef]
64. Krettek, C. MagicTube: New possibilities for completely internal bone segmental transport and optional lengthening: New additional module for motorized lengthening nails for treatment of large bone defects. *Unfallchirurg* **2018**, *121*, 884–892. [CrossRef]
65. Krettek, C.; El Naga, A. All Internal Segmental Bone Transport and Optional Lengthening with a Newly Developed Universal Cylinder-Kombi-Tube Module for Motorized Nails-Description of a Surgical Technique. *J. Orthop. Trauma* **2017**, *31* (Suppl. 5), S39–S41. [CrossRef] [PubMed]

66. Kirane, Y.M.; Fragomen, A.T.; Rozbruch, S.R. Precision of the PRECICE internal bone lengthening nail. *Clin. Orthop. Relat. Res.* **2014**, *472*, 3869–3878. [CrossRef] [PubMed]
67. Paley, D. PRECICE intramedullary limb lengthening system. *Expert Rev. Med. Devices* **2015**, *12*, 231–249. [CrossRef]
68. Schiedel, F.M.; Vogt, B.; Tretow, H.L.; Schuhknecht, B.; Gosheger, G.; Horter, M.J.; Rödl, R. How precise is the PRECICE compared to the ISKD in intramedullary limb lengthening? Reliability and safety in 26 procedures. *Acta Orthop.* **2014**, *85*, 293–298. [CrossRef] [PubMed]

Disclaimer/Publisher's Note: The statements, opinions and data contained in all publications are solely those of the individual author(s) and contributor(s) and not of MDPI and/or the editor(s). MDPI and/or the editor(s) disclaim responsibility for any injury to people or property resulting from any ideas, methods, instructions or products referred to in the content.

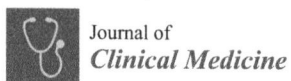

Article

Clinical Outcome of Carbon Fiber Reinforced Polyetheretherketone Plates in Patients with Proximal Humeral Fracture: One-Year Follow-Up

Patrick Ziegler [1], Sven Maier [2,*], Fabian Stuby [3], Tina Histing [2], Christoph Ihle [2], Ulrich Stöckle [4] and Markus Gühring [5]

1. Department of Trauma and Reconstructive Surgery, Klinik Gut, 7500 St. Moritz, Switzerland
2. Department of Trauma and Reconstructive Surgery, BG Unfallklinik Tuebingen, Eberhard Karls University Tuebingen, Schnarrenbergstrasse 95, 72076 Tuebingen, Germany
3. BG Trauma Center, Department for Traumatology, Orthopedics and Surgery, 82418 Murnau am Staffelsee, Germany; fabian.stuby@bgu-murnau.de
4. Center for Musculoskeletal Surgery, Charité University Medicine Berlin, 10117 Berlin, Germany
5. Kronprinzenbau Klinik, 72764 Reutlingen, Germany
* Correspondence: smaier@bgu-tuebingen.de

Abstract: Background: Proximal humerus fractures are seen frequently, particularly in older patients. The development of new osteosynthesis materials is being driven by the high complication rates following surgical treatment of proximal humerus fractures. Plate osteosyntheses made of steel, titanium and, for several years now, carbon fiber-reinforced polyetheretherketone (CFR-PEEK) are used most frequently. Methods: A prospective, randomized study was conducted in order to evaluate whether there are differences in the functional postoperative outcome when comparing CFR-PEEK and titanium implants for surgical treatment of proximal humerus fractures. The primary outcome of shoulder functionality 1 year after surgery was measured with the DASH score, the Oxford Shoulder Score, and the Simple Shoulder Test. Results: Bony consolidation of the respective fracture was confirmed in all the patients included in the study within the scope of postoperative follow-up care. No significant differences in the DASH score, Oxford Shoulder Score, or Simple Shoulder Test were observed 1 year post-operatively when comparing the implant materials CFR-PEEK and titanium. Conclusions: There are no differences in terms of the functional outcome between CFR-PEEK plates and titanium implants 1 year after surgery. Studies on the long-term outcomes using CFR-PEEK plates in osteoporotic bone should be the subject of further research.

Keywords: proximal humeral fracture; PEEK; complications; postoperative outcomes

Citation: Ziegler, P.; Maier, S.; Stuby, F.; Histing, T.; Ihle, C.; Stöckle, U.; Gühring, M. Clinical Outcome of Carbon Fiber Reinforced Polyetheretherketone Plates in Patients with Proximal Humeral Fracture: One-Year Follow-Up. *J. Clin. Med.* **2023**, *12*, 6881. https://doi.org/10.3390/jcm12216881

Academic Editor: Moshe Salai

Received: 18 September 2023
Revised: 16 October 2023
Accepted: 24 October 2023
Published: 31 October 2023

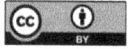

Copyright: © 2023 by the authors. Licensee MDPI, Basel, Switzerland. This article is an open access article distributed under the terms and conditions of the Creative Commons Attribution (CC BY) license (https://creativecommons.org/licenses/by/4.0/).

1. Introduction

Injuries to the shoulder are of great importance due to their high incidence and the heterogeneous patient population. Demographic changes with an aging society and a rising incidence of sports injuries are of importance. Proximal humerus fractures represent a common injury in humans and make up 4–5% of all fractures and up to 15% of fractures in patients over 65 years of age [1–4]. Despite numerous advances in surgical technology and innovations in the field of implants and osteosynthesis materials used in the last few decades, complication rates of up to 49% demonstrate the need for continuous improvement and further development of surgery–orthopedic care of proximal humerus fractures [5–8].

The goal when treating patients with proximal humerus fractures is complete restoration or improvement in musculoskeletal system functionality and attainment of an adequate quality of life. Various conservative and surgical treatments are available. In the context of surgical and head preservation treatment of proximal humerus fractures in adults, locking plate osteosynthesis and intramedullary nailing are the most common techniques. The introduction of locking implants and the resulting increased osteosynthesis stability improved results. Treatment with plates and open reduction and locking plate osteosynthesis became the standard surgical treatment for proximal humerus fractures [9–13]. With regards to materials selection and osteosynthesis properties, as well as surgical techniques, these procedures are subject to constant change with the aim of making treatment easier and improving the postoperative outcome. Frequent use of plate osteosyntheses historically showed high complication rates in the postoperative follow-up period [14–16]. Studies indicate that plate osteosynthesis can lead to complications requiring revision, e.g., secondary tilting of the fracture with subsequent screw penetration through the head (17%) [17–19]. These complications are especially prevalent in an elderly population with poor bone quality.

Plates made from carbon fiber-reinforced polyetheretherketone (CFR-PEEK) have been on the market for some years. The benefits of this thermoplastic material are radiolucency, no cold welding at the titanium screw–plate interface, and greater elasticity with the aim of increased micro-motion in the fracture gap. Although fewer secondary varus dislocations are described by Schliemann et al., the studies published to date do not show improved postoperative functional outcomes when using plates made of CFR-PEEK compared to titanium plates [20–23]. While increased elasticity compared to the titanium plate was confirmed in biomechanical studies, the question as to whether this elasticity offers an advantage in all fracture types is currently the source of much debate [23,24].

The aim of this study was to compare the postoperative outcome of patients with a proximal humerus fracture treated with a locking plate made from CRF-PEEK or titanium.

2. Materials and Methods

The study was registered at the German Register of Clinical Trials in Freiburg (DRKS00011376) and the protocol was approved by the local ethics committee (347/2016MP1). All patients included in this study gave consent to participation in writing.

Between October 2016 and June 2018, 76 patients treated for proximal humerus fractures at the BG Hospital Tübingen were included in the study and randomized to the titanium group or the CFR-PEEK group by means of a randomization list. There was no blinding of the patients, surgeons, or investigators.

The randomization list was generated before the start of the study using the "random number" feature of Office Excel 2016 (Microsoft Corporation©, Redmond, WA, USA). The corresponding results (PEEK/titanium) were placed in consecutively numbered envelopes. These were opened by the operating surgeon immediately before the surgical procedure.

The implants, made of carbon fiber-reinforced (CFR = carbon fiber reinforced) polyetheretherketone (PEEK), are characterized by a stiffness that is adapted to human bones. The CFR-PEEK plate consists of 55–60% carbon fiber. The random arrangement of these fibers within the plate contributes to the bone-adapted biomechanical properties described in the introduction. The remaining 40–45% of the plate is made of polyetheretherketone.

On the one hand, the new material allows interfragmentary micro-movements, which are intended to promote faster callus formations. On the other hand, the material is transparent to X-rays, which might lower the risk of primary unnoticed screw perforations. Furthermore, the rate of secondary screw perforations could also be reduced by adapting the stiffness of the implant to the bone. Similar to the PHILOS plate, the CFR-PEEK plate is adapted to the anatomical shape of the proximal humerus. There are seven screw holes in the proximal part of the plate so that screws can be inserted polyaxially. There are two types of plates available, which differ in the length of the part used to stabilize the shaft fragment. With the shorter version, three screws can be inserted into the shaft whereas the longer version allows stabilization to shaft with up to five screws. Titanium screws are used for the CFR-PEEK plate system, which has a core diameter of 4.0 mm in the head area and a core diameter of 3.5 mm in the shaft area. The CFR-PEEK plate offers the surgeon the opportunity to vary the insertion of the angle-stable screws with an angular deviation of up to 12°. This allows the screws to be placed individually to suit the anatomical conditions. Comparable with other modern plating systems, holes are provided for the attachment of suture cerclages for additional fragment stabilization.

The surgical procedure and osteosynthesis technique did not differ when using the CFR-PEEK and the PHILOS plate. The patients were positioned in beach chair position under full anesthesia. The anterolateral approach according to McKenzie was performed, characterized by the skin incision starting at the coracoid parallel to the axillary fold and the subsequent blunt cutting in the direction of the fibers of the deltoid muscle.

Under visualization of the fracture, the greater and lesser tuberosities were first addressed using non-absorbable sutures (FibreWire, Arthrex, Naples, FL, USA). The fracture fragments were then anatomically reduced and temporarily fixed using K-wires. The plate osteosynthesis was attached five to eight millimeters distal to the tip of the greater tuberosity and directly lateral to the bicipital groove. The plate was always fixed to the humeral shaft using a cortical screw and two angle-stable screws. Only angle-stable screws were used in the area of the humeral head. However, the number of these was variable and selected individually depending on the fracture. Furthermore, the FibreWires were fixed to the plate. The anatomical reduction and the correct implant position were checked intraoperatively using an image intensifier. All patients received a Gilchrist bandage for 7–10 days, which had to be worn permanently. In the following two weeks, the range of motion of the shoulder joint was increased to a maximum of 60° anteversion and abduction. External rotation movements and retroversion were not allowed. Anteversion and abduction were then limited to 90° and external rotation and retroversion to 20° for another two weeks. After this time, the glenohumeral joint was released to its full range of motion with a limited weight-bearing of the operated arm of 15 kg for 6 weeks postoperatively.

Bilateral or previous humerus fractures, head-split fractures, patients with cuff arthropathies, nerve or vascular injuries, thrombophilia, severe cardiac or pulmonary disease, and alcohol or drug abuse were all exclusion criteria. The results for bony consolidation and early postoperative outcomes have already been published by Ziegler et al. [25].

In addition to assessing the functional outcome, demographic data such as age, gender, body mass index, fracture type, and co-morbidities were also recorded. Functional outcome was determined using the DASH score, Simple Shoulder Test, and the Oxford Shoulder Score at 6 weeks, 12 weeks, 6 months, and 12 months post-operative. The scores described are accepted analysis methods that are used frequently in the literature.

Sample size planning was based on an assumed mean difference between the DASH scores of 5 points with a range of ±18 points. Based on a desired power of 80%, a sample size of n = 30 patients per group (30 CFR-PEEK and 30 titanium) was calculated. For planning, the independent two-sample t-test was used.

The 2 study groups were treated with 2 different plates: The locking CFR-PEEK plate (PEEKPower Humeral Fracture Plate, Arthrex, Naples, FL, USA) and a locking titanium plate (Depuy Synthes, Proximal Humerus Internal Locking System—PHILOS, West Chester, PA, USA). More detailed information on the surgical procedure and post-op follow-up can be found in the previously published paper from the working group [25].

Statistics

All obtained data were documented descriptively. Continuous variables were reported as means ± standard deviation. For dichotomous/categorical variables, frequencies and percentage shares, respectively, were reported. For the comparison of baseline characteristics, a two-sided significance level was used.

The statistical analysis was performed using SPSS (Version 24, SPSS Inc., Chicago, IL, USA). The independent two-sample t-test was used to analyze potential differences between the two groups with respect to the primary endpoint. The postoperative head–shaft angle measurements were evaluated using repeated measures analysis of variance. Potential preoperative differences between the two groups were calculated using the independent samples t-test (age, BMI), Fisher's exact test (comorbidities), or the chi-squared test (sex, fracture type, ASA classification). Values of $p < 0.05$ were regarded as significant.

All patients for whom data from at least one follow-up time point were available were included in the analysis. Missing data were not replaced. As a sensitivity analysis with respect to the primary endpoint (DASH), the independent two-sample t-test was used with the method of multiple imputations ($n = 100$), based on all randomized patients. The t-test was applied to 2 independent samples in order to identify possible significant differences in the functional outcome. The distribution of the independent samples was a result of the respective plate treatment type (CFR-PEEK; titanium). The significance level was set at $p < 0.05$.

3. Results

A total of 54 patients were included 1 year postoperatively in this prospective, randomized study. The average age was 62.65 ± 11.34 years (Table 1). The distribution of fracture severity based on the Neer classification showed a comparable number of II part fractures in both groups and a higher number of III part fractures with a simultaneously lower number of IV part fractures in the CFR-PEEK group compared with the titanium group (Table 1). Of the 54 patients, 29 (53.57%) were treated with a CRF-PEEK plate and 25 (46.43%) with a titanium plate.

Table 1. Demographic data age (a), gender (b), fracture classification (c).

	(a)		
	Average	Standard Deviation	Median
Age Overall Collective (1-Year-Follow-Up)	62.65	11.34	61
Age Titanium Collective (1-Year-Follow-Up)	62.80	9.79	62
Age PEEK Collective (1-Year Follow-Up)	62.52	12.53	61
	(b)		
Gender	PEEK		Titanium
Female	24 (82.8%)		21 (84.0%)
Male	5 (17.2%)		4 (16.0%)
	(c)		
Neer-Classification	PEEK		Titanium
2-Part	6 (20.7%)		3 (12.0%)
3-Part	19 (65.5%)		13 (52.0%)
4-Part	4 (13.8%)		9 (36.0%)

A total of 22 patients were lost to follow-up after 1 year. Two patients were already excluded intraoperatively due to a head-split component of the fracture. Two further patients had a second accident after surgery and required revision surgery. Eighteen patients declined further study participation without any reason. At the follow-up appointments 6 and 12 weeks post-op, the functional outcome of 63 patients ($n = 32$–50.80% CFR-PEEK; $n = 31$–49.20% titanium; follow-up rate 82.89%) could be analyzed. One-year outcomes could be obtained for 54 patients ($n = 29$–53.70% CFR-PEEK; $n = 25$–46.29% titanium, follow-up rate 71.05%). The two groups did not differ significantly in terms of distribution of age, BMI, handedness, or secondary disease, as defined by the ASA classification.

Functional Outcome

One year post-op, all patients demonstrated a significantly improved functional outcome compared with the previous follow-up examination at 6 weeks, 12 weeks, and 6 months post-op (Tables 2 and 3). The CFR-PEEK group reached 18.6 ± 14.7 points in the DASH Score, and the titanium group 23.9 ± 22.0 points. Similar results were also seen in the Simple Shoulder Test (71.5 ± 18.2 CFR-PEEK; 71.3 ± 22.8 titanium) and the Oxford Shoulder Score (38.4 ± 12.2 CFR-PEEK; 39.3 ± 8.6 titanium) (Table 2, Figure 1). No significant differences could be identified regarding treatment with the different plates.

Table 2. Differences in functional outcome at follow-up dates. ns: non-significant.

Questionnaire	Time Point	PEEK p-Value	Titan p-Value
OSS	6 w–12 m	<0.0001	<0.0001
	6 w–6 m	<0.0001	<0.0001
	6 w–12 w	<0.0001	<0.0001
	12 w–12 m	ns	0.0201
	12 w–6 m	ns	0.0358
SST	6 w–12 m	<0.0001	<0.0001
	6 w–6 m	<0.0001	<0.0001
	6 w–12 w	<0.0001	0.0001
	12 w–12 m	0.0185	0.0014
	12 w–6 m	ns	0.0363
DASH	6 w–12 m	<0.0001	<0.0001
	6 w–6 m	<0.0001	<0.0001
	6 w–12 w	0.0006	<0.0001
	12 w–12 m	0.0015	0.0264

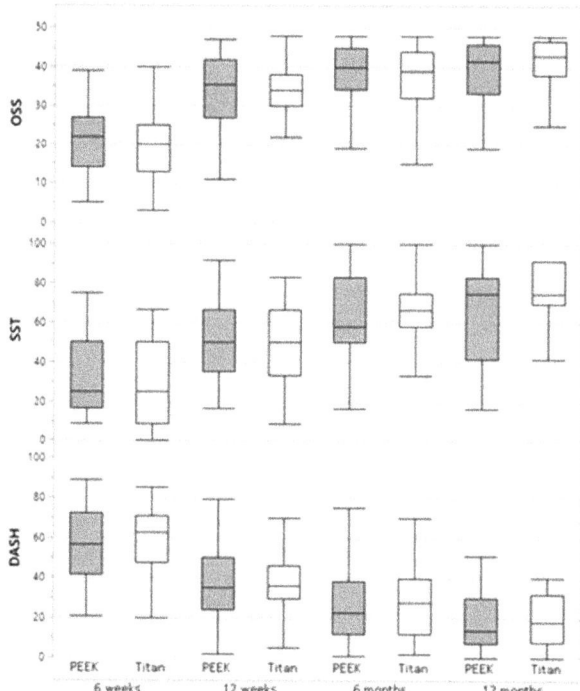

Figure 1. Differences in functional outcome regarding treatment with the different plates.

Table 3. Differences in functional outcome at follow-up dates.

Questionnaire	Time Point	PEEK		Titan	
		Mean ± SD	Median (Min–Max)	Mean ± SD	Median (Min–Max)
OSS	6 weeks	20.3 ± 9.8	20.5 (3.0–40.0)	20.4 ± 8.5	21.5 (3.0–39.0)
	12 weeks	33.8 ± 10.0	35.5 (11.0–47.0)	33.3 ± 6.5	34.0 (17.0–48.0)
	6 months	37.7 ± 8.8	40 (15.0–48.0)	38.6 ± 6.8	39.0 (19.0–48.0)
	12 months	38.4 ± 12.2	43 (22–48.0)	39.3 ± 8.6	42 (19.0–48.0)
SST	6 weeks	30.0 ± 20.8	29.2 (0.0–75.0)	29.4 ± 18.9	25.0 (0.0–75.0)
	12 weeks	54.9 ± 24.8	54.2 (8.3–91.7)	51.5 ± 16.5	50.0 (16.7–83.3)
	6 months	62.5 ± 22.3	61.8 (18.2–100)	65.0 ± 20.1	58.3 (16.7–100.)
	12 months	71.5 ± 18.2	75 (33.3–100)	71.3 ± 22.8	75 (16.7–100.)
DASH	6 weeks	56.5 ± 19.3	56.9 (20.7–88.9)	59.8 ± 15.6	62.5 (19.8–85.3)
	12 weeks	38.4 ± 21.4	35.1 (1.7–79.3)	37.7 ± 16.2	35.8 (5.2–73.3)
	6 months	27.5 ± 20.5	22.4 (1.0–81.5)	28.5 ± 17.9	27.6 (1.7–69.8)
	12 months	18.6 ± 14.7	13.8 (0.0–50.9)	23.9 ± 22.0	17.9 (0.0–78.4)

4. Discussion

This prospective, randomized study was conducted in order to evaluate whether the use of CFR-PEEK results in a change in the functional postoperative outcome compared to a titanium plate for the surgical treatment of proximal humerus fractures. Neither investigators nor patients could be blinded during the follow-up period. The study design did not allow for conclusions on the equivalence of the two interventions. That would have required a non-inferiority study design.

Since CFR-PEEK is radiotranslucent there is no superimposition of portions of the proximal humerus during intraoperative and postoperative imaging. Bony consolidation of the respective fracture was confirmed in all the patients included in the study within the scope of postoperative follow-up care. Within the scope of the functional outcome assessed using the DASH score, Oxford Shoulder Score, and the Simple Shoulder Test, no significant differences were detected between the implant materials CFR-PEEK and titanium for the treatment of proximal humerus fractures.

Various implants are available for the osteosynthetic treatment of proximal humerus fractures. Open reduction and stabilization with a locking plate are often the treatment of choice for multi-fragmented or displaced fractures of the proximal humerus [13,26]. The plates used for these fractures have different material properties. Plates made of steel, titanium, and CFR-PEEK are used most frequently. The cited advantages of CFR-PEEK over titanium or steel are radiolucency and no risk of screw–plate cold welding as is the case with titanium screw and plate combinations, i.e., the joining of two metallic workpieces of the same material at room temperature. In addition, the increased biomechanical elasticity of the CFR-PEEK plate may reduce stress-shielding at the plate–bone junction and offer a positive effect on bony consolidation through micro-motion.

An increase in the incidence of proximal humerus fractures has been observed in recent years. As demographic change and life expectancy continue to increase, the optimal treatment of proximal humerus fractures will become increasingly important. Therefore, treatment of proximal humerus fractures remains subject to constant change. Attempts are being made to reduce the high complication rates associated with the use of new implant materials. Complications such as primary screw perforation, misplacement of the plate, or loss of reduction due to lack of medical support can be avoided by optimizing the surgical technique. Thanks to the radiolucent nature of the CFR-PEEK plate, all screws used can be visualized without superimposition. Loss of reduction due to the high stiffness of titanium and steel locking plates may lead to failure at the bone–screw interface, particularly in osteoporotic bone. This occurrence can be reduced by the increased elasticity of the CFR-PEEK plate. Lill et al. examined the initial stiffness of various implants for the treatment of proximal humerus fractures [27]. They discovered that implants that are less stiff and more elastic seem to reduce peak stress at the bone–implant interface, making them suitable for fracture fixation in osteoporotic bone. Schliemann et al. documented less frequent secondary varus dislocations following treatment of a proximal humerus fracture with CFR-PEEK plate compared with an independent group which was surgically treated with titanium implants [22]. No statistically significant differences in terms of the functional postoperative outcome were found in our study population. This was also confirmed by other authors in further studies [21,28].

Studies on the long-term outcomes using CFR-PEEK plates in osteoporotic bone should be the subject of further research.

5. Conclusions

No significant differences could be detected in terms of functional outcome between CFR-PEEK plates and titanium implants 1 year after surgery. Studies on the long-term outcomes using CFR-PEEK plates in osteoporotic bone should be the subject of further research.

Author Contributions: All authors contributed to the study conception and design as well as the material preparation, data collection, and analysis. The first draft of the manuscript was written by P.Z. and all authors commented on further versions of the manuscript. All authors read and approved the final manuscript.

Funding: This study was financially supported by Arthrex. We acknowledge support from the Open Access Publication Fund of the University of Tübingen.

Institutional Review Board Statement: This trial was approved by the local ethics committee (University of Tübingen, 347/2016MP1) and was registered as a clinical trial (347/2016MP1). Informed consent was obtained from all individual participants included in the study.

Informed Consent Statement: Each participant gave his consent for the publication of the anonymized data.

Data Availability Statement: Data have not been deposited into a public repository but are available upon request.

Conflicts of Interest: P.Z., U.S., M.G. and F.S. received study support (third-party funding) from Arthex. T.H., S.M. and C.I. declare that no conflicts of interest exist.

Abbreviations

ASA	American Society of Anesthesiologists
BMI	Body Mass Index
DASH-Score	Disabilities of the Arm, Shoulder and Hand-Score
CFR-PEEK	carbon fiber reinforced polyetheretherketone
PHILOS	proximal humerus internal locking system

References

1. Baron, J.A.; Karagas, M.; Barrett, J.; Kniffin, W.; Malenka, D.; Mayor, M.; Keller, R.B. Basic epidemiology of fractures of the upper and lower limb among Americans over 65 years of age. *Epidemiology* **1996**, *7*, 612–618. [CrossRef]
2. Bell, J.E.; Leung, B.C.; Spratt, K.F.; Koval, K.J.; Weinstein, J.D.; Goodman, D.C.; Tosteson, A.N. Trends and variation in incidence, surgical treatment, and repeat surgery of proximal humeral fractures in the elderly. *J. Bone Jt. Surg.* **2011**, *93*, 121–131. [CrossRef]
3. Court-Brown, C.M.; McQueen, M.M. Global Forum: Fractures in the Elderly. *J. Bone Jt. Surg.* **2016**, *98*, e36. [CrossRef]
4. Passaretti, D.; Candela, V.; Sessa, P.; Gumina, S. Epidemiology of proximal humeral fractures: A detailed survey of 711 patients in a metropolitan area. *J. Shoulder Elb. Surg.* **2017**, *26*, 2117–2124. [CrossRef]
5. Gupta, A.K.; Harris, J.D.; Erickson, B.J.; Abrams, G.D.; Bruce, B.; McCormick, F.; Nicholson, G.P.; Romeo, A.A. Surgical management of complex proximal humerus fractures-a systematic review of 92 studies including 4500 patients. *J. Orthop. Trauma* **2015**, *29*, 54–59. [CrossRef] [PubMed]

6. Konigshausen, M.; Kubler, L.; Godry, H.; Citak, M.; Schildhauer, T.A.; Seybold, D. Clinical outcome and complications using a polyaxial locking plate in the treatment of displaced proximal humerus fractures. A reliable system? *Injury* **2012**, *43*, 223–231. [CrossRef] [PubMed]
7. Schliemann, B.; Siemoneit, J.; Theisen, C.; Kosters, C.; Weimann, A.; Raschke, M.J. Complex fractures of the proximal humerus in the elderly—Outcome and complications after locking plate fixation. *Musculoskelet. Surg.* **2012**, *96* (Suppl. 1), S3–S11. [CrossRef]
8. Schliemann, B.; Wähnert, D.; Theisen, C.; Herbort, M.; Kösters, C.; Raschke, M.J.; Weimann, A. How to enhance the stability of locking plate fixation of proximal humerus fractures? An overview of current biomechanical and clinical data. *Injury* **2015**, *46*, 1207–1214. [CrossRef] [PubMed]
9. Acklin, Y.P.; Stoffel, K.; Sommer, C. A prospective analysis of the functional and radiological outcomes of minimally invasive plating in proximal humerus fractures. *Injury* **2013**, *44*, 456–460. [CrossRef]
10. Brunner, F.; Sommer, C.; Bahrs, C.; Heuwinkel, R.; Hafner, C.; Rillmann, P.; Kohut, G.; Ekelund, A.; Muller, M.; Audigé, L.; et al. Open reduction and internal fixation of proximal humerus fractures using a proximal humeral locked plate: A prospective multicenter analysis. *J. Orthop. Trauma* **2009**, *23*, 163–172. [CrossRef]
11. Falez, F.; Papalia, M.; Greco, A.; Teti, A.; Favetti, F.; Panegrossi, G.; Casella, F.; Necozione, S. Minimally invasive plate osteosynthesis in proximal humeral fractures: One-year results of a prospective multicenter study. *Int. Orthop.* **2016**, *40*, 579–585. [CrossRef]
12. Handschin, A.E.; Cardell, M.; Contaldo, C.; Trentz, O.; Wanner, G.A. Functional results of angular-stable plate fixation in displaced proximal humeral fractures. *Injury* **2008**, *39*, 306–313. [CrossRef] [PubMed]
13. Tepass, A.; Blumenstock, G.; Weise, K.; Rolauffs, B.; Bahrs, C. Current strategies for the treatment of proximal humeral fractures: An analysis of a survey carried out at 348 hospitals in Germany, Austria, and Switzerland. *J. Shoulder Elb. Surg.* **2013**, *22*, e8–e14. [CrossRef]
14. Konrad, G.; Bayer, J.; Hepp, P.; Voigt, C.; Oestern, H.; Kääb, M.; Luo, C.; Plecko, M.; Wendt, K.; Köstler, W.; et al. Open reduction and internal fixation of proximal humeral fractures with use of the locking proximal humerus plate. Surgical technique. *J. Bone Jt. Surg.* **2010**, *92 Pt 1* (Suppl. 1), 85–95. [CrossRef] [PubMed]
15. Owsley, K.C.; Gorczyca, J.T. Fracture displacement and screw cutout after open reduction and locked plate fixation of proximal humeral fractures [corrected]. *J. Bone Jt. Surg.* **2008**, *90*, 233–240. [CrossRef]
16. Spross, C.; Platz, A.; Erschbamer, M.; Lattmann, T.; Dietrich, M. Surgical treatment of Neer Group VI proximal humeral fractures: Retrospective comparison of PHILOS(R) and hemiarthroplasty. *Clin. Orthop. Relat. Res.* **2012**, *470*, 2035–2042. [CrossRef] [PubMed]
17. Fu, T.; Xia, C.; Li, Z.; Wu, H. Surgical versus conservative treatment for displaced proximal humeral fractures in elderly patients: A meta-analysis. *Int. J. Clin. Exp. Med.* **2014**, *7*, 4607–4615. [PubMed]
18. Okike, K.; Lee, O.C.; Makanji, H.; Morgan, J.H.; Harris, M.B.; Vrahas, M.S. Comparison of locked plate fixation and nonoperative management for displaced proximal humerus fractures in elderly patients. *Am. J. Orthop.* **2015**, *44*, E106–E112.
19. Olerud, P.; Ahrengart, L.; Ponzer, S.; Saving, J.; Tidermark, J. Internal fixation versus nonoperative treatment of displaced 3-part proximal humeral fractures in elderly patients: A randomized controlled trial. *J. Shoulder Elb. Surg.* **2011**, *20*, 747–755. [CrossRef]
20. Padolino, A.; Porcellini, G.; Guollo, B.; Fabbri, E.; Kiran Kumar, G.N.; Paladini, P.; Merolla, G. Comparison of CFR-PEEK and conventional titanium locking plates for proximal humeral fractures: A retrospective controlled study of patient outcomes. *Musculoskelet. Surg.* **2018**, *102*, 49–56. [CrossRef]
21. Rotini, R.; Cavaciocchi, M.; Fabbri, D.; Bettelli, G.; Catani, F.; Campochiaro, G.; Fontana, M.; Colozza, A.; De Biase, C.F.; Ziveri, G.; et al. Proximal humeral fracture fixation: Multicenter study with carbon fiber peek plate. *Musculoskelet. Surg.* **2015**, *99* (Suppl. 1), S1–S8. [CrossRef]
22. Schliemann, B.; Hartensuer, R.; Koch, T.; Theisen, C.; Raschke, M.J.; Kösters, C.; Weimann, A. Treatment of proximal humerus fractures with a CFR-PEEK plate: 2-year results of a prospective study and comparison to fixation with a conventional locking plate. *J. Shoulder Elb. Surg.* **2015**, *24*, 1282–1288. [CrossRef] [PubMed]
23. Schliemann, B.; Seifert, R.; Theisen, C.; Gehweiler, D.; Wähnert, D.; Schulze, M.; Raschke, M.J.; Weimann, A. PEEK versus titanium locking plates for proximal humerus fracture fixation: A comparative biomechanical study in two- and three-part fractures. *Arch. Orthop. Trauma Surg.* **2017**, *137*, 63–71. [CrossRef] [PubMed]
24. Katthagen, J.C.; Schwarze, M.; Warnhoff, M.; Voigt, C.; Hurschler, C.; Lill, H. Influence of plate material and screw design on stiffness and ultimate load of locked plating in osteoporotic proximal humeral fractures. *Injury* **2016**, *47*, 617–624. [CrossRef] [PubMed]
25. Ziegler, P.; Maier, S.; Stockle, U.; Guhring, M.; Stuby, F.M. The Treatment of Proximal Humerus Fracture Using Internal Fixation with Fixed-angle Plates. *Dtsch. Arztebl. Int.* **2019**, *116*, 757–763. [CrossRef]
26. Arbeitsgemeinschaft der Wissenschaftlichen Medizinischen Fachgesellschaften. *S1 Leitlinie: Oberarmkopffraktur*; AWMF-Nr. 012-023; AWMF: Duesseldorfc, Germany, 18 October 2017.

27. Lill, H.; Hepp, P.; Korner, J.; Kassi, J.P.; Verheyden, A.P.; Josten, C.; Duda, G.N. Proximal humeral fractures: How stiff should an implant be? A comparative mechanical study with new implants in human specimens. *Arch. Orthop. Trauma Surg.* **2003**, *123*, 74–81. [CrossRef]
28. Katthagen, J.C.; Ellwein, A.; Lutz, O.; Voigt, C.; Lill, H. Outcomes of proximal humeral fracture fixation with locked CFR-PEEK plating. *Eur. J. Orthop. Surg. Traumatol.* **2017**, *27*, 351–358. [CrossRef]

Disclaimer/Publisher's Note: The statements, opinions and data contained in all publications are solely those of the individual author(s) and contributor(s) and not of MDPI and/or the editor(s). MDPI and/or the editor(s) disclaim responsibility for any injury to people or property resulting from any ideas, methods, instructions or products referred to in the content.

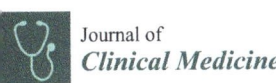

Article

Stabilization of Traumatic Iliosacral Instability Using Innovative Implants: A Biomechanical Comparison

Niklas Grüneweller [1], Julia Leunig [2], Ivan Zderic [2], Boyko Gueorguiev [2], Dirk Wähnert [1,†] and Thomas Vordemvenne [1,*,†]

1. Bielefeld University, Medical School and University Medical Center OWL, Protestant Hospital of the Bethel Foundation, Department of Trauma and Orthopedic Surgery, Burgsteig 13, 33617 Bielefeld, Germany; dirk.waehnert@evkb.de (D.W.)
2. AO Research Institute Davos, Clavadelerstrasse 8, 7270 Davos, Switzerland; julialeunig@icloud.com (J.L.); ivan.zderic@aofoundation.org (I.Z.)
* Correspondence: thomas.vordemvenne@evkb.de
† These authors contributed equally to this work.

Abstract: (1) Background: Demographic changes over the past decade have had a significant impact on pelvic ring fractures. They have increased dramatically in the orthogeriatric population. Surgeons are faced with implant fixation issues in the treatment of these fragility fractures. This study compares two innovative implants for stabilizing the iliosacral joint in a biomechanical setting. (2) Methods: An iliosacral screw with a preassembled plate allowing the placement of an additional short, angular stable screw in the ilium and a triangular fixation system consisting of a fenestrated ilium screw and an iliosacral screw quasi-statically inserted through the "fenestra" were instrumented in osteoporotic artificial bone models with a simulated Denis zone 1 fracture. Biomechanical testing was performed on a servo-hydraulic testing machine using increasing, synchronous axial and torsional sinusoidal cyclic loading to failure. (3) Results: The SI-Plate and TriFix showed comparable stiffness values. The values for fracture gap angle and screw tip cutout were significantly lower for the TriFix compared to the SI-Plate. In addition, the number of cycles to failure was significantly higher for the TriFix. (4) Conclusions: Implant anchorage and primary stability can be improved in iliosacral instability using the triangular stabilization system.

Keywords: dorsal pelvic ring; biomechanic; SI-plate; triangular fixation; iliosacral instability

1. Introduction

Fractures of the posterior pelvic ring are a major issue in trauma and orthogeriatric surgery. In the last few decades, the epidemiology of these injuries has changed considerably.

A recent analysis of the German Pelvic Trauma Registry showed that women are more often affected by pelvic fractures than men (incidence of 33.4/100,000 for men; 38.4/100,000 for women) [1]. In particular, the number of orthogeriatric patients suffering from pelvic fractures is increasing rapidly [2,3]. As a result, the majority of pelvic fractures today occur in elderly patients [4]. But it is not only the age and sex distribution of pelvic fractures that has changed. Fracture morphology has also changed dramatically. While the incidence of type A fractures decreased substantially (from 85% in 1991 to 44% in 2013), the incidence of type C fractures (from 7% in 1991 to 14% in 2013) and especially type B fractures (from 8% in 1991 to 42% in 2013) increased significantly [3].

Pelvic fractures, especially in the elderly, are very different from high-energy fractures in terms of symptoms and treatment. In the face of these dramatic demographic changes, the management of older patients is becoming increasingly important. The specific challenges of treating elderly patients include existing comorbidities, lack of physical fitness, and mental health conditions such as dementia [5]. In addition, reduced bone quality in this population is another major factor that makes it difficult to adequately treat patients

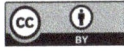

with fragility fractures of the pelvis [6]. A classification system was developed by Rommens and Hofmann to address the specific needs of patients suffering from these fragility fractures [2]. Many patients have comorbidities that put them at risk of complications and increased mortality [6]. As a result, there is no consensus on the indications for and type of surgical treatment of pelvic fragility fractures [5]. Both surgical and conservative treatment options have their benefits and risks. While conservative treatment puts patients at risk of pneumonia and urinary tract infection due to immobilization, operative treatment is associated with surgical complications such as hematoma and surgical site infection. In addition, the fragile bone increases the risk of further collapse with conservative treatment and implant loosening with surgical treatment [5].

Pain relief and early mobilization are the main goals in the treatment of fragility fractures of the pelvis. Any treatment should, therefore, be less invasive, aim to improve general health, and prevent further fragility fractures [7].

As a result, iliosacral screw osteosynthesis is now a well-established technique and is still considered the standard of care for many patients with fractures of the dorsal pelvic ring. This type of treatment is minimally invasive, provides adequate pain relief, and allows patient mobilization immediately after surgery [5,8]. A major disadvantage of this procedure is the reduced anchorage of the implant in the porous bone with the risk of screw loosening [9,10].

Several modifications aimed at increasing implant fixation have been introduced to address this major problem. Screw tip augmentation and screw-in-screw prototypes are two of these innovations [11–16]. In biomechanical comparisons, augmentation and screw-in-screw techniques have been shown to increase stability in osteoporotic bone and to prevent certain failure mechanisms, namely screw back-out [13,17].

The design and manufacture of new implants, especially those with connected parts, is more difficult and must take into account several aspects. It is well known that the implant material is crucial for bone-implant-load interaction (e.g., stress shielding) and can have an effect on tribocorrosion in connected implants [18]. Titanium alloys are widely used for orthopedic implants due to their superior strength-to-weight ratio, biocompatibility, and corrosion resistance. However, Ti-6Al-4V, in particular, does not have inherent tribocorrosion resistance. Therefore, it is necessary to eliminate or minimize metal-to-metal contact in motion areas. In pelvic implants, the washer head is such an area where minimal motion could occur. Due to the small contact area (screw head and washer) and the minimal motion, no clinical problems, such as aseptic loosening, have been reported. Implant areas with higher expected motion and larger contact areas such as a screw-in-screw (e.g., fenestrated iliac screw with iliosacral screw) have a higher potential for this problem. Measures such as polyethylene inlays have a dual effect: they reduce tribocorrosion by minimizing the metal-to-metal contact as well as by reducing motion.

The aim of this study was to compare the biomechanics of two implant configurations of an innovative modular implant system for stabilizing the dorsal pelvic ring. Two groups were compared in an artificial pelvis model. An iliosacral screw (Silony Medical AG, Frauenfeld, Switzerland) offering a double-threaded pedicle screw design for rapid insertion and improved primary stability with a pre-mounted plate (corresponding to an enlarged washer) and an additional angular stable plate screw was compared to a construct combining a uniquely designed fenestrated iliac screw (Silony Medical AG, Frauenfeld, Switzerland) with the above mentioned iliosacral screw providing an angular stable construct for the dorsal pelvic ring.

2. Materials and Methods

2.1. Implants

In this study, we used two different percutaneous implant configurations to stabilize the posterior pelvic ring. All implants were made from Ti6Al4V ELI, a well-known and widely used material for medical implants. Group I was stabilized with a 7.2 mm iliosacral screw with a pre-mounted plate (SI-plate, Silony Medical GmbH, Frauenfeld,

Switzerland). The plate allowed the placement of an additional short angular stable screw in the ilium (Figure 1). The iliosacral screw used for this study had a length of 100 mm. The angular stable locking was a 3.5 mm screw with a length of 20 mm. This iliosacral screw has been designed with biomedical needs in mind. Therefore, the double thread design is used to allow rapid insertion combined with good primary stability through some interfragmentary compression. The pre-mounted plate with the option of inserting a short, angular stable screw into the ilium secures the construct against unthreading and increases primary stability.

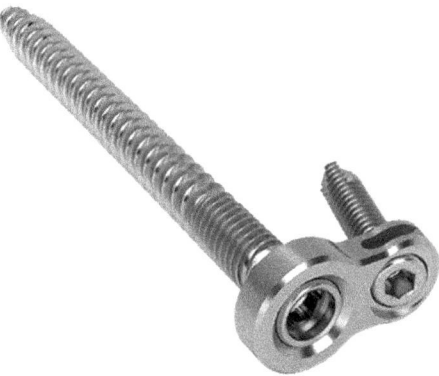

Figure 1. Picture of the SI-Plate, consisting of the double-threaded iliosacral screw with a pre-mounted plate that acts as a washer and provides the option of placing a short, angular stable screw for fixation in the ilium.

Group II was stabilized with the triangular fixation system (TriFix, Silony Medical GmbH, Frauenfeld, Switzerland). This system consists of a fenestrated iliac screw with a 9.2 mm diameter anterior screw portion and a 14 mm diameter fenestrated portion, and an iliosacral screw with a pre-mounted washer (Figure 2). The iliosacral screw is inserted through the "fenestra" of the ilium screw by using an aiming arm device. Due to a polyethylene inlay in the "fenestra", quasi-angular stable fixation is provided. The TriFix design allows stepwise and modular surgical treatment of the dorsal, pelvic ring according to the biomechanical needs of the fracture or instability. The primary stability of the construct is increased by the quasi-angle stable connection of the iliac screw and the iliosacral screw in combination with the additional medial support of the iliosacral screw. As mentioned above, the modular design allows for easy extension to spinopelvine stabilization.

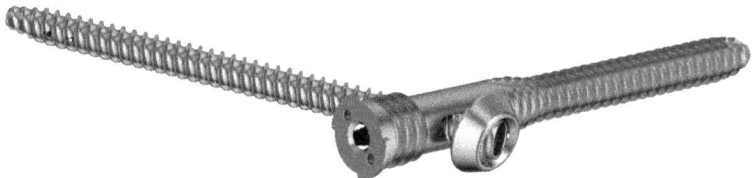

Figure 2. Image of the TriFix implant showing a fenestrated iliac screw and an iliosacral screw with a pre-mounted washer. This configuration provides an almost angular stable connection between the ilium and the iliosacral screw.

Actually, no connection between the pelvic ring and the lumbar spine was established in this study, but still, this iliac screw is referred to as the "TriFix" screw.

2.2. Bone Model

Sixteen artificial pelvises with simulated osteoporotic bone structure (LS4060, Synbone AG, Zizers, Switzerland) were used for this investigation. This bone model has already been successfully used in several biomechanical studies on the posterior pelvic ring [11,13].

2.3. Fracture Model and Instrumentation

On the right sacral side of each model, a vertical paraforaminal osteotomy was performed in Denis classification zone 1 using a band saw. A custom-made cutting guide was used to achieve consistent fracture lines. The symphysis and the left sacroiliac joint were then cut wide to disrupt the pelvic ring. The left hip bone was excluded from further use in this study [13]. The specimens were randomly assigned for instrumentation with an iliosacral screw plus locking screw (SI-plate) in Group I or with an iliosacral screw through a fenestrated ilium screw (TriFix) in Group II.

The SI joint was rigidly fixed in both groups using wood screws to simulate an ossified and fused joint, a common scenario in the elderly, and to concentrate the forces acting on the sacral fracture. The posterior pelvic ring fragments were anatomically reduced and instrumented in a standardized manner using custom-made drill guides to ensure standardized screw placement in each specimen for both groups. Instrumentation was carried out using the appropriate manufacturers' instruments and in accordance with the manufacturers' instructions. All specimens were instrumented by one experienced pelvic surgeon.

For the SI plate fixation in Group 1 (Figure 3), using a drill guide, a 3.2 mm guidewire was first inserted across the SI joint into the first sacral body under radiographic control. The guide wire was then over-drilled, followed by the insertion of a 100 mm long 7.2 mm fully threaded self-cutting cannulated SI with a pre-mounted plate. The screw was tightened according to the surgeons' best practice. The orientation of the plate was standardized posteriorly (9 o'clock orientation). After SI screw placement, the hole for the short-locking screw was prepared by drilling a 2.0 mm hole over the drill sleeve. A 20 mm head locking screw was then inserted and tightened at 4 Nm using a torque limiter.

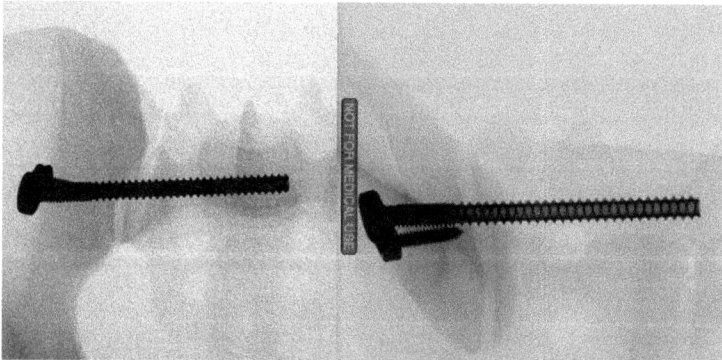

Figure 3. Radiograph of the SI plate fixation in two planes.

In Group 2 (Figure 4), the TriFix instrumentation began with the insertion of the iliac screw. A 3.2 mm guide wire was placed over the custom-made drill guide and inserted into the ilium under radiographic guidance from the posterior iliac spina. After correct wire placement, the screw hole was prepared by drilling and thread cutting. Afterward, the iliac screw was inserted over the guide wire to the correct depth. After that, an aiming device was mounted, allowing to interlock the ilium screw with the iliosacral screw. Afterward, the wire for the sacroiliac screw was placed using the mounted aiming arm and radiographic control. Once the correct position was achieved, the wire was over-drilled, and the 100 mm long 7.2 mm iliosacral screw was inserted. No additional locking screw was inserted into the sacroiliac screw plate in this case.

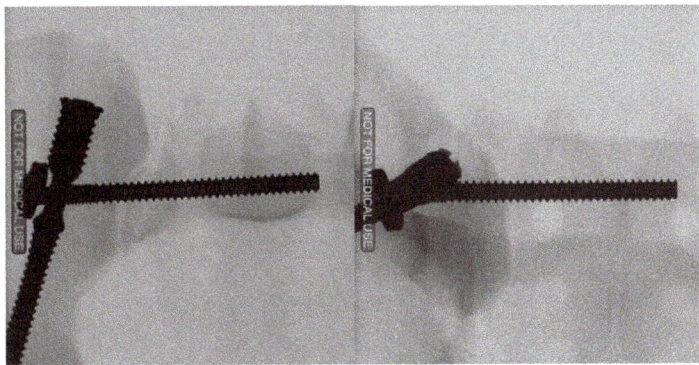

Figure 4. Radiograph of the TriFix fixation in two planes.

2.4. Biomechanical Testing

Biomechanical testing was performed on a biaxial servo-hydraulic testing machine (MTS 858 MiniBionix, MTS Systems Corp, Eden Prairie, MN, USA) equipped with a 5 kN/50 Nm load cell. The setup was adopted from previous studies [13]. Pre-tests were conducted to achieve a clinically relevant failure mode. Therefore, a muscular preload had to be included to prevent the pelvis from bending.

Each specimen was aligned in an upright standing position with its distal portion secured to the machine base using a vice and X-Y table (Figure 5). The latter facilitated the mounting of the specimen by mediolateral and anteroposterior sliding and was clamped in place during the test.

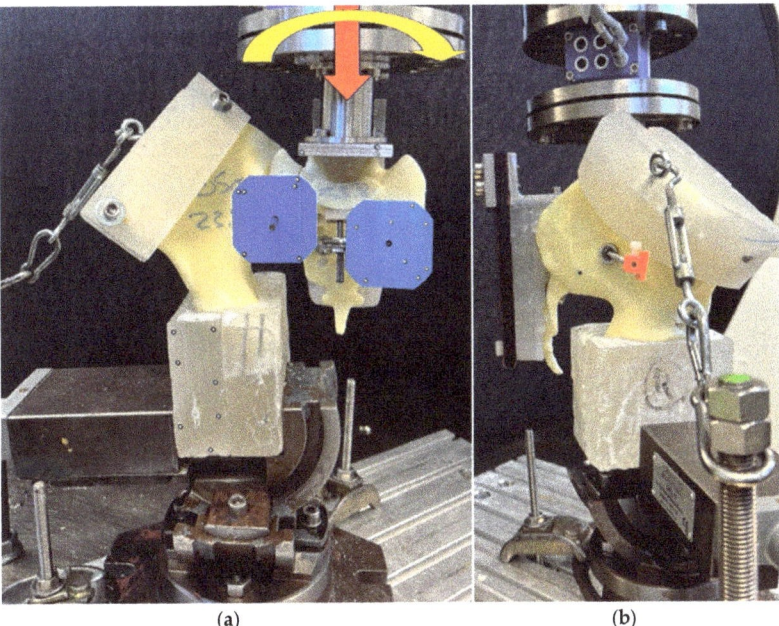

(a)   (b)

Figure 5. Test setup with a specimen mounted for biomechanical testing with colored arrows visualizing the loading directions. View from (**a**) anterior and (**b**) lateral.

The proximal part of the specimen was attached to the load cell and machine actuator via an L-shaped frame, which was secured to the posterior aspect of the sacrum with screws through the foramina. Muscle tension was simulated via a turnbuckle connecting the machine base with the iliac crest. For that purpose, a PMMA block was attached to the iliac crest and served as an anchor for the turnbuckle. Optical markers were attached to the sacrum medial and lateral to the fracture and to the iliosacral screw.

A muscular preload of 15 N was applied prior to biomechanical testing. The loading protocol commenced with a quasi-static axial compression ramp from 15 N to 100 N at a rate of 8.5 N/s, followed by synchronous axial and torsional sinusoidal cyclic loading to failure at 2 Hz. During the cyclic test, the axial load was progressively increased at a rate of 0.05 N/cycle from its initial peak value of 100 N. Torsional loading started at 0.5 Nm in external rotation with an increment of 0.00025 Nm/cycle. Test stop criteria were set at 30 mm actuator displacement with respect to its position at test start.

2.5. Data Evaluation and Statistics

Machine data in terms of axial displacement (mm) and axial load (N), as well as torsional angle (°) and torque (Nm), were recorded from the machine controllers at 128 Hz. The initial stiffness was calculated from the rising slope of the load-displacement curve of the quasi-static test ramp within a load range of 30–60 N.

Two optical cameras (Aramis SRX, GOM GmbH, Braunschweig, Germany) continuously recorded the marker positions at 50 Hz for motion tracking, with a resolution of 12 megapixels and a maximum acceptance error of 0.004 mm. Based on the motion tracking data, the fracture gap opening between the two initially reduced osteotomy surfaces of the medial and lateral sacral fragments relative to each other was calculated as a combined rotational movement in the coronal and transverse plane and defined as a gap angle. In addition, the movement of the SI-screw tip perpendicular to its axis within the sacrum was calculated as the screw tip cutout. The margins of these two parameters were evaluated at three time points after 2000, 4000, and 6000 cycles with respect to the corresponding values at the third test cycle to consider specimens' settling. A screw tip cutout of 2 mm was defined as the failure criterion, and the corresponding numbers of cycles until its fulfillment were calculated together with the corresponding load. All evaluations were performed under peak axial compressive loading. The evaluation algorithm was based on the publication of Zderic et al. [13].

Radiographs were taken in the anteroposterior direction at the beginning of the cyclic test and then every 500 cycles using a triggered C-arm (Siemens ARCADIS Varic, Siemens Medical Solutions AG, Erlangen, Germany) to determine the point of failure of the screw fixation and to investigate its mechanism.

Statistical analysis among the parameters of interest was performed using SPSS software (version 23, IBM SPSS, Chicago, IL, USA). The mean and standard deviation were calculated for each parameter of interest. Independent-sample t-tests and three-way General Linear Model (GLM) Repeated Measures (RM) tests were performed to detect significant differences between the two study groups for cross-sectional (initial stiffness, cycles to failure) and longitudinal (values at 2000, 4000, and 6000 cycles) data, respectively. p values < 0.05 were considered significant.

3. Results

3.1. Stiffness

The mean initial construct stiffness was 62.6 N/mm (SD 20.3 N/mm) for the SI-plate group and 49.7 N/mm (SD 17.1 N/mm) for the TriFix group. This difference of approximately 26% was statistically not significant ($p = 0.245$).

3.2. Fracture Gap-Angle and Screw Tip Cutout

Figure 6 shows the mean values for the two parameters evaluated over the first 6000 cycles at three intermittent time points, namely fracture gap angle and screw tip cutout, for both groups separately. For both parameters, the TriFix was associated with significantly lower values compared to the SI-plate ($p = 0.019/0.011$). The difference for the fracture gap angle was +72% at 2000 cycles, +71% at 4000 cycles, and +98% at 6000 cycles for the SI plate compared to the TriFix. The difference for the screw tip cutout was +98% at 2000 cycles, +92% at 4000 cycles, and +65% at 6000 cycles for the SI plate compared to the TriFix.

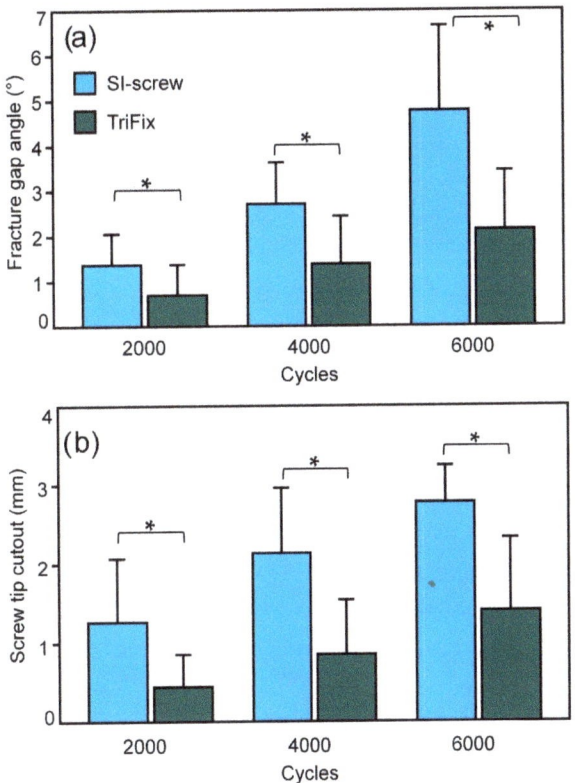

Figure 6. Fracture gap-angle (**a**) and screw tip cutout (**b**) are shown at intermittent time points after 2000, 4000, and 6000 cycles for each group separately in terms of mean and SD. Significant differences between the groups are marked with *.

In both groups, both the fracture gap-angle and screw tip cutout showed a significant increase over the number of cycles (all $p \leq 0.008$). The TriFix showed a 3-fold increase in fracture gap angle and the SI Plate 3.5-fold between cycles 2000 and 6000. In the screw tip cutout, the TriFix increased 2.6-fold, and the SI-Plate increased 2.2-fold between cycles 2000 and 6000.

3.3. Number of Cycles to Failure

The mean number of cycles to failure and the corresponding load at failure was 3399 cycles (SD 1583) and 270.0 N (SD 79.2 N) for the SI-screw, and 5747 cycles (SD 1389) and 387.4 N (SD 69.5 N) for the TriFix, respectively (Figure 7). This difference was statistically significant ($p = 0.017$). The TriFix showed a 69% increase in cycles to failure and a 44% increase in load to failure.

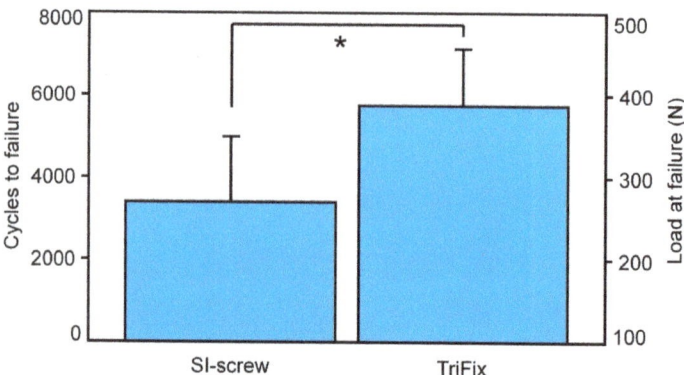

Figure 7. Mean number of cycles until failure with the standard deviation for both groups. Significant differences between the groups are marked with *.

3.4. Mode of Catastrophic Failure

Figures 8 and 9 show the catastrophic failure in the two groups. In addition to failing at the fracture plane, both groups also failed around the implants. In particular, fractures in the region of the entry points and implant trajectories were caused by the hard outer structure of the artificial bone material.

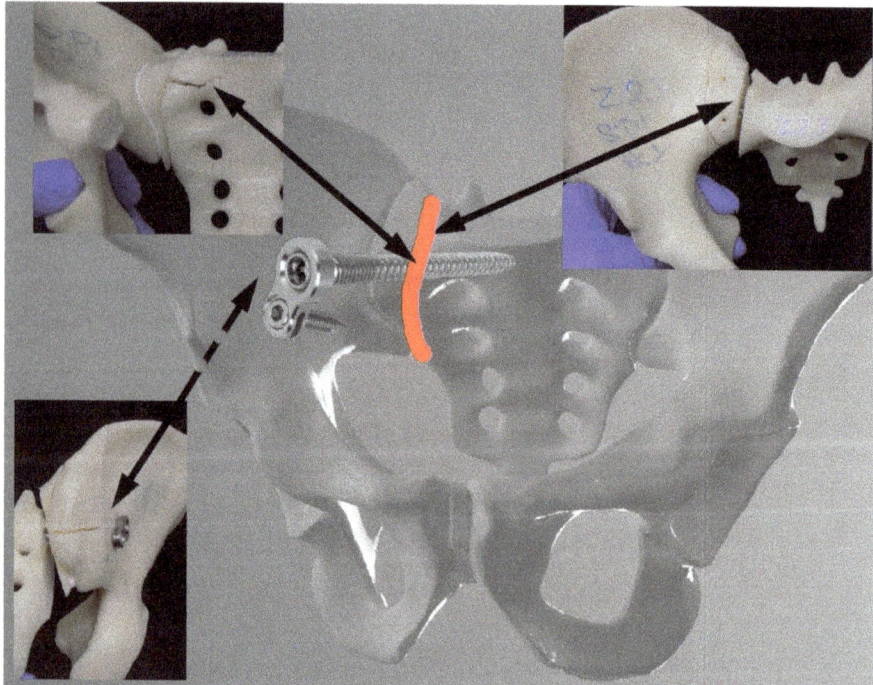

Figure 8. Failure pattern of the SI plate group projected onto a 3D pelvic model. The images show fractures of the sacrum and ilium and fracture gap dissociation. Red line = fracture line; dotted arrows indicate the location on the back of the model; sold arrows on the front.

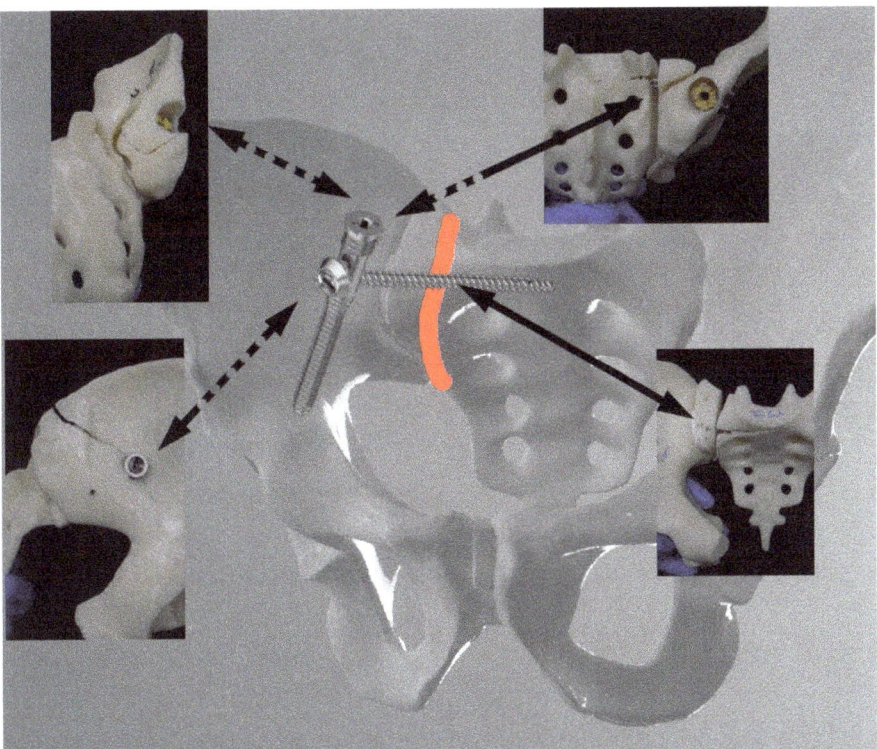

Figure 9. Failure pattern of the TriFix group projected onto a 3D pelvic model. The images show fractures of the sacrum and ilium, especially around the entry point of the ilium screw and fracture gap dissociation. Red line = fracture line; dotted arrows indicate the location on the back of the model; solid arrows on the front.

4. Discussion

Increased life expectancy in recent decades has led to an increased incidence of fragility fractures of the pelvic ring [3,4,19]. The mechanisms of trauma and the resulting treatment differ from other types of pelvic ring fracture. One standard operative treatment is iliosacral screw osteosynthesis. However, in osteoporotic bone, single iliosacral screw fixation may be mechanically inadequate and carries a high risk of screw loosening [9,20].

For this reason, the present study investigates two advanced percutaneous fixation options for the fracture stabilization of the dorsal pelvic ring in a biomechanical setup. In this study, we were able to demonstrate superior biomechanical characteristics of the TriFix fixation consisting of a fenestrated iliac screw and an iliosacral screw with a quasi-angle stable connection compared to an iliosacral screw with an additional short locking screw. In biomechanical testing, implant loosening parameters and number of cycles to failure showed significantly superior results for the TriFix stabilization.

This allows the implant to be selected according to the biomechanical requirements of the fracture, instability, and bone morphology. In young patients with good bone quality and the ability to unload or partial weight bear their leg, a standard iliosacral screw is sufficient. However, if any factor changes, such as the ability to unload the leg or the bone quality, the addition of a short, angular stable iliac screw is an option to increase stability and prevent construct loosening. If the fracture is more unstable and the bone quality is poor, the TriFix can provide even more stability to help prevent complications.

Several previous studies have focused on improving implant anchorage, particularly in osteoporotic bone and unstable fracture patterns. Loosening of the screw in the sacrum and unthreading of the screw are the two main failure mechanisms of iliosacral screws in osteoporotic dorsal pelvic ring fractures. Therefore, iliosacral screw augmentation with bone cement is one method to reduce sacral screw loosening [15,21]. Cement augmentation significantly improved sacral screw fixation [22–24]. Oberkirchner et al. compared iliosacral screws with and without cement augmentation in a human pelvic model. In their pull-out tests, the augmented groups showed significantly higher primary stability compared to the non-augmented groups [10]. In order to increase patient safety, the screw augmentation technique was changed from injecting cement prior to screw placement to a clinically viable procedure using cannulated iliosacral screws with perforations at the tip, allowing cement to be injected after successful screw placement [15,21,25].

To address the issue of unscrewing, Zderic et al. developed the screw-in-screw prototype, which allows the additional placement of a short 2.7 mm locking screw in the ilium through a threaded hole in the iliosacral screw head [13]. Their biomechanical comparison of this prototype implant with standard iliosacral screws shows successful prevention of loosening but also greater biomechanical stability in terms of cycles to failure, screw flexion, cut-through, and screw tilt [13]. These results clearly demonstrate the significant biomechanical advantages of an additional short iliac locking screw over a standard iliosacral screw. Therefore, we decided not to include a standard iliosacral group in our study.

The biomechanical principle of the TriFix construct consists of an iliac screw, which acts as a reinforced fixation anchor in the iliac bone, and an iliosacral screw, which are both connected in a quasi-angle stable manner. Anchoring in the TriFix screw moves the anchor point medially, and the polyethylene inlay increases the contact surface between the implants, both of which contribute to improved construct stability. The TriFix screw is equivalent to a reinforced fixation anchor in the iliac bone. Therefore, failures such as the washer penetration described are virtually impossible [26].

To the best of our knowledge, there are no techniques described to improve iliosacral screw anchoring in the iliac bone. However, it is possible to augment the tip of the iliosacral screws presented with polymethacrylate through the existing perforations at the tip of the screw. These two features allow the use of the TriFix constructs in patients with extremely poor bone quality and unstable fractures. Furthermore, the modularity of this system allows for a quick and easy extension to spinopelvic stabilization if required [27].

Although the pelvic models used in this study mimicked osteoporotic bone structure, catastrophic failures were observed in both groups, which are not known from the clinical situation and underline the strength of both constructs presented. However, the stability of the TriFix screw construct was significantly higher, with up to 70% more load cycles to failure compared to the SI plate group.

While implantation of the SI-Plate is mainly comparable to standard iliosacral screws, which can be performed in the supine or prone position, implantation of the TriFix screws requires the patient to be in the prone position. Surgeons may have to adapt to a new patient position, which may be seen as a disadvantage in the clinical setting. In our experience, the prone position is ideal for screw osteosynthesis of the dorsal, pelvic ring unless a supraacetabular external fixator is unavoidable. The clinical advantages of the implants used, particularly in terms of handling, have already been published [27].

There are also limitations to this study. An artificial pelvis model does not show physiological behavior, as mentioned above. In particular, the insertion of the iliac screw in the TriFix group differed from the clinical situation due to the brittle nature of the cortical bone. A study using cadaveric specimens may give an even more reliable result from a clinical point of view but would have the disadvantage of reduced comparability between the specimens used and the type of instrumentation due to different anatomical aspects and bone properties. However, several biomechanical studies were carried out using these bone models, allowing comparison of results between studies [12,13]. Therefore, we decided to use this osteoporotic artificial pelvis model. Another critical aspect is biomechanical testing, which can only investigate initial stability. However, cyclic loading is more informative than static failure testing. The setup used is comparable to several previous biomechanical studies and also allows for comparison of results, which is an advantage of the tests performed [12,13].

Clinical trials should be the next step in confirming the results of this preclinical biomechanical study.

5. Conclusions

Our results show that the primary stability and implant anchorage of osteosynthesis of the dorsal pelvic ring can be increased using the triangular fixation system and that the stiffness does not differ between the triangular fixation system and the SI plate group. Therefore, we conclude from the results of our biomechanical study that the use of the triangular fixation system has advantages, especially in weak bones and/or unstable fractures, which need to be confirmed in clinical trials.

Author Contributions: Conceptualization, N.G., B.G. and T.V.; Data curation, N.G., J.L. and B.G.; Formal analysis, J.L., I.Z. and D.W.; Funding acquisition, T.V.; Investigation, N.G., J.L., I.Z. and B.G.; Methodology, N.G., I.Z., D.W. and T.V.; Project administration, B.G., D.W. and T.V.; Resources, B.G., D.W. and T.V.; Software, J.L. and I.Z.; Supervision, I.Z. and T.V.; Writing—original draft, N.G., I.Z. and D.W.; Writing—review and editing, J.L., B.G. and T.V. All authors have read and agreed to the published version of the manuscript.

Funding: This research was funded by Silony Medial A.G. Biomechanical testing at the AO Research Institute Davos and artificial bone models were funded by Silony. All used implants and the necessary instruments have been provided by the manufacturer Silony Medical A.G.

Institutional Review Board Statement: Not applicable.

Informed Consent Statement: Not applicable.

Data Availability Statement: All data are available on request from the corresponding author.

Conflicts of Interest: N.G., J.L., I.Z., B.G. and D.W. declare no conflicts of interest. TV had the idea for the implant design and holds patent rights and royalties from Silony Medical GmbH. The funders had no role in the design of the study; in the collection, analyses, or interpretation of data; in the writing of the manuscript; or in the decision to publish the results.

References

1. Audretsch, C.K.; Siegemund, A.; Ellmerer, A.; Herath, S.C. Sex Differences in Pelvic Fractures-a Retrospective Analysis of 16 359 Cases From the German Trauma Registry. *Dtsch. Ärzteblatt Int.* **2023**, *120*, 221–222. [CrossRef]
2. Rommens, P.M.; Hofmann, A. The FFP-classification: From eminence to evidence. *Injury* **2023**, *54* (Suppl. S3), S10–S19. [CrossRef]
3. Rollmann, M.F.; Herath, S.C.; Kirchhoff, F.; Braun, B.J.; Holstein, J.H.; Pohlemann, T.; Menger, M.D.; Histing, T. Pelvic ring fractures in the elderly now and then—A pelvic registry study. *Arch. Gerontol. Geriatr.* **2017**, *71*, 83–88. [CrossRef]
4. Fuchs, T.; Rottbeck, U.; Hofbauer, V.; Raschke, M.; Stange, R. Beckenringfrakturen im Alter. *Der Unfallchirurg* **2011**, *114*, 663–670. [CrossRef]
5. Rommens, P.M.; Hofmann, A.; Kraemer, S.; Kisilak, M.; Boudissa, M.; Wagner, D. Operative treatment of fragility fractures of the pelvis: A critical analysis of 140 patients. *Eur. J. Trauma Emerg. Surg.* **2022**, *48*, 2881–2896. [CrossRef]
6. Maier, G.S.; Kolbow, K.; Lazovic, D.; Horas, K.; Roth, K.E.; Seeger, J.B.; Maus, U. Risk factors for pelvic insufficiency fractures and outcome after conservative therapy. *Arch. Gerontol. Geriatr.* **2016**, *67*, 80–85. [CrossRef]
7. Bukata, S.V.; Digiovanni, B.F.; Friedman, S.M.; Hoyen, H.; Kates, A.; Kates, S.L.; Mears, S.C.; Mendelson, D.A.; Serna, F.H., Jr.; Sieber, F.E.; et al. A guide to improving the care of patients with fragility fractures. *Geriatr. Orthop. Surg. Rehabil.* **2011**, *2*, 5–37. [CrossRef]
8. Hopf, J.C.; Krieglstein, C.F.; Müller, L.P.; Koslowsky, T.C. Percutaneous iliosacral screw fixation after osteoporotic posterior ring fractures of the pelvis reduces pain significantly in elderly patients. *Injury* **2015**, *46*, 1631–1636. [CrossRef]
9. Rommens, P.M.; Hofmann, A. Comprehensive classification of fragility fractures of the pelvic ring: Recommendations for surgical treatment. *Injury* **2013**, *44*, 1733–1744. [CrossRef]
10. Oberkircher, L.; Masaeli, A.; Bliemel, C.; Debus, F.; Ruchholtz, S.; Krüger, A. Primary stability of three different iliosacral screw fixation techniques in osteoporotic cadaver specimens-a biomechanical investigation. *Spine J.* **2016**, *16*, 226–232. [CrossRef]
11. Grechenig, S.; Gansslen, A.; Gueorguiev, B.; Berner, A.; Muller, M.; Nerlich, M.; Schmitz, P. PMMA-augmented SI screw: A biomechanical analysis of stiffness and pull-out force in a matched paired human cadaveric model. *Injury* **2015**, *46* (Suppl. S4), S125–S128. [CrossRef]

12. Lodde, M.F.; Katthagen, J.C.; Schopper, C.O.; Zderic, I.; Richards, G.; Gueorguiev, B.; Raschke, M.J.; Hartensuer, R. Biomechanical Comparison of Five Fixation Techniques for Unstable Fragility Fractures of the Pelvic Ring. *J. Clin. Med.* **2021**, *10*, 2326. [CrossRef]
13. Zderic, I.; Wagner, D.; Schopper, C.; Lodde, M.; Richards, G.; Gueorguiev, B.; Rommens, P.; Acklin, Y.P. Screw-in-screw fixation of fragility sacrum fractures provides high stability without loosening-biomechanical evaluation of a new concept. *J. Orthop. Res.* **2021**, *39*, 761–770. [CrossRef]
14. Guerin, G.; Laghmouche, N.; Moreau, P.E.; Upex, P.; Jouffroy, P.; Riouallon, G. Iliosacral screwing under navigation control: Technical note. *Orthop. Traumatol. Surg. Res.* **2020**, *106*, 877–880. [CrossRef]
15. König, M.A.; Hediger, S.; Schmitt, J.W.; Jentzsch, T.; Sprengel, K.; Werner, C.M.L. In-screw cement augmentation for iliosacral screw fixation in posterior ring pathologies with insufficient bone stock. *Eur. J. Trauma Emerg. Surg.* **2018**, *44*, 203–210. [CrossRef]
16. Ellmerer, A.E.; Küper, M.A.; Rollmann, M.F.; Herath, S.C.; Histing, T. Cement augmentation in pelvic ring fractures. *Unfallchirurgie* **2022**, *125*, 443–451. [CrossRef]
17. Suero, E.M.; Greiner, A.; Becker, C.A.; Cavalcanti Kussmaul, A.; Weidert, S.; Pfeufer, D.; Woiczinski, M.; Braun, C.; Flatz, W.; Bocker, W.; et al. Biomechanical stability of sacroiliac screw osteosynthesis with and without cement augmentation. *Injury* **2021**, *52*, 2707–2711. [CrossRef]
18. Chakkravarthy, V.; Manojkumar, P.; Lakshmanan, M.; Eswar Prasad, K.; Dafale, R.; Vadhana, V.C.; Narayan, R.L. Comparing bio-tribocorrosion of selective laser melted Titanium-25% Niobium and conventionally manufactured Ti-6Al-4 V in inflammatory conditions. *J. Alloys Compd.* **2023**, *952*, 169852. [CrossRef]
19. Oberkircher, L.; Ruchholtz, S.; Rommens, P.M.; Hofmann, A.; Bucking, B.; Kruger, A. Osteoporotic Pelvic Fractures. *Dtsch. Ärzteblatt Int.* **2018**, *115*, 70–80. [CrossRef] [PubMed]
20. Dudda, M.; Hoffmann, M.; Schildhauer, T.A. Sakrumfrakturen und lumbopelvine Instabilitäten bei Beckenringverletzungen. *Der Unfallchirurg* **2013**, *116*, 972–978. [CrossRef]
21. Höch, A.; Pieroh, P.; Henkelmann, R.; Josten, C.; Böhme, J. In-screw polymethylmethacrylate-augmented sacroiliac screw for the treatment of fragility fractures of the pelvis: A prospective, observational study with 1-year follow-up. *BMC Surg.* **2017**, *17*, 132. [CrossRef] [PubMed]
22. König, A.; Oberkircher, L.; Beeres, F.J.P.; Babst, R.; Ruchholtz, S.; Link, B.C. Cement augmentation of sacroiliac screws in fragility fractures of the pelvic ring-A synopsis and systematic review of the current literature. *Injury* **2019**, *50*, 1411–1417. [CrossRef] [PubMed]
23. Osterhoff, G.; Dodd, A.E.; Unno, F.; Wong, A.; Amiri, S.; Lefaivre, K.A.; Guy, P. Cement Augmentation in Sacroiliac Screw Fixation Offers Modest Biomechanical Advantages in a Cadaver Model. *Clin. Orthop. Relat. Res.* **2016**, *474*, 2522–2530. [CrossRef] [PubMed]
24. Collinge, C.A.; Crist, B.D. Combined Percutaneous Iliosacral Screw Fixation With Sacroplasty Using Resorbable Calcium Phosphate Cement for Osteoporotic Pelvic Fractures Requiring Surgery. *J. Orthop. Trauma* **2016**, *30*, e217–e222. [CrossRef]
25. Hack, J.; Krüger, A.; Masaeli, A.; Aigner, R.; Ruchholtz, S.; Oberkircher, L. Cement-augmented sacroiliac screw fixation with cannulated versus perforated screws—A biomechanical study in an osteoporotic hemipelvis model. *Injury* **2018**, *49*, 1520–1525. [CrossRef]
26. Crist, B.D.; Pfeiffer, F.M.; Khazzam, M.S.; Kueny, R.A.; Della Rocca, G.J.; Carson, W.L. Biomechanical evaluation of location and mode of failure in three screw fixations for a comminuted transforaminal sacral fracture model. *J. Orthop. Translat.* **2019**, *16*, 102–111. [CrossRef]
27. Gruneweller, N.; Wahnert, D.; Vordemvenne, T. Instability of the posterior pelvic ring: Introduction of innovative implants. *J. Orthop. Surg. Res.* **2021**, *16*, 625. [CrossRef]

Disclaimer/Publisher's Note: The statements, opinions and data contained in all publications are solely those of the individual author(s) and contributor(s) and not of MDPI and/or the editor(s). MDPI and/or the editor(s) disclaim responsibility for any injury to people or property resulting from any ideas, methods, instructions or products referred to in the content.

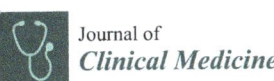

Article

Weak Points of Double-Plate Stabilization Used in the Treatment of Distal Humerus Fracture through Finite Element Analysis

Artur Kruszewski [1], Szczepan Piszczatowski [1,*], Piotr Piekarczyk [2], Piotr Cieślik [2] and Krzysztof Kwiatkowski [2]

[1] Faculty of Mechanical Engineering, Institute of Biomedical Engineering, Bialystok University of Technology, 45A Wiejska Street, 15-351 Bialystok, Poland; akruszewski69@gmail.com

[2] Department of Traumatology and Orthopedics, Military Institute of Medicine—National Research Institute, 128 Szaserów Street, 04-141 Warsaw, Poland; piotr@msnet.pl (P.P.); pcieslik@wim.mil.pl (P.C.); inst_ort@wim.mil.pl (K.K.)

* Correspondence: s.piszczatowski@pb.edu.pl

Citation: Kruszewski, A.; Piszczatowski, S.; Piekarczyk, P.; Cieślik, P.; Kwiatkowski, K. Weak Points of Double-Plate Stabilization Used in the Treatment of Distal Humerus Fracture through Finite Element Analysis. *J. Clin. Med.* **2024**, *13*, 1034. https://doi.org/10.3390/jcm13041034

Academic Editor: Christian von Rüden

Received: 21 December 2023
Revised: 31 January 2024
Accepted: 7 February 2024
Published: 11 February 2024

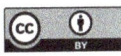

Copyright: © 2024 by the authors. Licensee MDPI, Basel, Switzerland. This article is an open access article distributed under the terms and conditions of the Creative Commons Attribution (CC BY) license (https://creativecommons.org/licenses/by/4.0/).

Abstract: Background: Multi-comminuted, intra-articular fractures of the distal humerus still pose a challenge to modern orthopedics due to unsatisfactory treatment results and a high percentage (over 50%) of postoperative complications. When surgical treatment is chosen, such fractures are fixed using two plates with locking screws, which can be used in three spatial configurations: either parallel or one of two perpendicular variants (posterolateral and posteromedial). The evaluation of the fracture healing conditions for these plate configurations is unambiguous. The contradictions between the conclusions of biomechanical studies and clinical observations were the motivation to undertake a more in-depth biomechanical analysis aiming to indicate the weak points of two-plate fracture stabilization. Methods: Research was conducted using the finite element method based on an experimentally validated model. Three variants of distal humerus fracture (Y, λ, and H) were fixed using three different plate configurations (parallel, posterolateral, and posteromedial), and they were analyzed under six loading conditions, covering the whole range of flexion in the elbow joint (0–145°). A joint reaction force equal to 150 N was assumed, which corresponds with holding a weight of 1 kg in the hand. The biomechanical conditions of bone union were assessed based on the interfragmentary movement (IFM) and using criteria formulated by Steiner et al. Results: The IFMs were established for particular regions of all of the analyzed types of fracture, with distinction to the normal and tangential components. In general, the tangential component of IFM was greater than normal. A strong influence of the elbow joint's angular position on the IFM was observed, with excessive values occurring for flexion angles greater than 90°. In most cases, the smallest IFM values were obtained for the parallel plaiting, while the greatest values were obtained for the posteromedial plating. Based on IFM values, fracture healing conditions in particular cases (fracture type, plate configuration, loading condition, and fracture gap localization) were classified into one of four groups: optimal bone union (OPT), probable union (PU), probable non-union (PNU), and non-union (NU). Conclusions: No plating configuration is able to ensure distal humerus fracture union when the full elbow flexion is allowed while holding a weight of 1 kg in the hand. However, flexion in the range of 0–90° with such loadings is acceptable when using parallel plating, which is a positive finding in the context of the early rehabilitation process. In general, parallel plating ensures better conditions for fracture healing than perpendicular plate configurations, especially the posteromedial version.

Keywords: distal humerus; fracture healing; stabilization; osteosynthesis; biomechanics; interfragmentary movement

1. Introduction

Distal humeral fractures (DHF) represent about 30% of the fractures involving the humerus [1,2], and they are the cause of about 37% of all elbow surgeries [3]. The gold standard in DHF surgical treatment is open reduction and internal fixation (ORIF), which uses two locking plates and a set of screws [4,5]. However, the use of double-plating in DHF osteosynthesis still results in a high complication rate, estimated to affect over 50% of all operated patients [6–9]. The most common complications are the need for reoperation due to, for example, deep infection or painful implant (20.8–49%); non-union, occurring when the fracture is not clinically or radiographically united after 6 months of fixation (4.1–9.3%); stiffness of the elbow joint, diagnosed, for example, when the patient cannot achieve a 30°–130° arc (19–46.5%); or degenerative changes, e.g., osteoarthritis (9–21.1%) or heterotrophic ossifications (5.1–21.8%). In this situation, elbow arthroplasty is increasingly used as an alternative, though much more radical, DHF treatment method [10]. Postoperative complications after the use of double-plating may have various causes and result from the course of the procedure itself, the specificity of the surgical approach, or coexisting diseases. However, non-union, limitations in joint movement, and heterotrophic ossifications are probably related to the insufficient stability of the bone fragments and improper joint movement during early postoperative rehabilitation. It is known, however, that stabilization should provide stable-enough fixation to obtain a union. It also should allow for an early rehabilitation process, as movement is essential for success in the final treatment due to the fact that the elbow is intolerant to immobilization [11–13].

Nowadays, there are two popular plating techniques used to treat distal humerus fractures. The first one involves parallel plating with medial and lateral plates [14,15], while the other involves perpendicular plating [16] and has two available options: "posterolateral", with medial and posterolateral plates, and "posteromedial", with lateral and posteromedial plates. Parallel plating is the consequence of earlier reports of unsatisfactory results among patients with perpendicular plating (the standard proposed by AO/ASIF) [17]. However, the optimal plate configuration still remains controversial.

Biomechanical studies attempted to assess the stability of the fixation of distal humerus fractures, and they were based primarily on the evaluation of the global stiffness of the bone–plate system. Most of the discussed studies indicated the advantage of parallel plating [18–20]. Both perpendicular configurations usually ensure the necessary stiffness of the fixation as well, but in general, their mechanical parameters are worse than those of parallel plating [21,22]. As a result, some contradictions can be noticed between the conclusions formulated in biomechanical studies and clinical observations. However, better clinical results are reported in the case of perpendicular plating [23–26], which is inconsistent with the fact that the parallel plating is indicated to guarantee more rigid stabilization. It seems that the biomechanical studies did not encompass all clinically important aspects of the problem. Ambiguities in the assessment of plate configurations may largely result from limitations of the testing method, such as oversimplified loading conditions (for example, only axial or bending loadings) [27,28]. The other problem is the lack of realistic analysis of interfragmentary movement in multi-comminuted fractures and the assessment of fixation only on the basis of global stiffness [21,27]. It is well known, however, that for proper bone union, it is crucial to stabilize all bone fragments to avoid their mutual movement, and the assessment of global stiffness does not provide a realistic evaluation of the union conditions when it comes to the particular bone fragments. All of these limitations may be the reason for the abovementioned contradictions between the biomechanical and clinical assessment of particular DHF stabilization methods. This was the motivation to undertake the present research.

The aim of the present study is to present a more comprehensive evaluation of biomechanical conditions of distal humerus fracture healing and, based on the results obtained, provide an indication of the weak points of particular variants of double-plating for such fractures. This analysis should allow for more optimal DHF treatment by raising awareness of the choice in plate configuration and introducing necessary restrictions during fracture healing and rehabilitation.

2. Materials and Methods

In order to achieve the above-presented research goal and taking into account the limitations of previous analyses, three main assumptions were made when planning the experiment. (1) The interfragmentary movement (IFM) of particular pairs of bone fragments should be used to calculate the local stiffness of the bone union and thus assess the biomechanical conditions of fracture healing based on Steiner's analysis [29]. (2) Research should be conducted based on realistic geometrical structures of typical DHFs present in clinical practice. (3) Finally, loading conditions occurring throughout the entire range of elbow flexion–extension should be taken into consideration.

Both parallel and perpendicular plate configurations, distinguishing the latter's posteromedial (PM) and posterolateral (PL) versions, were used as the objects of the research.

Modeling and numerical simulation were performed using the finite element method (FEM) as the main research method. However, a laboratory experiment was undertaken using an artificial humeral bone and testing machine to validate the numerical models and to obtain some parameters for numerical simulations (Figure 1).

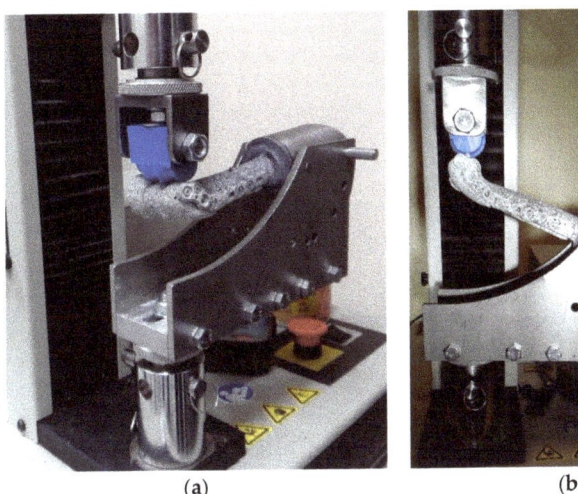

(a) (b)

Figure 1. Measuring station consisting of the MTS Insight 1 kN testing machine, a special clamping device, and the ARAMIS digital image correlation system: (**a**) general view; (**b**) side view of the device enabling the loading of the sample at various angles.

The same geometry of the humerus was used, both in the experimental and the numerical studies, using composite humeral bone (Sawbones Europe AB, Malmo, Sweden, 4th Gen., Composite, 17 PCF Solid Foam Core, Large). The three geometric variants of the fracture most frequently occurring in clinical practice were included (Figure 2) and marked Y, λ, and H according to the DHF classification proposed by Jupiter and Mehne [30]. The modeled gap between the particular bone fragments was about 1.6 mm wide.

Particular models of the fractured bone were fixed using the VariAx Elbow Plate System (Stryker, Portage, MI, USA) made of titanium alloy, reproducing the three above-mentioned spatial plating configurations: parallel, posteromedial, and posterolateral. The number and localization of the screws connecting the plates to the bone were modeled based on their implantation in clinical practice. General rules for inserting screws according to AO guidelines in perpendicular plating and principles for the optimization of stability postulated by O'Driscoll, applicable mainly for parallel plating, were used for the screw placement [14,27]. An example of the screw arrangements is presented in Figure 3.

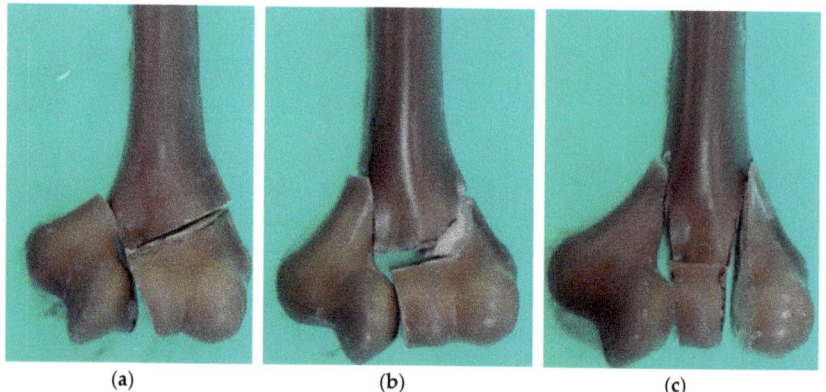

Figure 2. Three types of DHFs included in the study, determined based on Jupiter and Mehne's classification: (**a**) Y fracture, (**b**) λ fracture, and (**c**) H fracture.

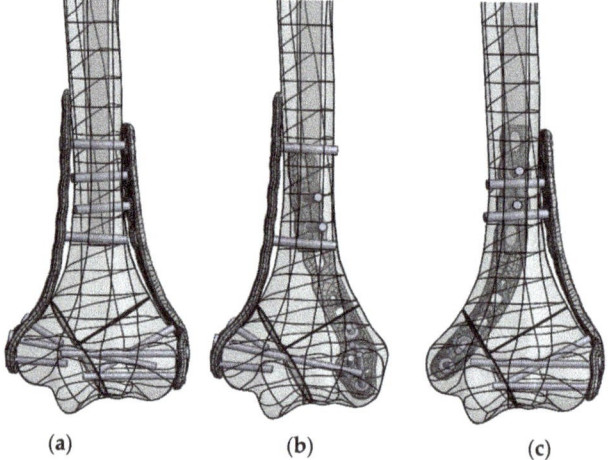

Figure 3. Placement of plates and screws in the Y-type fracture for the following plate configurations: (**a**) parallel, (**b**) posterolateral, and (**c**) posteromedial.

For the numerical analysis, bone models and particular plates were scanned using an optical scanner (Atos Core 200, GOM, Braunschweig, Germany), and their finite element models were obtained using CAD/CAE software (ANSYS Workbench 2021 R1, Canonsburg, PA, USA). The screws connecting the plates to the bone model were simplified in the numerical analysis and modeled without threads. The screws in the area of the humeral shaft were modeled as a cylinder with a diameter of 2.75 mm, which corresponds to the core diameter of the screw used in experimental setup with an outer thread diameter of 3.5 mm; those intended for the distal end of the humerus were modeled as cylinders with a diameter of 2 mm, which corresponds to the core diameter of the screw with an outer thread diameter of 2.7 mm.

Discretization was performed using the 10-node tetrahedral element Solid187. Convergence of the solution was ensured by diminishing the size of the elements up until the change in the maximum equivalent stress did not exceed 5%. The final models consisted of 380–420 thousands of elements and 230–280 thousands of nodes (Figure 4).

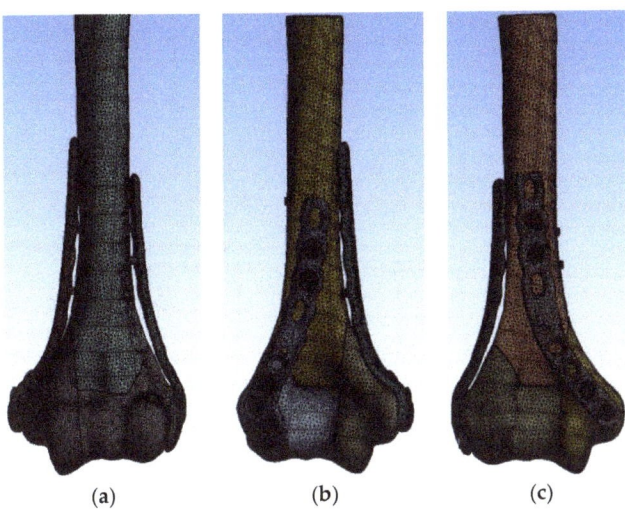

Figure 4. FEM model for λ fracture fixed with (**a**) parallel, (**b**) posterolateral, and (**c**) posteromedial plate configurations.

2.1. Loads and Boundary Conditions

During the laboratory experiment (Figure 1), the bone was mounted using special equipment in six different angular positions in relation to the load axis of the testing machine. This way, it was possible to reconstruct variable directions for the joint reaction force (JRF) vector in the humeroulnar joint during the elbow flexion movement in its entire range (0–145°). The loading directions for particular joint angles were assumed based on Kincaid and An's analysis [31] (Table 1). In all cases, the same value of JRF, equal to 150 N, was used, which corresponds to the loads occurring when holding a weight of approximately 1 kg in the hand with the elbow flexed at a 90° angle.

Table 1. Direction of JRF in sagittal plane in the humeroulnar joint for the whole range of elbow flexion.

Angle of the Elbow Flexion	0°	* 1	30°	60–90°	120°	145°
JRF direction	−20°	0°	10°	43°	63°	95°

[1] The symbol * indicates the unknown elbow position ensuring the direction of the JRF in agreement with the long humeral axis (JRF = 0°).

The value of the displacements of the testing machine's compressing upper plate, recorded during the laboratory experiment for particular loading directions, was used as kinematic boundary condition used in the numerical simulations. In order to validate the numerical model, the displacements of selected points located on the plates were recorded during the laboratory experiment using the digital image correlation (DIC) technique, and then they were compared with their numerically determined values. The obtained differences did not exceed 3.5%.

2.2. Material Properties

The material model took into account the heterogeneous structure of the humerus, which was divided into cortical and spongy tissue. The bone shaft was built of cortical tissue with a reconstructed medullary cavity. In the epiphyseal and metaphyseal regions, the external part was modeled as cortical bone, while the internal part was modeled as spongy bone. The thickness of the outer layer corresponding to the cortical tissue in this region was about 2 mm. The values of the material parameters used in the model were as follows (elastic modulus; Poisson coefficient): cortical bone (16.7 Gpa; 0.34), spongy bone (0.155 Gpa; 0.34) [32], and titanium alloy (110 Gpa; 0.30).

2.3. Interfragmentary Movement

A set of points was evenly distributed around the circumference of each pair of bone fragments in the models, where the points located on one side of the fracture gap had their counterparts on the other side (Figure 5). Then, the displacements of each point in the local coordinate system were determined and the mutual displacements between the pairs of points were calculated, distinguishing between displacements in the normal and tangential directions. The values of the mutual displacements for all pairs of points around particular fracture gaps are provided in Table S1 in Supplementary Material. Assuming that the risk of non-union is determined by the least favorable conditions occurring in the entire fracture gap, the greatest value of the mutual displacements between all pairs of points located in particular region of interest (ROI) were taken for further analyses, named the interfragmentary movement (IFM). Four ROIs were defined: ROI M: the fracture gap between the shaft and the medial bone fragment; ROI L: the fracture gap between the shaft and the lateral bone fragment; ROI S: the fracture gap between the shaft and the trochlea (only in λ- and H-type fractures); and ROI T: the fracture gaps inside the trochlea region. In H-type fractures, the IFM for ROI T was taken as the largest displacement value in the whole trochlea region (Figure 5c).

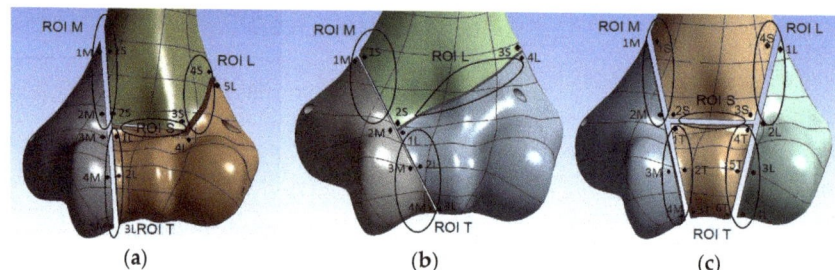

Figure 5. Pairs of points and their distribution in individual bone fragments in fractures: (**a**) λ; (**b**) Y; and (**c**) H. Front view; analogous pairs of points are marked on the back side (not visible).

2.4. Assessment of the Biomechanical Conditions of Fracture Healing

With the research aim of identifying weak points of fracture fixation using particular plate configurations, we assumed that the assessment of the biomechanical conditions of fracture healing should indicate cases with high risk of bone non-union. On the other hand, it is known that bone union should occur in cases where the level of interfragmentary movement remains within a certain range of values, ensured by the appropriate stiffness of the stabilization. Based on Steiner's analyses, it was assumed that the optimal axial stiffness of the stabilization promoting bone union should be in the range between 1000 N/mm (lower limit) and 2500 N/mm (upper limit) [29]. In the case of the elbow joint's reaction force equaling 150 N during the test, the optimal value of the axial component of IFM should be in the range of 0.06–0.15 mm. In turn, the lower limit of the bone-plating stiffness in the tangential direction should reach 400 N/mm for a gap of 1 mm. When the load value is equal to 150 N, the upper limit of the acceptable tangential component of IFM is 0.375 mm. We assumed that the optimal conditions for bone union (OPT) occur when the axial component of IFM remains in the range of 0.06–0.15 mm while the tangential component is below 0.375 mm. The previously mentioned research also shows that IFM values lower and higher than the normal optimal value could delay bone union, but they do not always lead to bone non-union. The coexisting range of the tangential IFM is, however, crucial. For this reason, we assumed that the normal component of IFM outside of the optimal range (below 0.06 mm or in the range of 0.15–0.375 mm) together with its tangential component below 0.375 mm would ensure a potentially non-optimal biomechanical condition, but bone union is still probable (classified as "probable union"—PU). An increase in IFM of over 0.375 mm could be treated as an increased risk of non-union, and those results are evaluated as a "probable non-union"—PNU. According to Steiner's analyses, the limit of tangential stiffness for a wider fracture gap (3 mm) decreases to 300 N/mm, which results in a greater limit of IFM equal to 0.5 mm. In this context, we assumed that fracture stabilization ensuring an IFM value below 0.5 mm (in any direction) cannot be treated as a cause of bone non-union when the loading is equal to 150 N. This way, contrary to the above assumption, IFM values higher than 0.5 mm were assumed to be a biomechanical condition with reasonable risk of bone non-union (NU).

Finally, in order to assess the biomechanical condition of fracture union, particular cases (combinations of plate configurations, loading directions, fracture type, and ROI) were classified into one of four groups based on the obtained IFM values and the assumptions presented above (Figure 6):

- Optimal bone union (OPT)—the value of the normal component of IFM within the range of 0.06–0.15 mm and the value of the tangential component of IFM below 0.375 mm;
- Probable union (PU)—the value of normal displacements in the range of 0–0.06 mm or 0.15–0.375 mm and the value of tangential displacements below 0.375 mm;
- Probable non-union (PNU)—the value of both tangential and normal displacements greater than 0.375 mm but below 0.5 mm;
- Non-union (NU)—the value of normal or tangential displacements greater than 0.5 mm.

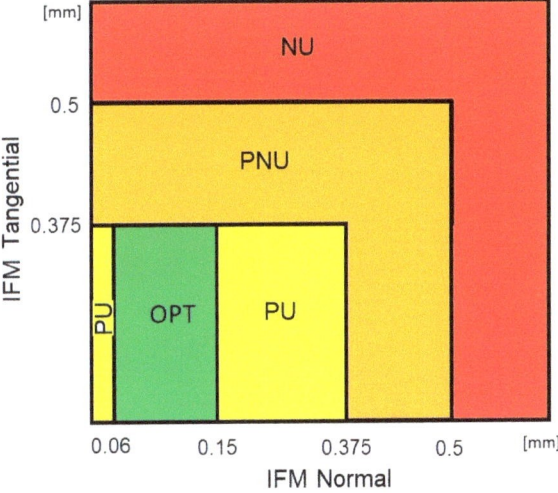

Figure 6. Criteria for assessing the biomechanical conditions of fracture healing for a 150 N load acting on the bone-plating system: OPT—optimal bone union conditions; PU—high probability of achieving bone union; PNU—probable non-union; NU—very high risk of non-union.

Summing up the presented methodology, it is worth noting that the basis of the research was the numerical analysis with use of the finite element method, carried out using models validated on the basis of experimental results. It should be emphasized that nine combinations of the bone–plate system (three variants of the DHF, fixed with one of three plate configurations) were analyzed under loads acting in six directions corresponding to the full range of elbow flexion. The analysis resulted in fifty-four spatial variants of the model. The biomechanical conditions of fracture healing were evaluated based on the values of interfragmentary movement determined in four regions of interest, covering the entire fracture region. The fracture union conditions were classified based on Steiner's analyses as optimal (OPT), highly probable union (PU), probable non-union (PNU), and risk of non-union (NU).

3. Results

Taking into account the analyzed variants of the model discussed above (including fracture types, plate configurations, and loading directions) as well as the four regions of interest (Figure 5) and two components of interfragmentary movement (normal and tangential), a substantial dataset was obtained for analysis. For this reason and for a concise presentation, the results are shown mainly in graph form. This should allow for comparative analyses of the influence of particular factors on IFM values. Additionally, the most important findings are briefly described after graphical presentation. For clarity, the same range of IFM values is maintained on all graphs. In the second part of the presentation of the results, particular variants of the model are classified in terms of their assessed biomechanical bone union conditions based on the IFM values obtained using the methodology discussed earlier (Figure 6).

Then, the IFM values obtained for the three analyzed fractures, all spatial plate configurations, and the six loading conditions (JRF directions) are presented in Figure 7 (tangential component) and Figure 8 (normal component).

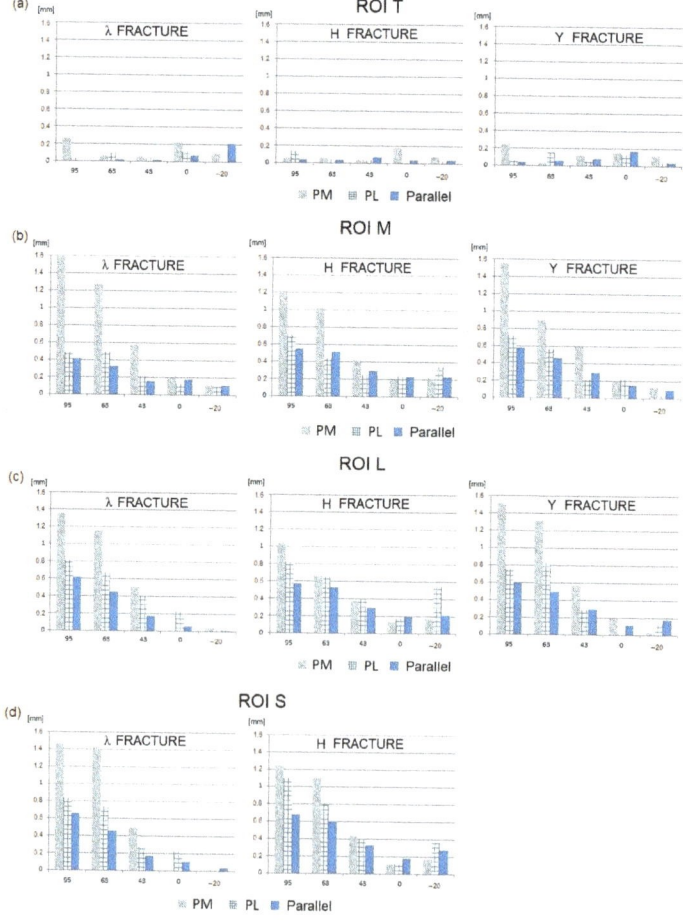

Figure 7. IFMs in the tangential direction for three plate configurations with respect to the JRF direction: (**a**) ROI T; (**b**) ROI M; (**c**) ROI L; and (**d**) ROI S.

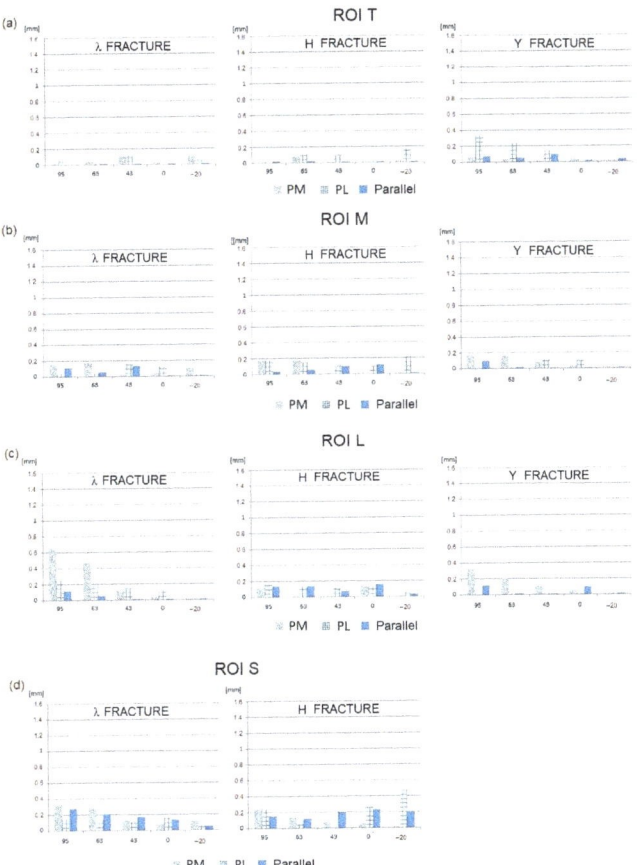

Figure 8. IFMs in the normal direction for the three plate configurations with respect to the JRF direction: (**a**) ROI T; (**b**) ROI M; (**c**) ROI L; and (**d**) ROI S.

Analyzing the presented results of the numerical research, the following phenomena can be observed:

- In general, the tangential components of IFMs are significantly greater than the normal components.
- The smallest IFMs, both tangential and normal, are observed for the parallel plate configuration in the majority of fracture types and elbow joint flexion angles.
- In most cases, the largest IFMs are observed for posteromedial (PM) stabilization.
- The angular position of the elbow joint and the related direction of the joint force reaction has a very strong influence on the value of IFM. It can be observed that the maximum IFM values occur when the elbow joint is almost fully flexed (JRF direction 63–95°; joint angle 120–145°) in all plating configurations and all types of fractures.
- For elbow joint angles in the range of 0–90° (JRF direction −20–43°), the IFM values are relatively low. In this angular range, the differences in the IFM values obtained for different plating configurations and different types of fractures are somewhat unclear.

The mutual displacements of bone fragments also depend on the type of fracture, although this effect is not as pronounced as in the case of the elbow flexion angle (or JRF direction) and the spatial configuration of the plates. The influence of the type of fracture on the IFM value results primarily from its position in the space of individual fracture gaps in relation to the line of screw insertion and the localization of the particular plates.

Based on both the normal and tangential IFM component values in a particular ROI, biomechanical conditions of fracture healing were evaluated for all cases (analyzing combinations of plate configurations, elbow angles, and fracture types). These are presented in Table 2.

Table 2. Assessment of the biomechanical conditions of bone union in the case of distal humerus fracture based on the criteria presented in Figure 6. Non-union is highlighted in red, probable non-union is highlighted in orange, high probability of achieving bone union is highlighted in yellow, while optimal conditions for union are highlighted in green.

Region (ROI)	Joint Reaction	Joint Angle	Plating Configuration		
			PM	PL	Parallel
λ Fracture					
T	−20	0°	OPT	PU	PU
	10	30°	PU	PU	PU
	43	60–90°	PU	PU	PU
	63	120°	PU	PU	PU
	95	145°	PU	OPT	PU
S	−20	0°	PU	OPT	OPT
	10	30°	OPT	OPT	OPT
	43	60–90°	PNU	OPT	PU
	63	120°	NU	NU	PU
	95	145°	NU	NU	NU
M	−20	0°	PU	PU	PU
	10	30°	PU	PU	PU
	43	60–90°	PNU	PU	OPT
	63	120°	NU	PNU	OPT
	95	145°	NU	PNU	PNU
L	−20	0°	PU	PU	PU
	10	30°	PU	OPT	PU
	43	60–90°	PNU	OPT	PU
	63	120°	NU	NU	PNU
	95	145°	NU	NU	NU
H Fracture					
T	−20	0°	PU	OPT	OPT
	10	30°	PU	OPT	PU
	43	60–90°	PU	PU	PU
	63	120°	OPT	PU	PU
	95	145°	OPT	PU	PU
M	−20	0°	PU	OPT	PU
	10	30°	PU	OPT	PU
	43	60–90°	PNU	OPT	PU
	63	120°	NU	PNU	PNU
	95	145°	NU	NU	NU
L	−20	0°	PU	PU	PU
	10	30°	PU	PU	OPT
	43	60–90°	PNU	OPT	OPT
	63	120°	NU	NU	NU
	95	145°	NU	NU	NU
S	−20	0°	PU	PU	PU
	10	30°	PU	PU	PU
	43	60–90°	PNU	PU	PU
	63	120°	NU	NU	PNU
	95	145°	NU	NU	NU

Table 2. *Cont.*

Region (ROI)	Joint Reaction	Joint Angle	Plating Configuration		
			PM	PL	Parallel
		Y Fracture			
T	−20	0°	PU	PU	OPT
	10	30°	PU	PU	OPT
	43	60–90°	PU	OPT	PU
	63	120°	PU	PU	PU
	95	145°	OPT	PU	PU
M	−20	0°	PU	PU	PU
	10	30°	PU	PU	PU
	43	60–90°	NU	PU	PU
	63	120°	NU	NU	PNU
	95	145°	NU	NU	NU
L	−20	0°	PU	PU	PU
	10	30°	OPT	PU	PU
	43	60–90°	OPT	PU	PU
	63	120°	NU	NU	NU
	95	145°	NU	NU	NU

Analyzing the obtained results, we can conclude that the following cases are classified as having a high risk of bone non-union:

- All variants of the fracture gap except in the trochlear region (i.e., the S, M, and L regions) in all types of fractures (λ, Y, and H) stabilized in a perpendicular configuration, both posterolateral (PL) and posteromedial (PM), for an elbow flexion angle equal to or greater than 120°;
- All variants of the fracture gap except in the trochlear region (i.e., the S, M, and L regions) in all types of fractures (λ, Y, and H) stabilized in a parallel configuration, for the maximum elbow joint flexion angle (145°),
- The fracture gap between the lateral fragment and the shaft (region L) in Y- and H-type fractures when they are stabilized in a parallel configuration, and when the elbow joint is flexed to 120°;
- The fracture gap between the medial fragment and the shaft (region M) in Y-type fractures with stabilization in a posteromedial (PM) configuration, for an elbow flexion angle of 60–90°.

The positive exception to the above rules is the fracture gap between the medial fragment and the shaft (region M):

- In the case of a λ-type fracture stabilized in a posterolateral (PL) or parallel configuration, the chance of union is not eliminated in the entire angular range of the loading direction;
- In the case of an H-type fracture stabilized in a posterolateral (PL) configuration, a high probability of non-union is obtained only for the maximum elbow flexion (145°).

A reasonable probability of non-union (PNU) also occurs in the following instances:

- In the case of stabilization in a posteromedial (PM) configuration for all types of fractures and all fracture gaps, for elbow joint flexed at 60° or 90°, with the exception of the gap between the lateral fragment and the shaft (ROI L) in a Y-type fracture;
- In the case of stabilization in a parallel configuration, for the elbow joint flexed at 120° in following situations:
    - In the gap between the medial fragment and the shaft (ROI M) for Y- and H-type fractures;
    - In the gap between the lateral fragment and the shaft (ROI L) for λ-type fractures;
    - In the gap between the trochlea and the shaft (ROI S) for H-type fractures.

In conclusion, based on the presented results, none of the stabilization variants provide the conditions necessary to achieve the union of intra-articular, multi-comminuted distal humerus fractures if a full range of motion is allowed in the elbow joint. Excessive mobility at the distal end of the humerus relative to the shaft of the bone is visible when the elbow joint is fully flexed in virtually every type of fracture and plate configuration. When the plating is used in a perpendicular configuration, this effect also occurs when the elbow is flexed at 120°, and in the posteromedial configuration, in some cases, it occurs even at 60° of flexion.

4. Discussion

The aim of this study was to indicate the weak points of the stabilization used during the surgical treatment of distal humerus fractures. These results should allow for the better understanding of the frequently occurring serious complications observed in clinical practice during fracture healing. It is possible to state that this aim was achieved. In the summary of the results presented above, we justify the clinical problems in DHF stabilization. The source of the problem may be excessive interfragmentary movement occurring when the full range of elbow joint flexion is allowed, together with the joint loading reaching 150 N. We show that, in this situation, none of the stabilization variants provide the sufficient fixation stability necessary to achieve the union of intra-articular, multi-comminuted distal humerus fractures. As mentioned earlier, ensuring an appropriate level of bone fragment mutual displacement is one of the key conditions for achieving proper bone union [33,34]. In this situation, the excessive mutual displacement of the fragments may result in bone non-union, causing frequent complications in DHF treatment [7,8,35]. Helfet et al. [36] analyzed the treatment outcomes of patients with previous distal humerus fracture non-union. They noted that 75% of cases were the result of failed internal fixation. Failure to adhere to the rigid stabilization of the lateral and medial column of the distal humerus with fixator plates can dramatically increase the rate of non-union complications by up to 75% [37].

It should be emphasized that this effect in the presented results was achieved by allowing for a relatively small reaction value in the joint, corresponding to lifting approximately 1 kg with the hand. This effect is seen for all stabilization cases, regardless of the type of fracture. This effect becomes more significant when the plates are used in a perpendicular configuration, especially when the posteromedial (PM) version is chosen. In this case, the presented results indicate a high risk of non-union even if a flexion of 60 degrees is allowed. This is consistent with the observations presented by Ku et al. [12] and Shin et al. [23], who indicated a higher rate of non-union in the case of stabilization in a perpendicular configuration. Excessive mobility at the distal end of the humerus relative to the shaft of the bone can result when the plates are used in a perpendicular configuration since the plates work asymmetrically. This leads to an increase in the mutual displacement of bone fragments, especially in their tangential component. The results for the posteromedial configuration are worse than those for the posterolateral configuration due to the lower stiffness of the posterior plate used in particular variants of the perpendicular plating system. This is influenced by unfavorable posteromedial plate geometry and its position in relation to the loading direction. Penzkofer et al. [18] presented a similar effect indicating worse healing conditions when using a posteromedial plate orientation for a flexed elbow joint.

Some clinical results indicate a relatively lower overall rate of complications when using plates in a perpendicular configuration. This is most likely due to the lower invasiveness of this surgical technique. At the same time, there is reason to state that when a perpendicular configuration is used, the most serious complication, i.e., the non-union of a broken bone, is more common [7]. While the installation of a perpendicular plate configuration itself carries a lower risk of complications, e.g., related to damage to nerves or blood vessels, the plating system may not provide sufficiently stable conditions for the union of the bone fragments.

We obtained relatively better results for stabilization with a parallel plate configuration, although this variant also does not ensure proper union conditions when movement is allowed throughout the entire range of elbow flexion. These better results obtained with a parallel configuration may be due to the more favorable space orientation in the plates, which are positioned parallel to each other and preferably in relation to the direction of the acting force (larger cross-sectional dimension of the plates set parallel to the plane of the force action). This effect is consistent with the results presented by Zha et al. [28]. It is also worth noting that the parallel arrangement of the plates allows for the use of maximum-length screws connecting the plates to as many bone fragments as possible, which additionally reduces their mutual displacement. This is consistent with the clinical results reported in the literature. O'Driscol [14] analyzed the clinical outcomes of humerus fractures and concluded that the parallel plate arrangement provided better fracture stabilization than the perpendicular configuration. Jung et al. [17] pointed out that it is possible to use the triangular stabilization technique for two-column reconstruction only with the use of parallel plates. This method ensures a mechanical connection between the lateral and the medial columns through the trochlea. This is described as effective and reliable in the treatment of intra-articular fractures of the distal humerus. This technique should increase the chance to obtain adequate stabilization in both the trochlea region and the medial and lateral columns. However, as mentioned earlier, based on the presented results, even parallel plating is not able to guarantee bone union when the elbow joint is loaded whilst close to full flexion, especially for the lateral column (ROI L).

The presented assessment of the bone union conditions was conducted based on the values of permissible stabilization stiffness established by Steiner et al. [29]. It should be noted that the upper limit of IFM calculated this way was equal to 0.5 mm. This value is lower than that obtained in other studies [38,39]. However, it must be emphasized that the calculated limit of IFM results directly from the force value taken into consideration in the research (150 N). In fact, this load can increase significantly during the healing process, for example, as a result of improper rehabilitation or uncontrolled events. Moreover, the presented IFMs in unfavorable cases significantly exceeded the permissible values, especially in the case of their tangential components (Figure 7), reaching the level of 1.05–1.60 mm. This makes the risk of non-union very high. This effect especially occurs in cases where the fracture plane is approximately parallel to the plane of the load action, which makes it easy for bone fragments to slide against each other. In this context, all fracture gaps extending along the sagittal plane should be treated as particularly unfavorable.

Based on the presented results, we recommend that in the period before bone union, full flexion of the elbow joint should not be allowed, unless this movement is performed passively. When using a perpendicular plate configuration (especially the posteromedial version), an even wider range motion in the elbow joint should be restricted. This result can be correlated with the commonly observed complication of the elbow joint having a limited range of motion after fracture healing, usually limited to the range of 99° [15] to 110° [7]. The fear of fracture destabilization and necessity of reoperation likely lead to a preventive limitation of motion in the early stages of the treatment. However, movement is essential for the success of the final treatment since the elbow is intolerant to immobilization [11–13]. The presented analysis results show that active flexion/extension can be safe even when lifting a 1 kg weight, provided that appropriate rules are followed. When a parallel plate configuration is used, elbow flexion/extension should be limited to the range of 0–90 degrees. However, even such limited movement can be beneficial during early rehabilitation since muscle strength returns faster and the range of motion returns earlier when weight training is applied. A perpendicular configuration allows for early rehabilitation with the use of external loads in a more limited range of motion, with a flexion/extension angle in the range of 0–30°. This knowledge can result in the modification of rehabilitation protocols, allowing for the earlier application of external loads, which can be positive in view of clinical treatment results. In addition, a wider range of motion greater than the presented limits is still possible, but should be performed without any external load.

This study has several limitations which need to be acknowledged. A constant value for the elbow force was used for various flexion angles, whilst the joint reaction varies during flexion/extension. Varus/valgus loadings were also neglected. Bone screws were modeled as fully bonded to both the plate and the bone tissue, disregarding the risk of screws loosening. The analyses were limited to the chosen method of screw placement. In clinical practice, the surgeon may use other lengths, numbers, and placements of screws, which can change the stiffness of the bone fragment fixation. The present analysis correspond to the early stage of fracture healing when no union between bone fragments is present and with the specific implants configurations that have been described in our manuscript. The research concept was focused on finding the weak points of particular plate configurations rather than proving the reliability of bone fusion in other cases.

5. Conclusions

The assessment of the mutual displacement of bone fragments made it possible to find the weak point of particular plate configurations. The main conclusions are as follows:

(1) No plating configuration is able to ensure DHF union when the full range of motion in the elbow (0–145°) is allowed while holding a weight of 1 kg in the hand.
(2) Elbow flexion in the range of 0–90°, lifting a weight of 1 kg, is allowed when using parallel plating, which is a positive finding in view of early rehabilitation.
(3) Better conditions for fracture healing are ensured when parallel plating is used. Worse conditions occur when perpendicular plating is used, especially the posteromedial version. In this case, the active elbow flexion should be limited to about 30°.

Supplementary Materials: The following supporting information can be downloaded at: https://www.mdpi.com/article/10.3390/jcm13041034/s1, Table S1: Mutual displacements of bone blocks in the fractured distal humerus.

Author Contributions: Conceptualization, A.K., K.K. and S.P.; methodology, S.P. and P.P.; software, A.K.; validation, A.K., S.P. and P.C.; formal analysis, P.P. and S.P.; investigation, A.K., S.P., P.P., P.C. and K.K.; resources, S.P.; data curation, A.K.; writing—original draft preparation, A.K.; writing—review and editing, S.P.; visualization, A.K.; supervision, S.P.; project administration, S.P.; funding acquisition, S.P. and P.P. All authors have read and agreed to the published version of the manuscript.

Funding: This research was funded by the Polish Ministry of Science and Higher Education as a part of project WI/WM-IIB/5/2023.

Institutional Review Board Statement: Not applicable.

Informed Consent Statement: Not applicable.

Data Availability Statement: The datasets generated during and/or analyzed during the current study are available from the corresponding author on reasonable request.

Conflicts of Interest: The authors declare no conflicts of interest.

References

1. Court-Brown, C.M.; Clement, N.D.; Duckworth, A.D.; Biant, L.C.; McQueen, M.M. The changing epidemiology of fall-related fractures in adults. *Injury* **2017**, *48*, 819–824. [CrossRef]
2. Bergdahl, C.; Ekholm, C.; Wennergren, D.; Nilsson, F.; Möller, M. Epidemiology and patho-anatomical pattern of 2,011 humeral fractures: Data from the Swedish Fracture Register. *BMC Musculoskelet. Disord.* **2016**, *17*, 159. [CrossRef]
3. Claessen, F.M.A.P.; Braun, Y.; van Leeuwen, W.F.; Dyer, G.S.; van den Bekerom, M.P.J.; Ring, D. What factors are associated with a surgical site infection after operative treatment of an elbow fracture? *Clin. Orthop. Relat. Res.* **2016**, *474*, 562–570. [CrossRef] [PubMed]
4. Goel, D.P.; Pike, J.M.; Athwal, G.S. Open reduction and internal fixation of distal humerus fractures. *Oper. Tech. Orthop.* **2010**, *20*, 24–33. [CrossRef]
5. Steinitz, A.; Sailer, J.; Rikli, D. Distal humerus fractures: A review of current therapy concepts. *Curr. Rev. Musculoskelet. Med.* **2016**, *9*, 199–206.

6. Rueadi, T.P.; Murphy, W.E. *AO Principle of Fracture Management*; AO Publishing Switzerland: Davos, Switzerland, 2009. [CrossRef]
7. Yetter, T.R.; Weatherby, P.J.; Somerson, J.S. Complications of articular distal humeral fracture fixation: A systematic review and meta-analysis. *J. Shoulder Elb. Surg.* **2021**, *30*, 1957–1967. [CrossRef] [PubMed]
8. Han, S.H.; Park, J.S.; Baek, J.H.; Kim, S.; Ku, K.H. Complications associated with open reduction and internal fixation for adult distal humerus fractures: A multicenter retrospective study. *J. Orthop. Surg. Res.* **2022**, *17*, 399. [CrossRef] [PubMed]
9. Patel, S.S.; Mir, H.R.; Horowitz, E.; Smith, C.; Ahmed, A.S.; Downes, K.; Nydick, J.A. ORIF of distal humerus fractures with modern pre-contoured implants is still associated with a high rate of complications. *Indian J. Orthop.* **2022**, *54*, 570–579. [CrossRef] [PubMed]
10. Vauclair, F.; Goetti, P.; Nguyen, N.T.; Sanchez-Sotelo, J. Distal humerus nonunion: Evaluation and management. *EFORT Open Rev.* **2020**, *5*, 289–298. [CrossRef]
11. Leung, B.; McKee, M.; Peach, C.; Matthews, T.; Arnander, M.; Moverley, R.; Murphy, R.; Phadnis, J. Elbow arthroplasty is safe for the management of simple open distal humeral fractures. *J. Shoulder Elb. Surg.* **2022**, *31*, 1005–1014. [CrossRef]
12. Ku, K.H.; Baek, J.H.; Kim, M.S. Risk Factors for Non-Union after Open Reduction and Internal Fixation in Patients with Distal Humerus Fractures. *J. Clin. Med.* **2022**, *11*, 2679. [CrossRef]
13. Savvidou, O.D.; Zampeli, F.; Koutsouradis, P.; Chloros, G.D.; Kaspiris, A.; Sourmelis, S.; Papagelopoulos, P.J. Complications of open reduction and internal fixation of distal humerus fractures. *EFORT Open Rev.* **2018**, *3*, 558–567. [CrossRef]
14. O'Driscoll, S.W. Optimizing stability in distal humeral fracture fixation. *J. Shoulder Elb. Surg.* **2005**, *14*, S186–S194. [CrossRef]
15. Sanchez-Sotelo, J.; Torchia, M.E.; O'Driscoll, S.W. Complex distal humeral fractures: Internal fixation with a principle-based parallel-plate technique. *J. Bone Joint Surg. Am.* **2008**, *90*, 31–46. [CrossRef] [PubMed]
16. Got, C.; Shuck, J.; Biercevicz, A.; Paller, D.; Mulcahey, M.; Zimmermann, M.; Blaine, T.; Green, A. Biomechanical comparison of parallel versus 90-90 plating of bicolumn distal humerus fractures with intra-articular comminution. *J. Hand Surg. Am.* **2012**, *37*, 2512–2518. [CrossRef] [PubMed]
17. Jung, S.W.; Kang, S.H.; Jeong, M.; Lim, H.S. Triangular fixation technique for bicolumn restoration in treatment of distal humerus intercondylar fracture. *Clin. Orthop. Surg.* **2016**, *8*, 9–18. [CrossRef] [PubMed]
18. Penzkofer, R.; Hungerer, S.; Wipf, F.; Oldenburg, G.; Augat, P. Anatomical plate configuration affects mechanical performance in distal humerus fracture. *Clin. Biomech.* **2010**, *25*, 972–978. [CrossRef] [PubMed]
19. Schwartz, A.; Oka, R.; Odell, T.; Mahar, A. Biomechanical comparison of two different periarticular plating systems for stabilization of complex distal humerus fracture. *Clin. Biomech.* **2006**, *21*, 950–955. [CrossRef] [PubMed]
20. Arnander, M.W.; Reeves, A.; MacLeod, I.A.; Pinto, T.M.; Khaleel, A.A. Biomechanical comparison of plate configuration in distal humerus fractures. *J. Orthop. Trauma* **2008**, *22*, 332–336. [CrossRef] [PubMed]
21. Zalavras, C.G.; Papasoulis, E. Intra-articular fractures of the distal humerus-a review of the current practice. *Int. Orthop.* **2018**, *42*, 2653–2662. [CrossRef]
22. Koonce, R.C.; Baldini, T.H.; Morgan, S.J. Are conventional reconstruction plates equivalent to precontoured locking plates for distal humerus fracture fixation? A biomechanics cadaver study. *Clin. Biomech.* **2012**, *27*, 697–701. [CrossRef] [PubMed]
23. Shin, S.J.; Sohn, H.S.; Do, N.H. A clinical comparison of two different double plating methods for intraarticular distal humerus fracture. *J. Shoulder Elb. Surg.* **2010**, *19*, 2–9. [CrossRef] [PubMed]
24. Puchwein, P.; Wildburger, R.; Archan, S.; Guschla, M.; Tanzer, K.; Gumpert, R. Outcome of type C (AO) distal humeral fractures: Follow-up of 22 patients with bicolumnar plating osteosynthesis. *J. Shoulder Elb. Surg.* **2011**, *20*, 631–636. [CrossRef]
25. Reising, K.; Hauschild, O.; Strohm, P.C.; Suedkamp, N.P. Stabilization of articular fractures of the distal humerus: Early experience with a novel perpendicular plate system. *Injury* **2009**, *40*, 611–617. [CrossRef]
26. Schmidt-Horlohe, K.H.; Bonk, A.; Wilde, P.; Becker, L.; Hoffmann, R. Promising results after a treatment of simple and complex distal humerus type C fractures by angular-stable double-plate osteosynthesis. *J. Orthop. Trauma* **2013**, *99*, 531–541. [CrossRef]
27. Varady, P.; Rüden, C.; Greinwald, M.; Hungerer, S.; Pätzold, R.; Augat, P. Biomechanical comparison of anatomical plating systems for comminuted distal humeral fractures. *Int. Orthop.* **2017**, *41*, 1709–1714. [CrossRef]
28. Zha, Y.; Hua, K.; Huan, Y.; Chen, C.; Sun, W.; Ji, S.; Xiao, D.; Gong, M.; Jiang, X. Biomechanical comparison of three internal fixation configurations for low transcondylar fractures of the distal humerus. *Injury* **2023**, *54*, 362–369. [CrossRef] [PubMed]
29. Steiner, M.; Claes, L.; Ignatius, A.; Simon, U.; Wehner, T. Numerical Simulation of Callus Healing for Optimization of Fracture Fixation Stiffness. *PLoS ONE* **2014**, *9*, e101370. [CrossRef]
30. Jupiter, J.B.; Mehne, D.K. Fractures of the distal humerus. *Orthopedics* **1992**, *15*, 825–833. [CrossRef]
31. Kincaid, B.L.; An, K.N. Elbow joint biomechanics for preclinical evaluation of total elbow prosthese. *J. Biomech.* **2013**, *46*, 2331–2341. [CrossRef]
32. Sawbones. Available online: https://www.sawbones.com/catalog/biomechanical.html?cat=72_composite-bones (accessed on 1 May 2023).
33. Claes, L.; Meyers, N.; Schülke, J.; Reitmaier, S.; Klose, S.; Ignatius, A. The mode of interfragmentary movement affects bone formation and revascularization after callus distraction. *PLoS ONE* **2018**, *13*, e0202702. [CrossRef] [PubMed]
34. Augat, P.; Hollensteiner, M.; von Rüdenb, C. The role of mechanical stimulation in the enhancement of bone healing. *Injury* **2021**, *52*, S78–S83. [CrossRef] [PubMed]
35. Luciani, A.M.; Baylor, J.; Akoon, A.; Grandizio, L.C. Controversies in the Management of Bicolumnar Fractures of the Distal Humerus. *J. Hand Surg.* **2023**, *48*, 177–186. [CrossRef] [PubMed]

36. Helfet, D.L.; Kloen, P.; Anand, N.; Rosen, H.S. Open reduction and internal fixation of delayed unions and nonunions of fractures of the distal part of the humerus. *J. Bone Joint Surg.* **2003**, *85*, 33–40. [CrossRef]
37. Ring, D.; Jupiter, J.B. Fracture–dislocation of the elbow. *Hand Clin.* **2002**, *18*, 55–63. [CrossRef]
38. Ferrara, F.; Biancardi, E.; Touloupakis, G.; Bibiano, L.; Ghirardelli, S.; Antonini, G.; Crippa, C. Residual interfragmentary gap after intramedullary nailing of fragility fractures of the humeral diaphysis: Short and midterm term results. *Acta Biomed.* **2019**, *90*, 432–438.
39. Baltov, A.; Mihail, R.; Dian, E. Complications after interlocking intramedullary nailing of humeral shaft fractures. *Injury* **2014**, *45* (Suppl. S1), S9–S15. [CrossRef]

Disclaimer/Publisher's Note: The statements, opinions and data contained in all publications are solely those of the individual author(s) and contributor(s) and not of MDPI and/or the editor(s). MDPI and/or the editor(s) disclaim responsibility for any injury to people or property resulting from any ideas, methods, instructions or products referred to in the content.

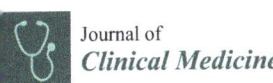

Article

Long-Term Outcomes Following Single-Stage Reamed Intramedullary Exchange Nailing in Apparently Aseptic Femoral Shaft Nonunion with Unsuspected Proof of Bacteria

Simon Hackl [1,2,*], Christian von Rüden [2,3,†], Katharina Trenkwalder [2,4], Lena Keppler [1], Christian Hierholzer [5] and Mario Perl [6,†]

1. Department of Trauma Surgery, BG Unfallklinik Murnau, 82418 Murnau, Germany
2. Institute for Biomechanics, Paracelsus Medical University, 5020 Salzburg, Austria
3. Department of Trauma Surgery, Orthopedics and Hand Surgery, Weiden Medical Center, 92637 Weiden, Germany
4. Institute for Biomechanics, BG Unfallklinik Murnau, 82418 Murnau, Germany
5. Department of Trauma Surgery, University Hospital Zurich, 8091 Zurich, Switzerland
6. Department of Trauma and Orthopedic Surgery, University Hospital Erlangen, Friedrich-Alexander University Erlangen-Nürnberg, 91054 Erlangen, Germany
* Correspondence: simon.hackl@bgu-murnau.de; Tel.: +49-8841-480
† These authors contributed equally to this work.

Citation: Hackl, S.; von Rüden, C.; Trenkwalder, K.; Keppler, L.; Hierholzer, C.; Perl, M. Long-Term Outcomes Following Single-Stage Reamed Intramedullary Exchange Nailing in Apparently Aseptic Femoral Shaft Nonunion with Unsuspected Proof of Bacteria. *J. Clin. Med.* **2024**, *13*, 1414. https://doi.org/10.3390/jcm13051414

Academic Editor: Frank Schildberg

Received: 14 February 2024
Revised: 25 February 2024
Accepted: 27 February 2024
Published: 29 February 2024

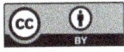

Copyright: © 2024 by the authors. Licensee MDPI, Basel, Switzerland. This article is an open access article distributed under the terms and conditions of the Creative Commons Attribution (CC BY) license (https://creativecommons.org/licenses/by/4.0/).

Abstract: Background: The aim of this study was to evaluate detection rates and risk factors for unsuspected proof of bacteria, as well as clinical and radiologic outcomes following femoral shaft nonunion without clinical signs of infection treated by a single-stage surgical revision procedure including reamed intramedullary exchange nailing. **Methods:** A retrospective cohort study was performed in a European level I trauma center between January 2015 and December 2022. Fifty-eight patients were included who underwent reamed intramedullary exchange nailing as a single-step procedure for surgical revision of posttraumatic diaphyseal femoral nonunion without any indications of infection in medical history and without clinical signs of local infection. Clinical details of the patients were analyzed and functional and radiologic long-term outcomes were determined. **Results:** In all patients, with and without proof of bacteria osseous, healing could be observed. The physical component summary of the SF-12 demonstrated significantly better results at least one year after the final surgical revision in case of a negative bacterial culture during exchange nailing. **Conclusions:** Clinical long-term outcomes demonstrated a trend towards better results following femoral shaft nonunion revision if there was no evidence for the presence of low-grade infected nonunion. In this case, a single-stage surgical procedure may be recommended.

Keywords: femur; fracture nonunion; outcome; septic; low-grade infection; intramedullary nail; SF-12; lower extremity functional scale (LEFS)

1. Introduction

Despite the ongoing development and optimization of surgical techniques and implants, impaired bone healing remains a challenging problem in fracture treatment, which is combined with a burden for the individual patient due to ongoing pain, as well as for society due to an enormous socioeconomic impact, such as therapy costs or productivity losses caused by relatively long treatment duration [1–5]. The reported prevalence of diaphyseal delayed union or nonunion of the femur reached up to 12.5%, mainly depending on the type of fracture stabilization [6,7]. It is a common consensus that the pathogenesis of nonunion is multifactorial and may be influenced, for example, by mechanical, metabolic and endocrine factors, as well as special medication such as non-steroidal anti-inflammatory drugs or the fracture pattern such as shaft fractures and the patient's age [1,8–12]. In addition, the occurrence of infection at the fracture site is of significant importance in the pathogenesis of nonunion [13]. Despite the eye-catching appearance and the quite obvious diagnosis of an acute infection, chronic infection often could be characterized by a lack of clinical and laboratory signs of infection and is usually limited to the zone of the osseous lesion. Chronic infection also includes low-grade infection, which is mainly caused by low-virulence organisms with the ability of biofilm formation [14–17]. Thus, the development of nonunion could be the only symptom of low-grade infection. The diagnosis of low-grade infection is therefore much more difficult than that of acute infection. Microbiological and histological analyses of tissue samples collected from the nonunion area are the only appropriate way to differentiate between aseptic and septic nonunion caused by low-grade infection [18,19]. This is more critical since the treatment concepts and the surgical management of aseptic and septic nonunion are almost opposite: Reamed intramedullary exchange nailing as a single-step procedure is the treatment of choice for aseptic diaphyseal nonunion of the femur and is combined with a high rate of osseous union [20–22]. In the case of septic nonunion, the treatment concept is in accordance with the therapy principles of chronic fracture-related infection and involves a multi-step procedure, including debridement with removal of the implant and eradication of infection combined with antimicrobial therapy, subsequent revision osteosynthesis and reconstruction of the bone and soft tissue defect is performed [23–28]. Considering that the occurrence of low-grade infection is associated with the absence of clinical signs of infection, surgical revision of these cases is mainly performed as a single-step procedure without focusing on an accurate debridement, as it would be recommended in case of fracture-related infection since septic nonunion has not been recognized primarily [29]. Currently, the clinical impact of low-grade infection as an underlying cause of femoral shaft nonunion in regard to the surgical revision is unclear. Thus, the aim of this study was to evaluate detection rates and risk factors for unsuspected proof of bacteria, as well as the clinical and radiologic long-term outcome in a patient cohort with femoral shaft nonunion without clinical signs of acute infection who underwent single-stage surgical revision procedure with reamed intramedullary exchange nailing. Therefore, clinical details of the patients, as well as preoperative C-reactive protein (CRP) and white blood cell (WBC) counts, were analyzed, and functional and radiologic long-term outcomes were determined.

2. Materials and Methods

A retrospective cohort study was performed in a European level I trauma center between January 2015 and December 2022. Fifty-eight patients were included who underwent reamed intramedullary exchange nailing as a single-step procedure for surgical revision of posttraumatic diaphyseal femoral nonunion without any indications for infection in medical history and without clinical signs of local infection, including pain at rest, redness, local hyperthermia, fever, persistent wound secretion and a sinus tract. If even a single parameter indicated a possible underlying infection, the patient was excluded from the study. In addition, patients treated with a surgical technique other than intramedullary nailing of a femoral shaft fracture were excluded from the study (Figure 1).

Clinical details of the patients are displayed in Table 1.

Table 1. Patients' data overview. Values are presented as mean standard deviation or as total number of patients.

Parameter	Number
Gender	
Male	45
Female	13
Age	46.3 ± 2.1 (range 18–81) years
Fracture location	
Proximal part of the femoral shaft	19
Middle part of the femoral shaft	27
Distal part of the femoral shaft	12

Table 1. Cont.

Parameter	Number
Fracture pattern according to the AO/OTA classification [1]	
Type A1	16
Type A2	17
Type A3	7
Type B1	3
Type B2	5
Type B3	3
Type C1	1
Type C2	3
Type C3	3
Initial soft tissue injury	
Closed fracture	50
Gustilo–Anderson open fracture classification I–III	8
Nonunion type	
Hypertrophic	40
Atrophic/Oligotrophic	18
Comorbidities	
Charlson comorbidity index	0.3 ± 0.1 (range 0–3) points
Nicotine abuse	12
Diabetes mellitus	6
Period of time between initial fracture fixation and nonunion revision	11.2 ± 1.0 (range 4–32) months

[1] AO Foundation/Orthopaedic Trauma Association.

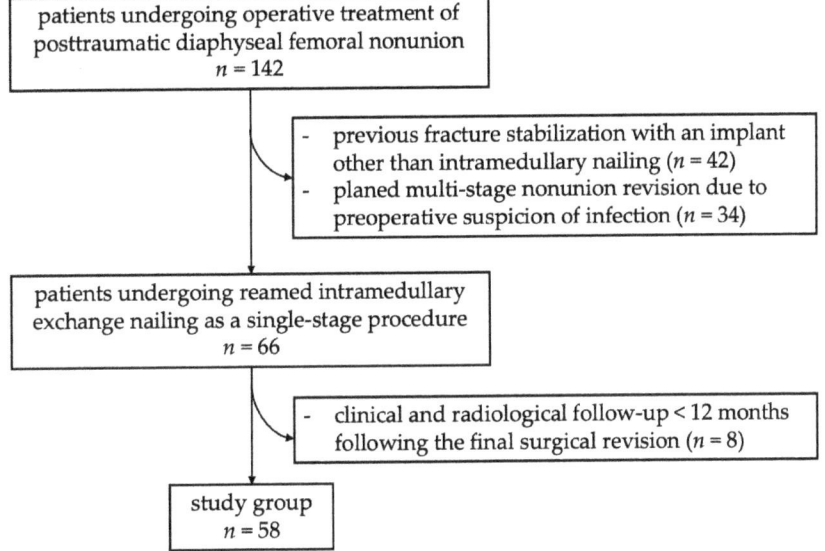

Figure 1. Overview of patients' inclusion process.

For the classification of the initial type of fracture, the AO/OTA classification was utilized. In the case of open fracture, the Gustilo–Anderson classification was used additionally [30]. The Carlson comorbidity index was used to objectify the morbidity of the study group [31]. Nonunion was defined clinically and radiologically after at least 6 months of missing osseous union during initial fracture treatment [32]. In 11 cases, diagnosis of nonunion was already made after 4 to 6 months due to a clear loss in progression of bone healing in regard to the current definition of the European Society of Tissue Regeneration in Orthopedics and Traumatology (ESTROT) [21,33]. Clinical signs of nonunion contained persistent instability in the fracture zone or inability to perform full weight bearing without pain. Radiographic evidence of nonunion was defined as the absence of osseous bridging in at least three of the four cortices as assessed on the antero-posterior and lateral views of conventional radiographs [34]. Whenever conventional radiographs were not conclusive enough to determine the diagnosis of nonunion, a computed tomography (CT) scan of the bony lesion was performed to clarify the presence of nonunion. Diagnosis of low-grade infection was made if at least two out of all four samples harvested during the surgical procedure demonstrated growth of bacteria in microbiological analysis and if clinical suggestive criteria for infection were missing [35].

2.1. Surgical Procedure

Surgical revision of diaphyseal femoral nonunion was performed in a standard manner and according to the diamond concept [36]. A preoperative single-shot microbiological prophylaxis using 1.5 g of cefuroxime was administered 30 min prior to the beginning of the surgical revision procedure. If contraindications concerning allergies existed, intravenous application of clindamycin was used. The patient was placed in a lateral position on a radiolucent operating table. The standard surgical procedure for diaphyseal femoral nonunion revision included the removal of the intramedullary nail used for initial fracture stabilization. Thereupon, a tissue sample on a dry swab (MASTASWAB, Mast Group Ltd., Bootle, UK), which was circulated 5 to 6 times around the part of the implant that had contact with the nonunion was gained for microbiological diagnostics. In the next step, a guide wire slightly bent at its tip was inserted into the femoral intramedullary canal and precisely positioned in the center–center position of the intercondylar region assessed by biplanar radiologic views. Then, stepwise reaming was carried out with the aim of osteogenic stimulus, as well as improving mechanical properties by inserting an intramedullary exchange nail with a larger diameter of at least 2 mm compared to the previous nail, plus a good cortical contact in the isthmus region and further microbiological diagnostics was performed using the initial graft material gained from intramedullary reaming [21,37,38]. For this purpose, one tissue sample with a swab that was circulated 5 to 6 times directly around the reaming graft material, and two tissue samples, each measuring at least 0.5 cm^3 of the reaming graft material, were harvested [19]. In summary, four samples were obtained for microbiological diagnostics consisting of one tissue sample on a swab from the interface between the implant and nonunion and one tissue sample on a swab, as well as two tissue samples from the reaming graft material [39]. After ensuring that no gap or dehiscence was left at the fracture site, a T2 femur nail (Stryker Co., Ltd., Kalamazoo, MI, USA) with the option of interfragmentary compression was inserted to its correct position and the guide wire was removed. Then, distal interlocking screws were inserted and the femoral torsion was assessed: The femoral condyles were imaged in a lateral view with a precise projection of both condyles. The c-arm X-ray machine was then adjusted and moved in a strictly parallel direction until it was centered over the region of the femoral head. If the projection of the femoral head was anterior to the axis of the femoral shaft at two-thirds of its circumference, the femoral torsion was considered acceptable [40]. After compression was applied to the nonunion site, proximal interlocking was performed. Postoperatively, patients received physiotherapy with permitted weight bearing as tolerated. If low-grade infection—defined by at least two out of four samples demonstrating bacterial growth and without clinical indications for infection—was observed, test-specific and calculated antimicrobial medication was applied for at least six weeks after nonunion revision without any further surgical interventions. In case of postoperative clinical and laboratory signs of infection, removal of the intramedullary nail and a two- or multi-staged surgical procedure for eradication of infection was started [16].

2.2. Diagnostic Procedure

The tissue samples harvested on dry swabs during nonunion revision were immediately placed in the sterile swab container filled with protective Amies agar gel medium and were directly transferred to the on-site microbiological laboratory. These tissue samples were streaked out on Columbia agar with 5% sheep blood (bioMérieux, Hazelwood, MO, USA), Chocolat agar (PolyViteX, bioMérieux, Hazelwood, MO, USA), MacConkey agar (bioMérieux, Hazelwood, MO, USA) and thioglycolate broth (bioMérieux, Hazelwood, MO, USA). Samples were incubated in 5% CO_2, as well as under anaerobic conditions at 37° Celsius for 48 h (short-term culturing). Morphologically distinct colony types were identified using a Vitek2 machine (bioMérieux Vitek Inc., Hazelwood, MO, USA) by MALDI-TOF mass spectrometry.

The tissue samples collected from the reaming graft material were directly inserted into a sterile containment prefilled with 9 mL of thioglycolate broth (bioMérieux, Hazelwood, MO, USA) and were immediately transferred to the on-site microbiological laboratory. After incubation in 5% CO_2, as well as under anaerobic conditions at 37° Celsius for at least 14 days (long-term culturing), the suspension was additionally streaked out on Columbia agar with 5% sheep blood (bioMérieux, Hazelwood, MO, USA). Morphologically distinct colony types were identified as analogous to short-term culturing.

Laboratory values for systemic inflammation consisting of CRP concentrations and WBC counts were determined. These parameters were measured in peripheral blood samples drawn at the time point of hospital admission no more than two days before surgical nonunion revision [41]. Quantifications were performed by the institutional hematological laboratory during the regular preoperative diagnostic workup. The limit of determination for CRP concentration was <0.4 mg/dL and the cut-off value was determined at 1.0 mg/dL.

2.3. Follow-Up

After being discharged from the hospital, patients were clinically and radiologically followed up in the outpatient department at regular intervals: 6 weeks, 3 months, 6 months, and at least 1 year after the final surgical revision. The patients' objective and subjective health status was assessed using the 12-item Short Form Survey (SF-12), which includes the mental component summary (MCS) and the physical component summary (PCS), as well as the Lower Extremity Functional Score (LEFS) [42,43].

2.4. Statistical Analysis and Ethical Standards

Statistical analysis was performed using IBM SPSS® Statistics 26.0 for Windows (IBM Co., Ltd., Armonk, New York, NY, USA). The results of this study are presented as mean values ± standard deviation (SD) or median. Significance was statistically calculated based on the Mann–Whitney U test and Fisher's exact test. Results were considered to be statistically significant with p-values < 0.05. G*Power 3.1 for Windows [44] was used to estimate the sample size. In regard to previous studies that compared the PCS of the SF-12 between femoral nonunion and normative group effect sizes (d) could be determined, which were between 1.35 and 2.55 [45–47]. Assuming the most unfavorable effect size (d) of 1.35, a sufficient power of 80% can be achieved with a sample size of 20 subjects and a probability of error (α) of 0.05. Written informed consent was given by all individuals participating in this study. The procedures involving human participants were in accordance with the bioethical standards of the institutional and national research committee (Bavarian Chamber of Physicians, ID 2017-162) and with the 1964 Helsinki Declaration and its following amendments.

3. Results

3.1. Rate of Low-Grade Infection in Femoral Shaft Nonunion

The study cohort consisted of 58 patients with apparently aseptic femoral shaft nonunion. Unsuspected proof of bacteria in at least two samples—followed by diagnosing low-grade infection—could be detected in the samples harvested during single-stage reamed intramedullary exchange nailing: in 10 cases (17%), positive bacterial cultures, meeting our criteria for low-grade infection, were detected following short-term culturing of the swabs and in 25 cases (43%) following long-term culturing of the tissue samples. The prevalence of cultured bacteria is presented in Table 2.

Table 2. Breakdown of organisms cultured.

Organism	Number of Isolates (Total $n = 29$)
Coagulase-negative *Staphylococcus* spp.	
Staphylococcus epidermidis	10
Staphylococcus capitis	3
Staphylococcus lugdunensis	3
Staphylococcus haemolyticus	2
Staphylococcus warneri	2
Staphylococcus hominis	1
Staphylococcus aureus	1
Streptococcus alactolyticus	1
Enterococcus faecalis	2
Pseudomonas aeruginosa	1
Pseudomonas fluorescenses	1
Cutibacterium acnes	2

In 21 patients, a single organism was isolated from tissue samples harvested during intramedullary exchange nailing, whereas in 4 patients, a mixed culture with two different bacteria was detected. Only one polymicrobial culture was associated with an open fracture. Bacterial cultures remained negative in 48 cases (83%) following short-term culturing, whereas after long-term culturing, only 33 patients (57%) with apparently aseptic femoral shaft nonunion still had negative bacterial cultures.

The patient group with at least two surprising positive bacterial cultures with the same pathogen and no preoperative clinical signs of infection (group P) consisted of 21 male and 4 female patients with a mean age of 42.8 ± 3.3 (range 18–74) years. The group without proof of bacteria (group N) was composed of 24 male and 9 female patients with a mean age of 48.9 ± 2.8 (range 21–81) years ($p = 0.162$). The time internal between initial traumatic fracture treatment and surgical nonunion revision was 11.1 ± 1.6 (range 4–32; median 10) months in group P versus 11.2 ± 1.2 (range 4–25; median 8) months in group N ($p = 0.951$).

3.2. Evaluation of Risk Factors for the Occurrence of Positive Bacterial Cultures and/or Nonunion

In analyzing potential risk factors for the occurrence of positive bacterial cultures and/or nonunion, there was no statistical difference between both groups regarding the following parameters: Nicotine abuse was documented in eight cases in group P and in four cases in group N ($p = 0.064$). Three patients both in group P and group N were suffering from diabetes mellitus ($p = 0.523$). In addition, the Charlson comorbidity index was 0.32 ± 0.14 points in group P and 0.36 ± 0.14 points in group N ($p = 0.831$). In 20 of the 58 patients analyzed, a documented and anamnestic use of non-steroidal anti-inflammatory drugs could be observed, whereas in group P seven cases and in group N thirteen cases were recorded ($p = 0.569$). Regarding injury, as well as nonunion-related factors for the occurrence of positive bacterial cultures, despite a tendency with regard to the complexity of fracture pattern, only a significant difference could be found in regard to open soft tissue injuries. However, due to the small number of cases in this subgroup analysis, the relevance for clinical practice has to be used with caution (Table 3).

Table 3. Evaluation of injury-related risk factors for the occurrence of positive bacterial cultures and/or nonunion. Values are presented as total number of patients.

Parameter	Group P (Positive Cultures)	Group N (Negative Cultures)	p-Value
Fracture location			
Proximal part of the femoral shaft	7	12	
Middle part of the femoral shaft	11	16	
Distal part of the femoral shaft	7	5	0.472
Fracture pattern according to the AO/OTA classification			
Type A	19	21	
Type B	1	10	
Type C	5	2	0.068
Initial soft tissue injury			
Closed fracture	19	31	
Gustilo–Anderson open fracture I–III	6	2	0.045
Nonunion type			
Hypertrophic	15	25	
Atrophic/Oligotrophic	10	8	0.199

3.3. Preoperative Systemic Inflammation Markers

Patients in group P demonstrated a mean concentration of the preoperative CRP of 1.4 ± 0.3 (range 0.4–5.9; median 0.8) mg/dL and patients in group N of 0.8 ± 0.1 (range 0.4–3.3; median 0.4) mg/dL ($p = 0.095$). Considering patients with CRP levels above the cut-off value of 1.0 mg/dL, with 9 cases each in both groups, no statistically significant difference could be observed there, too ($p = 0.477$). Preoperative values for WBC of 8.0 ± 0.4 (range 4.6–12.4; median 8.1)/nL in group P and of 7.4 ± 0.4 (range 3.1–11.3; median 7.0)/nL in group N did not show a statistic significant difference ($p = 0.249$). In addition, the potential diagnostic efficiency of CRP level was analyzed by the receiver operating characteristic (ROC) curve with an area under the curve (AUC) of 0.591 (Figure 2).

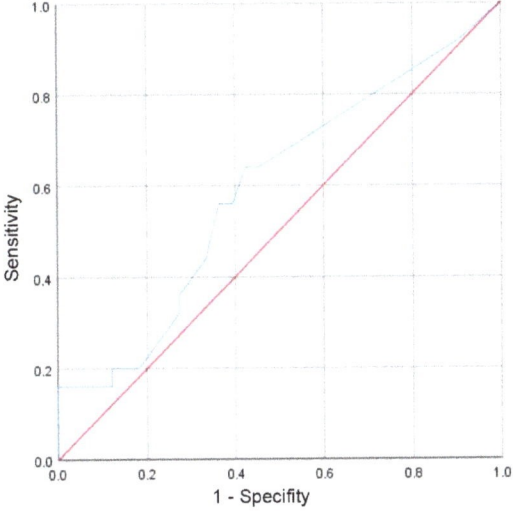

Figure 2. ROC curve of preoperative CRP values for diagnosis of positive bacterial culture. AUC = 0.591 (95% CI [0.441, 0.741]). Best possible cut-off value at CRP level of 0.6 mg/dL resulting in a sensitivity of 64% and a specificity of 58% (blue line: CRP; red line: reference line).

A Youden index calculation demonstrated the best possible cut-off value at a CRP level of 0.6 mg/dL with a sensitivity of 64% and a specificity of 58%, demonstrating that no clinically relevant cut-off value could be observed in this patient cohort. With an AUC of 0.563 and the best possible cut-off value at a WBC level of 7.3/nL (sensitivity: 67%; specificity: 55%), this inflammatory marker was also not suitable for a clinically relevant prediction.

3.4. Objective and Subjective Outcome

In all patients of both groups, a completed osseous healing could be observed. In group N osseous healing could be detected after 14.0 ± 2.0 (range 2–35; median 12) months and in group P after 15.3 ± 2.0 (range 2–32; median 17) months ($p = 0.651$). After exchange nailing in group N, 27 out of 33 patients (82%) healed without any further intervention, whereas 6 patients needed 1.3 ± 0.2 (range 1–2; median 1) additional surgical procedures to achieve osseous healing. In these patients, the following further procedures were performed: Three patients received a singular dynamization of the intramedullary nail, one patient received a further exchange nailing procedure to a larger diameter combined with bone grafting, and two patients underwent a dynamization of the intramedullary nail due to a lack of osseous healing repeating the exchanging nailing to a larger diameter nail, whereby in one of these two patients additional bone grafting was performed. In contrast, in group P, only 14 out of 25 patients (56%) healed after the exchange nailing procedure. However, none of these patients demonstrated fulminant systemic septic conditions after the exchange nailing procedure. Eleven patients needed 1.8 ± 0.2 (range 1–7; median 1) additional procedures for eradication of infection and achieving osseous healing. Hereby, the patients underwent the following further procedures: Seven patients received a debridement with a further exchange nailing procedure, three patients underwent debridement with the removal of the implant, followed by a further exchange nailing after negative bacterial cultures, and one patient received multiple debridements, followed by a further exchange nailing, due to ongoing delayed osseous healing dynamization of the intramedullary nail. In case of positive bacterial cultures and necessary additional surgical procedures, a collagen matrix loaded with either Gentamycin or Vancomycin was placed intramedullary—if one of these antibiotics was effective against the cultured microorganism. In summary, the different osseous healing rates in group N (82%) and in group P (56%) were statistically different ($p = 0.032$). Regarding the number of patients with additional further interventions, there was no significant difference in the positive bacterial growth that could be already detected after short-term culturing or only after long-term culturing (Figure 3).

In addition, regarding all data harvested, no clinically meaningful parameter could be found that leads to a statistically reliable statement if additional surgical procedures may be necessary following exchange nailing with unsuspected proof of bacteria. An example is provided here: CRP values in group P with additional surgical intervention were 1.5 ± 0.6 (range 0.4–5.9; median 0.6) mg/dl and CRP values in group P without additional surgical intervention were 1.3 ± 0.3 (range 0.4–4.5; median 0.9) mg/dL ($p = 0.789$); nonunion with initial open fractures in group P with additional surgical intervention were three cases and nonunion with initial open fractures in group P without additional surgical intervention were also three cases.

Regarding the objective outcome, represented by the LEFS, no statistically significant difference could be observed after the achievement of osseous healing in both groups. In contrast, the physical component summary of the SF-12, a display for the subjective outcome, demonstrated significantly better results at least one year after the final surgical revision in case of a negative bacterial culture during femur exchange nailing (Table 4).

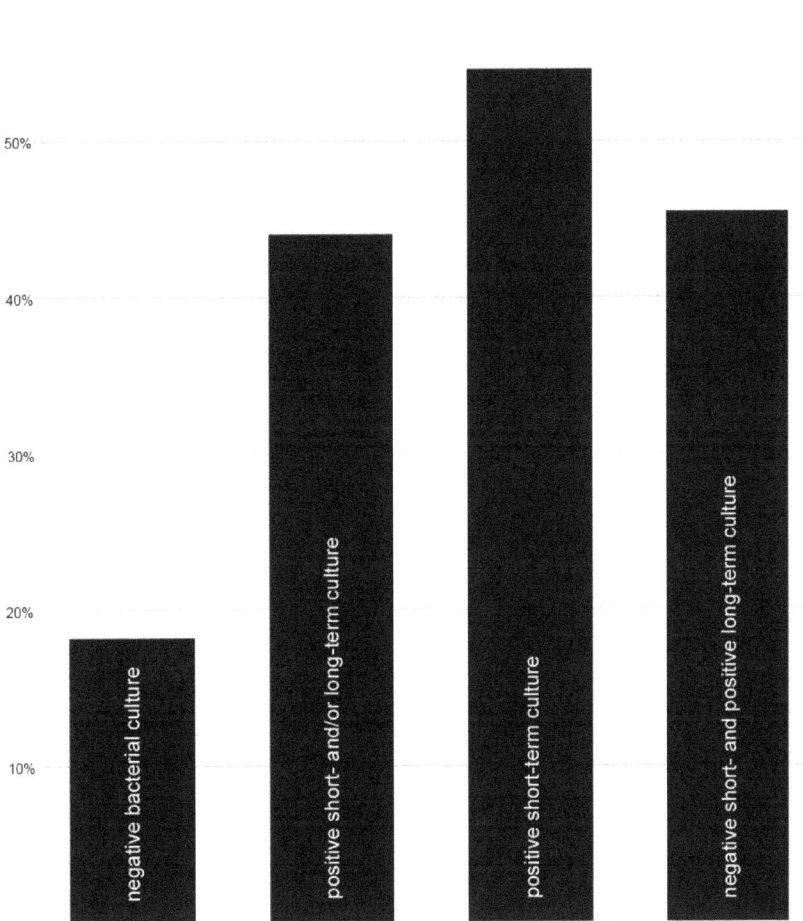

Figure 3. Patients with additional surgical interventions (%). Negative bacterial culture (n = 6 out of group N); positive short- and/or long-term culture (n = 11 out of group P); positive short-term culture (n = 6 out of 11 positive cultures); negative short- and positive long-term culture (n = 5 out of 11 positive cultures).

Table 4. Overview of the objective and subjective outcome at least one year after exchange nailing procedure. Values are presented as mean standard deviation.

Test Procedure	Group P (Positive Cultures)	Group N (Negative Cultures)	*p*-Value
LEFS	46.0 ± 5.1 points	51.6 ± 5.7 points	0.479
PCS of SF-12	35.6 ± 3.1 points	44.4 ± 2.6 points	0.040
MCS of SF-12	49.5 ± 3.2 points	50.1 ± 2.4 points	0.875

LEFS: best functional outcome with 80 points; SF-12: best possible outcome with 100 points.

Nevertheless, there was no statistically significant difference between patients without any further intervention (PCS of SF-12 42.3 ± 2.3 points) and those with additional surgical interventions (PCS of SF-12 35.9 ± 4.5 points; *p* = 0.205), regardless of whether there was proof of bacteria or not.

4. Discussion

Nonunion is defined as the failure of the bone to unite after the occurrence of a bone lesion that will not heal without further intervention, regardless of the length of treatment [32,48]. Despite the clinical appearance, 43% of the primarily aseptic categorized diaphyseal femur nonunion demonstrated positive bacterial cultures from intraoperative samples harvested during revision surgery, emphasizing the clinical relevance of low-grade infection. Although there are no acute clinical signs of infection, in almost every second patient with detection of bacterial growth additional surgical interventions are needed until osseous healing is reached, in contrast to only 20% of patients with negative bacterial cultures after single-stage reamed intramedullary exchange nailing.

Taking into account the period of time elapsed during nonunion development, it can be assumed that the infection responsible for the development of nonunion might potentially be chronic. Therefore, low-virulent bacteria including a mature biofilm on the fixation material must be assumed, which is in accordance with our findings of 21 coagulase-negative *Staphylococcus* spp. (CoNS) isolated from the total number of 29 bacterial isolates, as well as with other studies [49,50]. Thus, the basic principle in the treatment of chronic fracture-related infection with consistent removal of avital tissue and exchange of fixation material should be applied to septic femoral shaft nonunion [51,52]. Due to the insufficient addressing of the biomechanics that may underlie nonunion, implant retention is not expedient [17]. These principles are basically integrated into the single-stage reamed intramedullary exchange nailing, emphasizing the need to remove the previous osteosynthesis material [53,54] and aim for infection eradication to achieve nonunion healing, in combination with the avoidance of infection recurrence in the sense of chronic osteomyelitis after osseous healing, and, finally, the recovery of a sufficient regaining of function [55]. Nevertheless, the higher number of additional surgical revisions in case of positive bacterial culture necessary until osseous healing demonstrated in this study—44% of the femoral shaft nonunion with and 18% without proof of bacteria—is in accordance with the current multidisciplinary surgical treatment principles for septic diaphyseal femoral nonunion and could be also demonstrated by other studies analyzing nonunion at different locations, observing a revision rate in case of infected nonunion between 6 to 22% [56]. However, it is important to note that the final healing rates are similarly high.

On the other hand, 56% of diaphyseal femoral nonunion with unsuspected proof of bacteria healed after single-stage reamed intramedullary exchange nailing—in addition to test-specific antibiotic therapy—without any further intervention, which is, for example, comparable to diaphyseal tibial nonunion caused by low-grade infection [14]. These findings are in contrast to a study performed by Amorosa et al. analyzing the outcome of a single-stage treatment protocol for presumptive aseptic diaphyseal nonunion—including 87 cases of clavicular, humeral, radial, ulnar, femoral and tibial nonunion within 28.7% of the cases positive bacterial cultures—with a healing rate of 72% in cases of positive bacterial cultures and 93.6% in patients without proof of bacteria. However, no further information was given regarding the microbiological diagnostics, and also patients with at least one positive intraoperative culture were classified as infected [50]. In addition, the definition of nonunion varies widely in the literature, making it even more difficult to compare different studies [32]. Nevertheless, comparable results with a healing rate of 78% in cases of positive bacterial culture in presumed aseptic diaphyseal nonunion could be achieved by a single-stage surgical protocol—including nonunion revisions both with plate and nail fixation—described by Arsoy et al. [49].

In general, sufficient treatment of femoral shaft nonunion is a challenge for every trauma surgeon. The distinction between presumed aseptic and septic nonunion yields an additional complicating component in this regard. A tendency to develop septic nonunion was found with respect to the complexity of the fracture pattern, but the only significant risk factor for infection was an open fracture. This is in line with the known literature [51,57,58]. In addition, regarding all data harvested in the current study, no clinically meaningful parameter could be found that leads to a statistically reliable statement if additional surgical procedures may be necessary following exchange nailing with unsuspected proof of bacteria.

The development of septic nonunion occurs in two ways: On the one hand, an early infection can develop into manifest infectious nonunion if not treated optimally with antimicrobial agents alone. On the other hand, a pathogen of relatively low virulence can cause a low-grade infection. The current study could confirm that the rate of low-grade infection is relevant among femoral shaft nonunion and can be sufficiently detected after long-term culturing. This is in line with other studies demonstrating the importance of long-term culturing in contrast to short-term culturing (Table 5) [59–63].

Table 5. Literature overview of intraoperative germ detection in nonunion revisions in regard to the microbiological diagnostics.

Study	Inclusion Criteria	Number of Patients	Bacterial Detection Rate	
Gille et al. [62]	preoperatively aseptic classified tibial shaft nonunion	23	culturing for 14 days:	0%
Olszewski et al. [59]	nonunion without signs of infection but with risk factors for infection	453	culturing for 5 days:	20%
Dapunt et al. [60]	atrophic nonunion of long bones (32.7% with clinical signs of infection)	49	culturing for 2 days: culturing for 5 days: sonication and culturing for 14 days:	6.8% 10.2% 57.1%
Palmer et al. [61]	nonunion of long bones	34	culturing for 5 days:	23.5%

In addition, in accordance with our study, the rate of septic nonunion in patients with presumed aseptic nonunion is indicated between 0% to 37%. However, patients, regardless of the location of the nonunion and the type of initial fracture stabilization, were included [56]. Thus, it is even more interesting that patients treated by a soft tissue-preserving procedure as intramedullary nailing is assumed, presented such a high rate of positive bacterial cultures. To our knowledge, there are no further studies that provide an explanation for this: Possible reasons for up to 43% of positive bacterial cultures might be either a disturbed skin barrier because of the contusion during the initial trauma, difficulties in the initial fracture stabilization with damage to the soft tissue due to the fact that the majority of the included patients were secondary transferred to our Level I trauma center or a secondary hematogenous colonization of the atrophic nonunion area.

In contrast, a clinically relevant cut-off value for preoperative systemic inflammation markers (C-reactive protein, white blood cell count) could not be observed in the current patient cohort with unsuspected proof of bacteria, which is consistent with a study performed by Wang et al. that laboratory analysis of serum inflammatory markers is not an effective screening method for septic nonunion [64]. Thus, we cannot recommend ruling out the possibility of nonunion-caused low-grade infection preoperatively by a sole consideration of CRP values or WBC.

Next, this study highlighted the objective and subjective long-term clinical outcomes. Interestingly, there was no significant difference regarding the number of patients with additional further interventions following positive bacterial growth detected during short-term culturing compared to those with only positive long-term culturing. Furthermore, clinically meaningful parameters resulting in a statistically reliable statement on whether or not additional surgical procedures are mandatory, following reamed exchange nailing in all cases of septic femoral shaft nonunion with unsuspected proof of bacteria, could not be found. Regarding the objective outcome represented by the LEFS at least one year after the final surgical revision, statistically significant differences were not detected after osseous healing in both groups. These results confirm the available literature [22,65,66]. In contrast, the PCS of SF-12—as a tool for assessing physical functioning and pain—demonstrated a significantly worse outcome in the case of low-grade infection compared to the aseptic femoral shaft nonunion, with the values themselves being comparable to the current literature [67]. The finding is noteworthy because a subsequent surgical intervention does not significantly impact the Physical Component Summary of SF-12. This indicates that low-grade infection alone—even after complete osseous healing of the nonunion—has an effect on the outcome similar to fracture-related infection [68,69], which may be caused by chronic inflammation—although a significant increase in the acute-phase protein CRP was not detected in the current study—and highlights the importance of also addressing low-grade infected nonunion early on to achieve optimal outcomes.

In addition to the multifactorial cause of impaired fracture healing [36], there is also the complicating fact that with the currently available diagnostic methods, the reliable exclusion of germ detection is only possible by intraoperative sample collection—implicating that an additional surgical procedure seems to be necessary to gain samples for microbiology and histology diagnostics before the actual nonunion revision. This is why both the single-stage and the two-stage surgical procedure, including adequate sample collection for microbiological diagnostics in the first step and surgical nonunion revision in the second step, are reported to be sufficient options in the recent literature [70], with previous studies demonstrated that the positive evidence of germs in a single-stage procedure does not generally result in treatment failure [22,51]. Nevertheless, a surgical procedure in septic nonunion differs in part significantly from the surgical revision of an aseptic nonunion, due to the need to address the infection and resultant biofilm formation in addition to the "singular" failure of the bone to unite in aseptic nonunion, which is why the authors propose the following procedure: If the preoperative patient's history, as well as the clinical, laboratory and radiological examination, reveal indications of a possible underlying infectious event, further surgical revision is performed in the sense of a two-stage procedure with surgical specimen collection prior to definitive nonunion revision. Only if there is no indication for the presence of septic nonunion, the single-stage procedure is suggested. In this case, however, empirical antibiotic therapy should be initiated at the end of surgical nonunion revision until complete microbiological and histological diagnostics are obtained, while the frequency of intraoperative bacterial detection is relevant, even in the absence of preoperative signs of infection. In case of low-grade infected nonunion, following chronic fracture-related infection or periprosthetic infection, adjuvant test-appropriate systemic antibiotic therapy should be applied in addition to surgical therapy [71,72]. When a septic femoral shaft nonunion is present, there is no pressure to bring about an immediate definitive surgical treatment solution at any cost. Rather, the greatest possible care should be taken to optimize the patient prior to the surgical revision procedure. The main goal is to identify and treat potential risk factors that could delay or completely compromise nonunion healing.

Limitations of this study inherently include the retrospective study design. To our knowledge, this is one of only a few studies that focused exclusively on femur diaphysis using routine clinical diagnostics to demonstrate that the presence of unexpected evidence of bacteria has a relevant impact on daily clinical practice. The strength of the study is the large number of patients treated by the same surgical team at the same institution using a standardized treatment protocol.

5. Conclusions

The diagnosis of low-grade infection in femoral shaft nonunion remains challenging using routine clinical diagnostics such as preoperative systemic inflammatory markers or common risk factors because, despite an open soft tissue injury, no tools used in daily clinical practice could be identified for diagnosing low-grade infection. This is even more important since a worse subjective outcome in terms of physical function and pain has been observed in the case of low-grade infection—even after complete osseous healing of the femoral shaft nonunion. Furthermore, the probability of additional surgical interventions after the single-step procedure to achieve complete osseous healing is higher in cases of low-grade infected nonunion of the femoral shaft compared to aseptic femoral shaft nonunion.

Author Contributions: Conceptualization, S.H., C.H. and M.P.; methodology, S.H., C.v.R. and M.P.; validation, S.H. and L.K.; formal analysis, S.H. and K.T.; investigation, S.H. and L.K.; data curation, S.H. and L.K.; writing—original draft preparation, S.H. and C.v.R.; writing—review and editing, S.H., C.v.R., K.T., L.K., C.H. and M.P.; visualization, S.H. All authors have read and agreed to the published version of the manuscript.

Funding: This research received no external funding.

Institutional Review Board Statement: This study was conducted in accordance with the Declaration of Helsinki, and approved by the national research committee (Bavarian Chamber of Physicians, ID 2017-162).

Informed Consent Statement: Informed consent was obtained from all subjects involved in this study.

Data Availability Statement: The data presented in this study are available on request from the corresponding author. The data are not publicly available due to privacy.

Conflicts of Interest: The authors declare no conflicts of interest.

References

1. Vanderkarr, M.F.; Ruppenkamp, J.W.; Vanderkarr, M.; Holy, C.E.; Blauth, M. Risk factors and healthcare costs associated with long bone fracture non-union: A retrospective US claims database analysis. *J. Orthop. Surg. Res.* **2023**, *18*, 745. [CrossRef]
2. Medlock, G.; Stevenson, I.M.; Johnstone, A.J. Uniting the un-united: Should established non-unions of femoral shaft fractures initially treated with IM nails be treated by plate augmentation instead of exchange IM nailing? A systematic review. *Strategies Trauma Limb Reconstr.* **2018**, *13*, 119–128. [CrossRef]
3. Rupp, M.; Biehl, C.; Budak, M.; Thormann, U.; Heiss, C.; Alt, V. Diaphyseal long bone nonunions—Types, aetiology, economics, and treatment recommendations. *Int. Orthop.* **2018**, *42*, 247–258. [CrossRef]
4. Ekegren, C.L.; Edwards, E.R.; de Steiger, R.; Gabbe, B.J. Incidence, Costs and Predictors of Non-Union, Delayed Union and Mal-Union Following Long Bone Fracture. *Int. J. Environ. Res. Public Health* **2018**, *15*, 2845. [CrossRef] [PubMed]
5. Dahabreh, Z.; Dimitriou, R.; Giannoudis, P.V. Health economics: A cost analysis of treatment of persistent fracture non-unions using bone morphogenetic protein-7. *Injury* **2007**, *38*, 371–377. [CrossRef] [PubMed]
6. Tzioupis, C.; Giannoudis, P.V. Prevalence of long-bone non-unions. *Injury* **2007**, *38* (Suppl. 2), 3–9. [CrossRef] [PubMed]
7. Pihlajamäki, H.K.; Salminen, S.T.; Böstman, O.M. The treatment of nonunions following intramedullary nailing of femoral shaft fractures. *J. Orthop. Trauma* **2002**, *16*, 394–402. [CrossRef] [PubMed]
8. Quan, K.; Xu, Q.; Zhu, M.; Liu, X.; Dai, M. Analysis of Risk Factors for Non-union After Surgery for Limb Fractures: A Case-Control Study of 669 Subjects. *Front. Surg.* **2021**, *8*, 754150. [CrossRef] [PubMed]
9. Andrzejowski, P.; Giannoudis, P.V. The 'diamond concept' for long bone non-union management. *J. Orthop. Traumatol.* **2019**, *20*, 21. [CrossRef]
10. Hackl, S.; Hierholzer, C.; Friederichs, J.; Woltmann, A.; Bühren, V.; von Rüden, C. Long-term outcome following additional rhBMP-7 application in revision surgery of aseptic humeral, femoral, and tibial shaft nonunion. *BMC Musculoskelet. Disord.* **2017**, *18*, 342. [CrossRef] [PubMed]
11. Copuroglu, C.; Calori, G.M.; Giannoudis, P.V. Fracture non-union: Who is at risk? *Injury* **2013**, *44*, 1379–1382. [CrossRef] [PubMed]
12. Gelalis, I.D.; Politis, A.N.; Arnaoutoglou, C.M.; Korompilias, A.V.; Pakos, E.E.; Vekris, M.D.; Karageorgos, A.; Xenakis, T.A. Diagnostic and treatment modalities in nonunions of the femoral shaft: A review. *Injury* **2012**, *43*, 980–988. [CrossRef] [PubMed]
13. Wildemann, B.; Ignatius, A.; Leung, F.; Taitsman, L.A.; Smith, R.M.; Pesántez, R.; Stoddart, M.J.; Richards, R.G.; Jupiter, J.B. Non-union bone fractures. *Nat. Rev. Dis. Primers* **2021**, *7*, 57. [CrossRef] [PubMed]
14. Hackl, S.; Keppler, L.; von Rüden, C.; Friederichs, J.; Perl, M.; Hierholzer, C. The role of low-grade infection in the pathogenesis of apparently aseptic tibial shaft nonunion. *Injury* **2021**, *52*, 3498–3504. [CrossRef] [PubMed]
15. Brinker, M.R.; Macek, J.; Laughlin, M.; Dunn, W.R. Utility of Common Biomarkers for Diagnosing Infection in Nonunion. *J. Orthop. Trauma* **2021**, *35*, 121–127. [CrossRef]
16. Depypere, M.; Morgenstern, M.; Kuehl, R.; Senneville, E.; Moriarty, T.F.; Obremskey, W.T.; Zimmerli, W.; Trampuz, A.; Lagrou, K.; Metsemakers, W.J. Pathogenesis and management of fracture-related infection. *Clin. Microbiol. Infect.* **2020**, *26*, 572–578. [CrossRef]
17. Soumya, K.R.; Philip, S.; Sugathan, S.; Mathew, J.; Radhakrishnan, E.K. Virulence factors associated with Coagulase Negative Staphylococci isolated from human infections. *3 Biotech* **2017**, *7*, 140. [CrossRef]
18. Steinhausen, E. Low-Grade-Infekt. *Trauma Berufskrankh.* **2017**, *19*, 267–271. [CrossRef]
19. Mouzopoulos, G.; Kanakaris, N.K.; Kontakis, G.; Obakponovwe, O.; Townsend, R.; Giannoudis, P.V. Management of bone infections in adults: The surgeon's and microbiologist's perspectives. *Injury* **2011**, *42* (Suppl. 5), 18–23. [CrossRef]

20. Vaughn, J.E.; Shah, R.V.; Samman, T.; Stirton, J.; Liu, J.; Ebraheim, N.A. Systematic review of dynamization vs exchange nailing for delayed/non-union femoral fractures. *World J. Orthop.* **2018**, *9*, 92–99. [CrossRef]
21. Hierholzer, C.; Glowalla, C.; Herrler, M.; von Rüden, C.; Hungerer, S.; Bühren, V.; Friederichs, J. Reamed intramedullary exchange nailing: Treatment of choice of aseptic femoral shaft nonunion. *J. Orthop. Surg. Res.* **2014**, *9*, 88. [CrossRef]
22. Shroeder, J.E.; Mosheiff, R.; Khoury, A.; Liebergall, M.; Weil, Y.A. The outcome of closed, intramedullary exchange nailing with reamed insertion in the treatment of femoral shaft nonunions. *J. Orthop. Trauma* **2009**, *23*, 653–657. [CrossRef]
23. Rupp, M.; Walter, N.; Baertl, S.; Lang, S.; Lowenberg, D.W.; Alt, V. Terminology of bone and joint infection. *Bone Joint Res.* **2021**, *10*, 742–743. [CrossRef]
24. Morgenstern, M.; Kuehl, R.; Zalavras, C.G.; McNally, M.; Zimmerli, W.; Burch, M.A.; Vandendriessche, T.; Obremskey, W.T.; Verhofstad, M.H.J.; Metsemakers, W.J. The influence of duration of infection on outcome of debridement and implant retention in fracture-related infection. *Bone Joint J.* **2021**, *103-B*, 213–221. [CrossRef]
25. Foster, A.L.; Moriarty, T.F.; Trampuz, A.; Jaiprakash, A.; Burch, M.A.; Crawford, R.; Paterson, D.L.; Metsemakers, W.J.; Schuetz, M.; Richards, R.G. Fracture-related infection: Current methods for prevention and treatment. *Expert Rev. Anti-Infect. Ther.* **2020**, *18*, 307–321. [CrossRef]
26. Metsemakers, W.J.; Morgenstern, M.; Senneville, E.; Borens, O.; Govaert, G.A.M.; Onsea, J.; Depypere, M.; Richards, R.G.; Trampuz, A.; Verhofstad, M.H.J.; et al. General treatment principles for fracture-related infection: Recommendations from an international expert group. *Arch. Orthop. Trauma Surg.* **2020**, *140*, 1013–1027. [CrossRef]
27. Simpson, A.H.; Tsang, J.S.T. Current treatment of infected non-union after intramedullary nailing. *Injury* **2017**, *48* (Suppl. 1), 82–90. [CrossRef]
28. Ueng, S.W.; Wei, F.C.; Shih, C.H. Management of femoral diaphyseal infected nonunion with antibiotic beads local therapy, external skeletal fixation, and staged bone grafting. *J. Trauma* **1999**, *46*, 97–103. [CrossRef] [PubMed]
29. Prasarn, M.L.; Ahn, J.; Achor, T.; Matuszewski, P.; Lorich, D.G.; Helfet, D.L. Management of infected femoral nonunions with a single-staged protocol utilizing internal fixation. *Injury* **2009**, *40*, 1220–1225. [CrossRef] [PubMed]
30. Kim, P.H.; Leopold, S.S. In brief: Gustilo-Anderson classification. *Clin. Orthop. Relat. Res.* **2012**, *470*, 3270–3274. [CrossRef] [PubMed]
31. Charlson, M.E.; Pompei, P.; Ales, K.L.; MacKenzie, C.R. A new method of classifying prognostic comorbidity in longitudinal studies: Development and validation. *J. Chronic Dis.* **1987**, *40*, 373–383. [CrossRef]
32. Wittauer, M.; Burch, M.A.; McNally, M.; Vandendriessche, T.; Clauss, M.; Della Rocca, G.J.; Giannoudis, P.V.; Metsemakers, W.J.; Morgenstern, M. Definition of long-bone nonunion: A scoping review of prospective clinical trials to evaluate current practice. *Injury* **2021**, *52*, 3200–3205. [CrossRef] [PubMed]
33. Findeisen, S.; Schwilk, M.; Haubruck, P.; Ferbert, T.; Helbig, L.; Miska, M.; Schmidmaier, G.; Tanner, M.C. Matched-Pair Analysis: Large-Sized Defects in Surgery of Lower Limb Nonunions. *J. Clin. Med.* **2023**, *12*, 4239. [CrossRef] [PubMed]
34. Fisher, J.S.; Kazam, J.J.; Fufa, D.; Bartolotta, R.J. Radiologic evaluation of fracture healing. *Skeletal. Radiol.* **2019**, *48*, 349–361. [CrossRef] [PubMed]
35. Metsemakers, W.J.; Morgenstern, M.; McNally, M.A.; Moriarty, T.F.; McFadyen, I.; Scarborough, M.; Athanasou, N.A.; Ochsner, P.E.; Kuehl, R.; Raschke, M.; et al. Fracture-related infection: A consensus on definition from an international expert group. *Injury* **2018**, *49*, 505–510. [CrossRef]
36. Giannoudis, P.V.; Einhorn, T.A.; Marsh, D. Fracture healing: The diamond concept. *Injury* **2007**, *38* (Suppl. 4), 3–6. [CrossRef] [PubMed]
37. Onsea, J.; Pallay, J.; Depypere, M.; Moriarty, T.F.; Van Lieshout, E.M.M.; Obremskey, W.T.; Sermon, A.; Hoekstra, H.; Verhofstad, M.H.J.; Nijs, S.; et al. Intramedullary tissue cultures from the Reamer-Irrigator-Aspirator system for diagnosing fracture-related infection. *J. Orthop. Res.* **2021**, *39*, 281–290. [CrossRef]
38. Canadian Orthopaedic Trauma Society. Nonunion following intramedullary nailing of the femur with and without reaming. Results of a multicenter randomized clinical trial. *J. Bone Joint Surg. Am.* **2003**, *85*, 2093–2096. [CrossRef]
39. Peel, T.N.; Spelman, T.; Dylla, B.L.; Hughes, J.G.; Greenwood-Quaintance, K.E.; Cheng, A.C.; Mandrekar, J.N.; Patel, R. Optimal Periprosthetic Tissue Specimen Number for Diagnosis of Prosthetic Joint Infection. *J. Clin. Microbiol.* **2016**, *55*, 234–243. [CrossRef]
40. Friederichs, J.; von Rüden, C.; Hierholzer, C.; Bühren, V. Antegrade femoral intramedullary nailing in a lateral position. *Unfallchirurg* **2015**, *118*, 295–301. [CrossRef]
41. Stucken, C.; Olszewski, D.C.; Creevy, W.R.; Murakami, A.M.; Tornetta, P. Preoperative diagnosis of infection in patients with nonunions. *J. Bone Joint Surg. Am.* **2013**, *95*, 1409–1412. [CrossRef]
42. Ware, J.; Kosinski, M.; Keller, S.D. A 12-Item Short-Form Health Survey: Construction of scales and preliminary tests of reliability and validity. *Med. Care* **1996**, *34*, 220–233. [CrossRef]
43. Binkley, J.M.; Stratford, P.W.; Lott, S.A.; Riddle, D.L. The Lower Extremity Functional Scale (LEFS): Scale development, measurement properties, and clinical application. North American Orthopaedic Rehabilitation Research Network. *Phys. Ther.* **1999**, *79*, 371–383.
44. Faul, F.; Erdfelder, E.; Lang, A.G.; Buchner, A. G*Power 3: A flexible statistical power analysis program for the social, behavioral, and biomedical sciences. *Behav. Res. Methods* **2007**, *39*, 175–191. [CrossRef] [PubMed]

45. Brinker, M.R.; Trivedi, A.; O'Connor, D.P. Debilitating Effects of Femoral Nonunion on Health-Related Quality of Life. *J. Orthop. Trauma* **2017**, *31*, e37–e42. [CrossRef] [PubMed]
46. Moghaddam, A.; Thaler, B.; Bruckner, T.; Tanner, M.; Schmidmaier, G. Treatment of atrophic femoral non-unions according to the diamond concept: Results of one- and two-step surgical procedure. *J. Orthop.* **2016**, *14*, 123–133. [CrossRef] [PubMed]
47. Zeckey, C.; Mommsen, P.; Andruszkow, H.; Macke, C.; Frink, M.; Stübig, T.; Hüfner, T.; Krettek, C.; Hildebrand, F. The aseptic femoral and tibial shaft non-union in healthy patients—An analysis of the health-related quality of life and the socioeconomic outcome. *Open Orthop. J.* **2011**, *5*, 193–197. [CrossRef] [PubMed]
48. Perren, S.M.; Fernandez, A.; Regazzoni, P. Understanding Fracture Healing Biomechanics Based on the "Strain" Concept and its Clinical Applications. *Acta Chir. Orthop. Traumatol. Cech.* **2015**, *82*, 253–260. [CrossRef] [PubMed]
49. Arsoy, D.; Donders, J.C.E.; Kleeblad, L.J.; Miller, A.O.; Henry, M.W.; Wellman, D.S.; Helfet, D.L. Outcomes of Presumed Aseptic Long-Bone Nonunions With Positive Intraoperative Cultures Through a Single-Stage Surgical Protocol. *J. Orthop. Trauma* **2018**, *32* (Suppl. 1), 35–39. [CrossRef] [PubMed]
50. Amorosa, L.F.; Buirs, L.D.; Bexkens, R.; Wellman, D.S.; Kloen, P.; Lorich, D.G.; Helfet, D.L. A single-stage treatment protocol for presumptive aseptic diaphyseal nonunions: A review of outcomes. *J. Orthop. Trauma* **2013**, *27*, 582–586. [CrossRef] [PubMed]
51. Hackl, S.; Trenkwalder, K.; Militz, M.; Augat, P.; Stuby, F.M.; von Rüden, C. Infected nonunion: Diagnostic and therapeutic work-up. *Unfallchirurgie* **2022**, *125*, 602–610. [CrossRef]
52. Bonicoli, E.; Piolanti, N.; Giuntoli, M.; Polloni, S.; Scaglione, M. Septic femoral shaft non-union treated by one-step surgery using a custom-made intramedullary antibiotic cement-coated carbon nail: Case report and focus on surgical technique. *Acta Biomed.* **2020**, *91*, e2020176.
53. Wu, C.C. Aseptic femoral nonunion treated with exchange locked nailing with intramedullary augmentation cancellous bone graft. *J. Orthop. Surg. Res.* **2022**, *17*, 339. [CrossRef]
54. Ding, P.; Chen, Q.; Zhang, C.; Yao, C. Revision with Locking Compression Plate by Compression Technique for Diaphyseal Nonunions of the Femur and the Tibia: A Retrospective Study of 54 Cases. *Biomed Res. Int.* **2021**, *2021*, 9905067. [CrossRef] [PubMed]
55. Bose, D.; Kugan, R.; Stubbs, D.; McNally, M. Management of infected nonunion of the long bones by a multidisciplinary team. *Bone Joint J.* **2015**, *97-B*, 814–817. [CrossRef] [PubMed]
56. Wagner, R.K.; van Trikt, C.H.; Visser, C.E.; Janssen, S.J.; Kloen, P. Surprise positive culture rate in the treatment of presumed aseptic long-bone nonunion: A systematic review with meta-analysis of 2397 patients. *Arch. Orthop. Trauma Surg.* **2024**, *144*, 701–721. [CrossRef] [PubMed]
57. Fang, C.; Wong, T.M.; Lau, T.W.; To, K.K.; Wong, S.S.; Leung, F. Infection after fracture osteosynthesis—Part I. *J. Orthop. Surg.* **2017**, *25*, 2309499017692712. [CrossRef] [PubMed]
58. Zalavras, C.G.; Marcus, R.E.; Levin, L.S.; Patzakis, M.J. Management of open fractures and subsequent complications. *J. Bone Joint Surg. Am.* **2007**, *89*, 884–895. [CrossRef] [PubMed]
59. Olszewski, D.; Streubel, P.N.; Stucken, C.; Ricci, W.M.; Hoffmann, M.F.; Jones, C.B.; Sietsema, D.L.; Tornetta, P. Fate of Patients With a "Surprise" Positive Culture After Nonunion Surgery. *J. Orthop. Trauma* **2016**, *30*, e19–e23. [CrossRef] [PubMed]
60. Dapunt, U.; Spranger, O.; Gantz, S.; Burckhardt, I.; Zimmermann, S.; Schmidmaier, G.; Moghaddam, A. Are atrophic long-bone nonunions associated with low-grade infections? *Ther. Clin. Risk Manag.* **2015**, *11*, 1843–1852. [CrossRef] [PubMed]
61. Palmer, M.P.; Altman, D.T.; Altman, G.T.; Sewecke, J.J.; Ehrlich, G.D.; Hu, F.Z.; Nistico, L.; Melton-Kreft, R.; Gause, T.M.; Costerton, J.W. Can we trust intraoperative culture results in nonunions? *J. Orthop. Trauma* **2014**, *28*, 384–390. [CrossRef]
62. Gille, J.; Wallstabe, S.; Schulz, A.P.; Paech, A.; Gerlach, U. Is non-union of tibial shaft fractures due to nonculturable bacterial pathogens? A clinical investigation using PCR and culture techniques. *J. Orthop. Surg. Res.* **2012**, *7*, 20. [CrossRef]
63. Tiemann, A.; Hofmann, G.O.; Krukemeyer, M.G.; Krenn, V.; Langwald, S. Histopathological Osteomyelitis Evaluation Score (HOES)—An innovative approach to histopathological diagnostics and scoring of osteomyelitis. *GMS Interdiscip. Plast. Reconstr. Surg. DGPW* **2014**, *3*, Doc08. [CrossRef]
64. Wang, S.; Yin, P.; Quan, C.; Khan, K.; Wang, G.; Wang, L.; Cui, L.; Zhang, L.; Zhang, L.; Tang, P. Evaluating the use of serum inflammatory markers for preoperative diagnosis of infection in patients with nonunions. *Biomed Res. Int.* **2017**, *2017*, 9146317. [CrossRef]
65. Wu, C.C. Exchange nailing for aseptic nonunion of femoral shaft: A retrospective cohort study for effect of reaming size. *J. Trauma* **2007**, *63*, 859–865. [CrossRef]
66. Hak, D.J.; Lee, S.S.; Goulet, J.A. Success of exchange reamed intramedullary nailing for femoral shaft nonunion or delayed union. *J. Orthop. Trauma* **2000**, *14*, 178–182. [CrossRef]
67. Johnson, L.; Igoe, E.; Kleftouris, G.; Papachristos, I.V.; Papakostidis, C.; Giannoudis, P.V. Physical Health and Psychological Outcomes in Adult Patients with Long-bone Fracture Non-unions: Evidence Today. *J. Clin. Med.* **2019**, *8*, 1998. [CrossRef]
68. Maurer, E.; Walter, N.; Baumgartner, H.; Histing, T.; Alt, V.; Rupp, M. Quality of life after fracture-related infection of the foot. *Foot Ankle Surg.* **2022**, *28*, 1421–1426. [CrossRef]
69. Iliaens, J.; Onsea, J.; Hoekstra, H.; Nijs, S.; Peetermans, W.E.; Metsemakers, W.J. Fracture-related infection in long bone fractures: A comprehensive analysis of the economic impact and influence on quality of life. *Injury* **2021**, *52*, 3344–3349. [CrossRef] [PubMed]
70. Rupp, M.; Bärtl, S.; Lang, S.; Walter, N.; Alt, V. Fracture-related infections after intramedullary nailing: Diagnostics and treatment. *Unfallchirurgie* **2022**, *125*, 50–58. [CrossRef] [PubMed]

71. Bernard, L.; Arvieux, C.; Brunschweiler, B.; Touchais, S.; Ansart, S.; Bru, J.P.; Oziol, E.; Boeri, C.; Gras, G.; Druon, J.; et al. Antibiotic Therapy for 6 or 12 Weeks for Prosthetic Joint Infection. *N. Engl. J. Med.* **2021**, *384*, 1991–2001. [CrossRef] [PubMed]
72. Depypere, M.; Kuehl, R.; Metsemakers, W.J.; Senneville, E.; McNally, M.; Obremskey, W.T.; Zimmerli, W.; Atkins, B.L.; Trampuz, A.; Fracture-Related Infection Consensus Group. Recommendations for Systemic Antimicrobial Therapy in Fracture-Related Infection: A Consensus From an International Expert Group. *J. Orthop. Trauma* **2020**, *34*, 30–41. [CrossRef] [PubMed]

Disclaimer/Publisher's Note: The statements, opinions and data contained in all publications are solely those of the individual author(s) and contributor(s) and not of MDPI and/or the editor(s). MDPI and/or the editor(s) disclaim responsibility for any injury to people or property resulting from any ideas, methods, instructions or products referred to in the content.

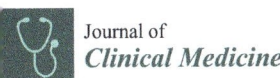

Article

Balance and Weight Distribution over the Lower Limbs Following Calcaneal Fracture Treatment with the Ilizarov Method

Marcin Pelc [1], Krystian Kazubski [2], Wiktor Urbański [3], Paweł Leyko [2], Joanna Kochańska-Bieri [4], Łukasz Tomczyk [5], Grzegorz Konieczny [6] and Piotr Morasiewicz [2,*]

1. Institute of Medical Sciences, University of Opole, Witosa 26, 45-401 Opole, Poland
2. Department of Orthopaedic and Trauma Surgery, Institute of Medical Sciences, University of Opole, Witosa 26, 45-401 Opole, Poland
3. Department of Neurosurgery, Wrocław Medical University, Borowska 213, 50-556 Wroclaw, Poland
4. Universitätsspital CH, University of Basel, Petersgraben 4, 4031 Basel, Switzerland
5. Department of Food Safety and Quality Management, Poznan University of Life Sciences, Wojska Polskiego 28, 60-637 Poznan, Poland
6. Faculty of Health and Physical Culture Sciences, Witelon Collegium State University, Sejmowa 5A, 59-220 Legnica, Poland

* Correspondence: morasp@poczta.onet.pl

Citation: Pelc, M.; Kazubski, K.; Urbański, W.; Leyko, P.; Kochańska-Bieri, J.; Tomczyk, Ł.; Konieczny, G.; Morasiewicz, P. Balance and Weight Distribution over the Lower Limbs Following Calcaneal Fracture Treatment with the Ilizarov Method. *J. Clin. Med.* **2024**, *13*, 1676. https://doi.org/10.3390/jcm13061676

Academic Editor: Hiroyuki Katoh

Received: 19 January 2024
Revised: 29 February 2024
Accepted: 13 March 2024
Published: 14 March 2024

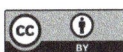

Copyright: © 2024 by the authors. Licensee MDPI, Basel, Switzerland. This article is an open access article distributed under the terms and conditions of the Creative Commons Attribution (CC BY) license (https://creativecommons.org/licenses/by/4.0/).

Abstract: Background: The biomechanical outcomes of intra-articular calcaneal fracture treatment have not been fully explored. The purpose of this study was to analyze pedobarographic assessments of balance and body weight distribution over the lower limbs in patients following calcaneal fracture treatment with the Ilizarov method and to compare the results with those of a control group. **Materials and Methods**: The data for our retrospective study came from cases of intra-articular calcaneal fractures treated with the Polish modification of the Ilizarov method in the period between 2021 and 2022. The experimental group (21 patients; 7 women, 14 men) included Sanders classification calcaneal fractures type 2 ($n = 3$), type 3 ($n = 5$), and type 4 ($n = 13$). The control group comprised 21 sex-matched healthy volunteers, with no significant differences from the experimental group in terms of age or BMI. The examination included an assessment of balance and weight distribution over the lower limbs. The device used was a FreeMED MAXI pedobarographic platform (SensorMedica). **Results**: The mean displacement of the center of gravity in the experimental group was significantly higher at 1307.31 mm than in the control group (896.34 mm; $p = 0.038$). The mean area of the center of gravity was not significantly different between the groups. An analysis of weight distribution over the operated and uninjured limb in the experimental group and the non-dominant and dominant limb, respectively, in the control group revealed no significant differences. We observed no significant differences in the percentage of weight distribution over the lower limbs between the operated limb in the experimental group and the non-dominant limb in the control group, or between the uninjured limb in the experimental group and the dominant limb in the control group. **Conclusions**: The use of the Ilizarov method in calcaneal fracture treatment helps normalize the percentage weight distribution in the lower limbs, with the results comparable with those obtained in the healthy control group. The mean displacement of the center of gravity was worse in the experimental group than in controls; whereas the mean area of the center of gravity was comparable between the two groups. Treatment of calcaneal fractures with the Ilizarov method does not help achieve completely normal static parameters of lower-limb biomechanics. Patients treated for calcaneal fractures with the Ilizarov method require longer and more intense rehabilitation and follow-up.

Keywords: balance; weight distribution; biomechanics; Ilizarov method; intra-articular; calcaneal fractures

1. Introduction

Fractures of the calcaneus account for approximately 2% of all fractures and for 50–60% of tarsal fractures [1–5]. The intra-articular and comminuted fractures of the calcaneus that require surgical treatment constitute approximately 75% of all calcaneal fractures [1–4]. There is no gold standard for the treatment of intra-articular and comminuted fractures of the calcaneus [1–4,6–13]. In the past, most calcaneal fractures were treated either by closed reduction and cast immobilization or by bone fragment repositioning and fixation with a few Kirschner wires or Steinmann pins [2,6,10]. Technological advancement has popularized the technique of open reduction and internal plate fixation of calcaneal fractures [1–4,6,7]; however, the necessary large incision has been associated with a high risk of complications, including delayed wound healing, infections, skin and soft tissue necrosis, fixation material-induced irritation, or loss of fixation (14–33%) [1–3,6,7].

One of the techniques used in calcaneal fracture management is the Ilizarov method [2–14]. Due to the high risk of complications and the complexity of the required surgical technique, calcaneal fractures have always posed a challenge for orthopedic surgeons [1–4,6,7,9–13]. Earlier papers on the topic dealt primarily with the clinical [2–7,10,12], radiological [2–5,9,10,13], and functional [2,3,6,9,10,13] outcomes of treating calcaneal fractures with external fixators and the Ilizarov method.

The growing use of various implants (Kirschner wires, Schanz pins) to complement the Ilizarov method may increase the risk of complications, such as peri-implant infections, delayed wound healing, or skin and soft-tissue necrosis [2,4]. The techniques for intra-articular calcaneal fracture management reported to date include the use of the Ilizarov method along with the insertion of at least three Kirschner wires into the foot [2,3,5–9,12–14]. The modified approach to intra-articular calcaneal fractures with the use of an Ilizarov fixator conducted in a center in Wrocław, Poland, requires the insertion of a single Kirschner wire into the foot [4].

The biomechanical outcomes of intra-articular calcaneal fracture treatment have not been fully explored. Such fractures result in bone fragment displacement, which alters the overall shape and three-dimensional structure of the calcaneus and of the whole foot [1,2,4,6]. One of the purposes of surgical treatment in intra-articular calcaneal fractures is to restore the shape and three-dimensional structure of both the calcaneus and the whole foot, in order to normalize kinetic and static parameters of the lower limbs [1,2,4,6]. Any abnormalities in the three-dimensional structure of the calcaneus and foot may lead to asymmetric load distribution in the foot, which causes pain, as well as accelerates tissue degeneration [4]. Post-traumatic deformities and changes in three-dimensional structure of the calcaneus and foot may adversely affect gait, balance, and weight distribution over the lower limbs [1,2,4,6,15–25].

Normal gait function is largely dependent on the anatomical bony structure of the foot [5–7,14]. Apart from the standard clinical and radiological assessments following lower-limb surgery, it is very important to also evaluate biomechanical parameters [15–25]. Pedobarography helps assess balance parameters and the distribution of loads on the lower limbs [15–23,26–37]. Pedobarography is an accepted method for examining the statics and dynamics of musculoskeletal issues [15–34,36]. Pedobarography is a useful, reproducible, objective, and comparable assessment method in the treatment of musculoskeletal pathologies [15–23,26–29,34–36]. Unfortunately, there is a lack of available literature on lower-limb biomechanics assessments following calcaneal fracture treatment with the Ilizarov method. The authors of earlier papers on calcaneal fracture treatment have only assessed gait following an open reduction and internal plate fixation approach [22–25]. The assessed parameters included also the mean contact area, peak pressures in the forefoot and hindfoot, and total contact time in patients with calcaneal fractures treated with an open reduction and internal plate fixation approach [33,34]. There have been no studies to assess the balance and weight distribution over the lower limbs following calcaneal fracture treatment. The studies conducted so far included assessments of balance and weight distribution over the lower limbs following lengthening and corrective corticotomy procedures on the thigh and leg with the Ilizarov method, ankle joint arthrodesis procedures, or tibial nonunion treatment with the Ilizarov method [15–18].

We hypothesized that calcaneal fracture treatment with the Ilizarov method would help restore normal balance and weight distribution over the lower limbs. The purpose of this study was to analyze pedobarographic assessments of balance and body weight distribution over the lower limbs in patients following calcaneal fracture treatment with the Ilizarov method and to compare the results with those of a control group of healthy individuals.

2. Materials and Methods

The data for our retrospective study came from patients with intra-articular calcaneal fractures treated with the Polish modification of the Ilizarov method in the period between 2021 and 2022. The study inclusion criteria were as follows: intra-articular calcaneal fracture treated with the Polish modification of the Ilizarov method, a follow-up period of over 2 years after treatment completion, complete medical and radiological records, complete pedobarographic assessment records, patient's written informed consent, and the absence of lower-limb comorbidities. The study exclusion criteria were as follows: calcaneal fracture treatment with a method different than the Ilizarov method, a follow-up period of less than 2 years, incomplete medical and/or radiographic records, incomplete pedobarographic assessment records, other lower-limb injuries, lower-limb comorbidities, and a lack of consent. All patients were informed of the voluntary nature of study participation and the possibility of withdrawing from the study at any time. This study was approved by the local ethics committee (UO/0023/KB/2023).

Application of the inclusion and exclusion criteria yielded 21 patients (7 women, 14 men), aged from 25 to 67 years (mean age 47 years), with a body mass index of 24–40 (mean 28), height of 152–188 cm (mean 171 cm), body weight of 61–130 kg (mean 81 kg). The control group comprised 21 sex-matched healthy volunteers, with no significant differences from the experimental group in terms of age, demographics, BMI, or physical activity levels.

The experimental group included Sanders classification calcaneal fractures type 2 ($n = 3$), type 3 ($n = 5$), and type 4 ($n = 13$). Each of the evaluated patients was operated on by the same surgeon, who used the Polish modification of the Ilizarov method for calcaneal fracture treatment [4] (verbal accounts by P. Koprowski and L. Morasiewicz).

The external fixator used for calcaneal fracture treatment in accordance with the Polish modification of the Ilizarov method was composed of two fully circular rings, which were fixed to crural bones with Kirschner wires, and one half-ring, which was fixed to the calcaneus with a single Kirschner wire (Figure 1).

All surgical procedures were conducted with a closed approach, without an open access to the calcaneus. Once the two full rings were mounted on the leg, one Kirschner wire was inserted (under fluoroscopy) into the calcaneal bone fragment that was both the most proximal and the most dorsal. Subsequently, the half-ring was positioned behind the foot and fixed to a Kirschner wire inserted into the calcaneus. The half-ring was then connected with the distal leg ring by means of two connectors (Figure 2).

Each connector was composed of two perpendicular, threaded rods (Figure 2). Once the fixator was mounted on the leg and foot, the calcaneal fracture was reduced under fluoroscopy. Ligamentotaxis via this modified Ilizarov fixator allowed a closed, indirect reduction in the calcaneal fracture. On day one after surgery, the patients began walking with two elbow crutches, with partial weight bearing on the treated limb. Gradually, the patients were allowed to bear more and more weight on the operated foot, to the extent of their pain tolerance. All patients underwent the same rehabilitation protocol and were scheduled for periodic follow-up visits in an outpatient setting. The follow-up visits included clinical examination and radiological imaging. The fixator was removed once clinical and radiological evidence of bone union was observed.

The clinical examination included assessments of balance (Figure 3) and weight distribution over the lower limbs (Figure 4).

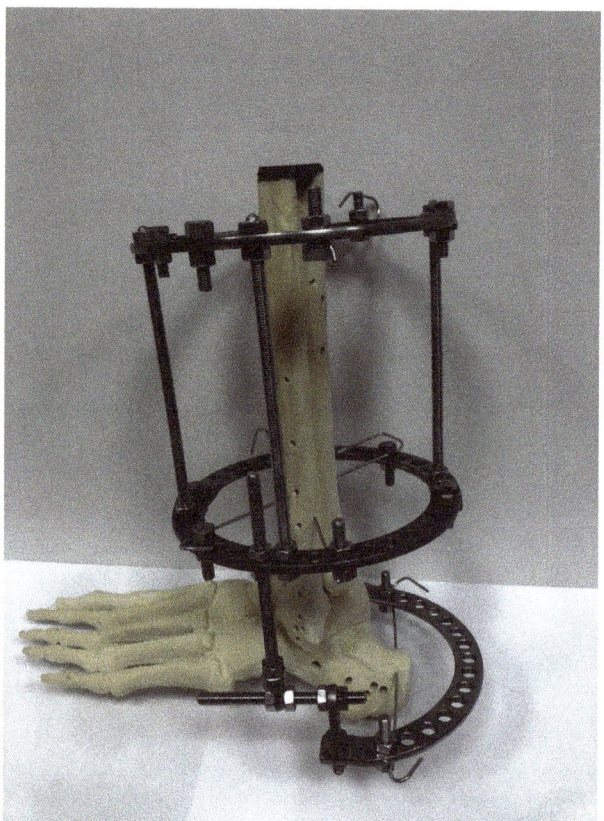

Figure 1. A three-dimensional model of the Polish modification of an Ilizarov fixator for calcaneal fracture treatment.

The device used was a FreeMED MAXI pedobarographic platform manufactured by SensorMedica (Guidonia Montecelio, Rome, Italy). The pedobarographic assessment set includes a platform measuring 63.5 × 70 cm (total active sensor area of 50 × 60 cm), two inactive mats measuring 70 × 100 cm each, and a computer with appropriate software, Figure 5.

The platform can measure pressures of up to 150 N/cm^2 with a minimum acquisition frequency of 300 Hz in real time. The 3000 square resistive sensors coated in 24-carat gold, each with a durability of 1,000,000 cycles, ensure high accuracy and reproducibility of measurements [26–29,35,36].

Each study subject had received detailed instructions on the measurement procedure. During pedobarographic and posturographic assessments, each subject was asked to make corrective adjustments to his or her posture. The measurements were taken while the subjects had their eyes open and were standing on both lower limbs, with their feet positioned freely in a physiological position (with an external rotation of 5–10°) [30]. The mean duration of balance assessments was 51.2 s. Weight distribution was recorded following a 5-second stabilization after a subject stepped onto the platform. The subjects were advised to maintain an upright posture, with their arms hanging symmetrically along the torso, and to keep their eyes fixed on one point on the wall in front of them at their eye level. Each subject underwent the measurement three times, and the mean value of the three was used in further analyses. The measurements were recorded via

FreeSTEP software, V.2.02.006. Subsequently, the results were exported onto a spreadsheet and analyzed statistically.

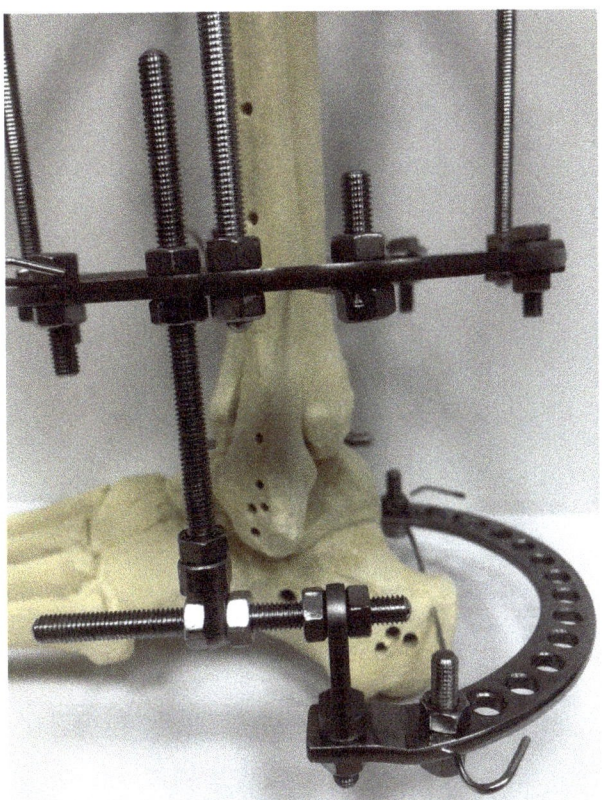

Figure 2. Detailed structure of an Ilizarov fixator.

Balance was assessed based on center-of-gravity displacement. This parameter was expressed as the total distance (in millimeters) traversed by the center of gravity over the course of the evaluation [15–17,27]. Balance assessment was also based on the surface area determined by maximum displacements of the center of gravity and defined as the area (in mm^2) enclosed by the points of maximum center-of-gravity displacement in all directions over the course of the evaluation [15–17,27].

Weight distribution over the lower limbs was expressed in percentage values. In the experimental group, we assessed the load on the uninjured and the treated lower limb and calculated the proportion of weight distribution on the forefoot and hindfoot of either limb. The dominant limbs in the control group of healthy individuals were compared with the uninjured limbs of treated individuals, and the non-dominant limbs of control individuals were compared with the operated limbs of treated individuals [15,16,18]. The results obtained in the experimental group of patients with calcaneal fractures treated with the Ilizarov method were compared with those obtained in the control group of healthy volunteers.

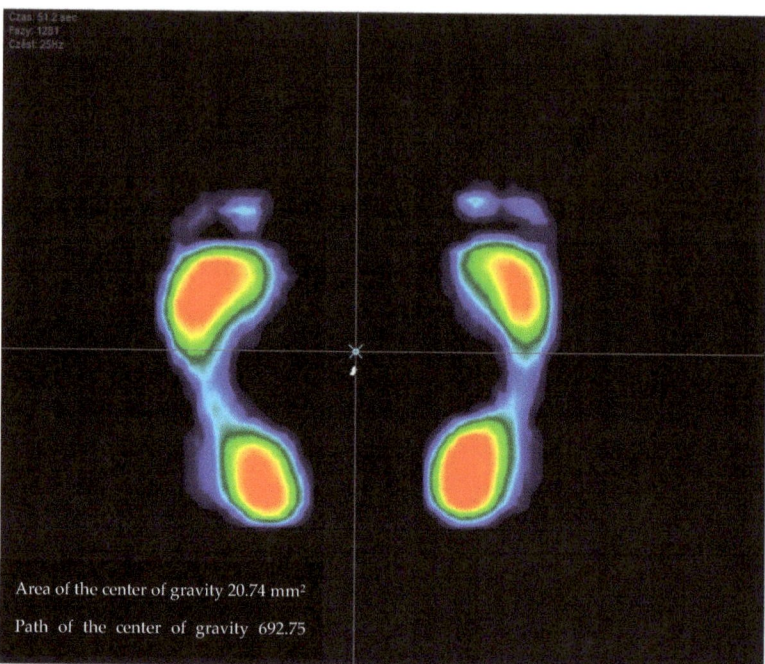

Figure 3. Image of balance test.

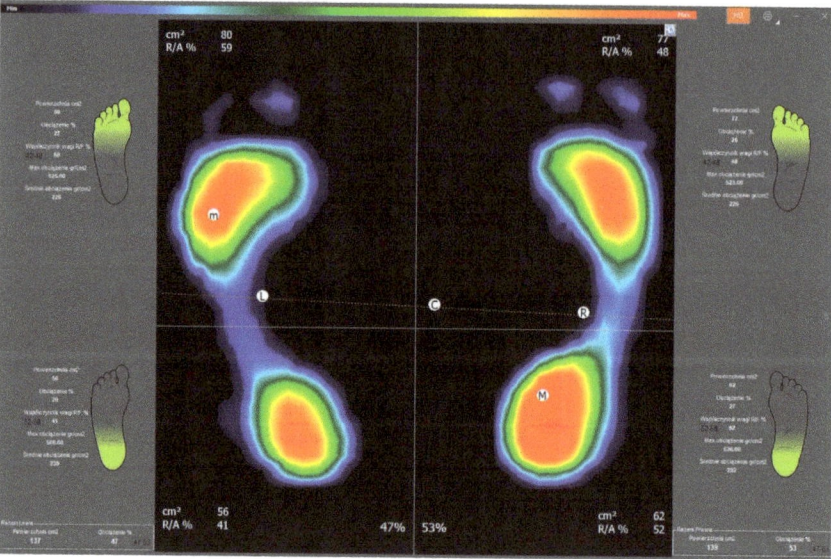

Figure 4. Image of the percentage weight distribution over the limbs. Color map of the pressures: red to dark green—from the area of the highest to the lowest level of pressure; blue—foot perimeter.

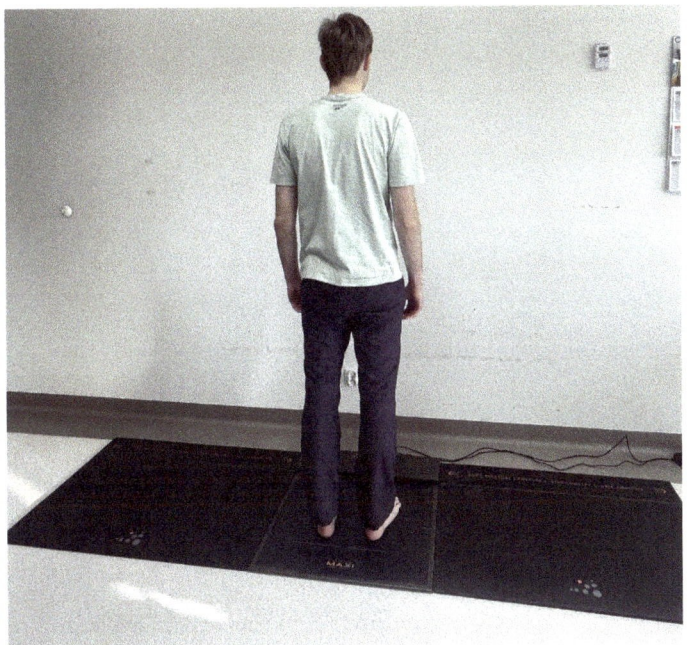

Figure 5. SensorMedica pedobarographic platform.

Statistical Analysis

Data were statistically analyzed using Statistica 13.1. The Shapiro–Wilk test was used to check for normality of distribution. Continuous variables were reported as mean (±SD). A Levene's test was performed to assess the homogeneity of variance within the two repeat sets of measurements. Inter-group comparisons of continuous variables were made with Student's *t*-test. The level of statistical significance was set at $p < 0.05$.

3. Results

The mean displacement of the center of gravity in the experimental group was significantly higher at 1307.31 mm than in the control group (896.34 mm; $p = 0.038$), (Figure 6, Table 1). The mean area of the center of gravity was 162.77 mm² in the experimental group and 96.67 mm² in the control group. This difference between groups was not statistically significant (Table 1).

Table 1. Path of center of gravity and area of the center of gravity.

Analyzed Variable	Patients	Control Group	*p*-Value *
	Mean ± Standard Deviation		
Area of the center of gravity [mm^2]	162.77 ± 132.85	96.67 ± 73.89	0.324
Path of the center of gravity [mm]	1307.31 ± 372.33	896.34 ± 272.89	0.038

* Student's *t*-test.

An analysis of weight distribution over the operated and uninjured limb in the experimental group and the non-dominant and dominant limb, respectively, in the control group revealed no significant differences (Table 2).

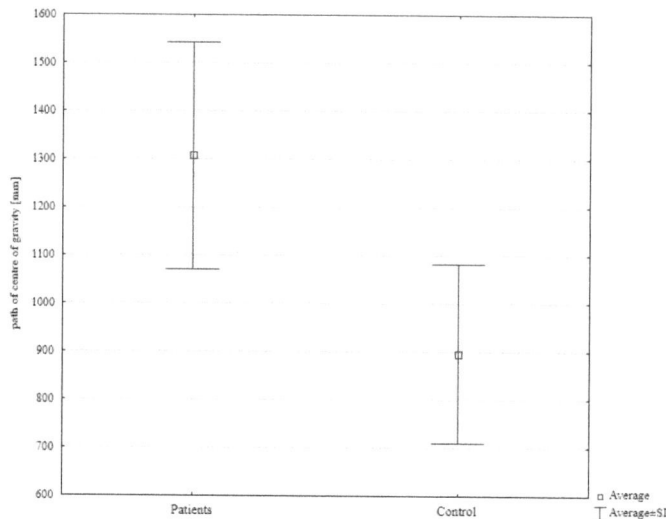

Figure 6. Path of the center of gravity in the experimental group compared with that in the control group.

Table 2. Body weight distribution in patients after treatment and in controls.

Loads on Limb	Control Group	Patients after Surgery
	Mean ± Standard Deviation	
OL [%]	47.16 ± 2.97	46.01 ± 5.67
NOL [%]	52.83 ± 13.72	53.11 ± 7.23
p-value *	0.715	0.077
OL forefoot [%]	23.66 ± 3.7	19.22 ± 4.79
NOL forefoot [%]	26.41 ± 4.75	25.33 ± 6.57
p-value *	0.128	0.038
OL hindfoot [%]	23.5 ± 3.06	27.66 ± 6.34
NOL hindfoot [%]	26.41 ± 4.81	27.77 ± 4.54
p-value *	0.090	0.966

OL—operated limb; NOL—non-operated limb. * Student's t-test.

Nonetheless, it is worth noting that patients treated with the Polish modification of the Ilizarov method tended to bear significantly less weight on the forefoot of the operated limb (19.22%) in comparison with that of the uninjured limb (25.33%), $p = 0.038$ (Table 2, Figure 7). We observed no significant differences in the proportion of weight borne on the hindfoot in the two study groups (Table 2).

The forefoot of the operated limbs in the experimental group also bore significantly less weight (19.22%) than that in the non-dominant limbs in the control group (23.66%), $p = 0.026$, (Table 3, Figure 8).

Table 3. Body weight distribution in the two groups.

Analyzed Variable	Patients	Control Group	p-Value *
	Mean ± Standard Deviation		
OL [%]	46.01 ± 5.67	47.16 ± 2.97	0.668
NOL [%]	53.11 ± 7.23	52.83 ± 13.72	0.390
OL forefoot [%]	19.22 ± 2.79	23.66 ± 2.71	0.026
OL hindfoot [%]	27.66 ± 5.34	23.5 ± 3.06	0.060
NOL forefoot [%]	25.33 ± 6.57	26.41 ± 4.75	0.666
NOL hindfoot [%]	27.77 ± 4.54	26.42 ± 4.81	0.519

OL—operated limb; NOL—non-operated limb. * Student's t-test.

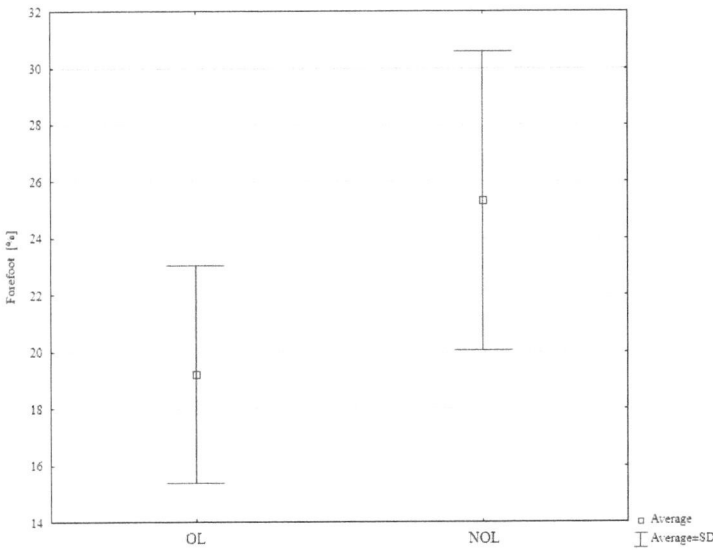

Figure 7. Weight distribution in the forefoot of the operated and the uninjured limbs.

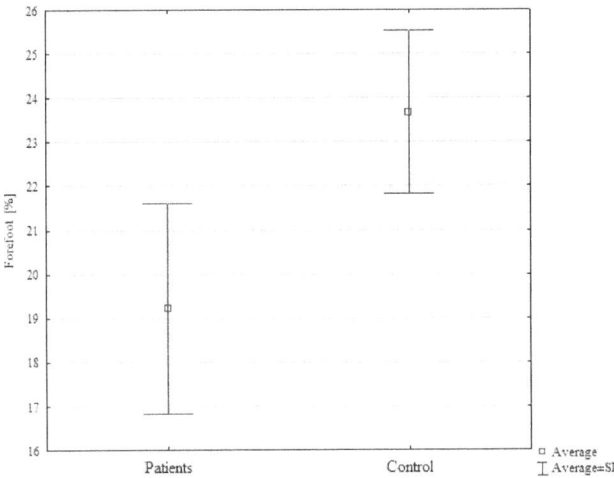

Figure 8. A comparison of weight distribution in the forefoot of the operated limb in the experimental group and that of the non-dominant limb in the control group.

We observed no significant differences in the percentage of weight distribution between the operated limb in the experimental group and the non-dominant limb in the control group, or between the uninjured limb in the experimental group and the dominant limb in the control group (Table 3). Moreover, these compared pairs of limbs showed no significant differences in terms of any other analyzed parameters (Tables 2 and 3).

4. Discussion

This paper presents our assessment of balance and weight distribution over the lower limbs following calcaneal fracture treatment with the Polish modification of the Ilizarov external fixator. We observed no differences in the percentage distribution of weight over the lower limbs between any of the following pairs of compared limbs: the operated and uninjured limbs in the experimental group; the operated limb in the experimental group and the non-dominant limb in the control group; and the uninjured limb in the experimental group and the dominant limb in the control group. The analysis of balance showed some of the results to be significantly poorer in the group of calcaneal fracture patients than in the group of healthy volunteers, which partly supports our hypothesis. The mean displacement of the center of gravity in the experimental group was not as good as that in the control group, whereas the mean area of the center of gravity was comparable in both groups.

Intra-articular calcaneal fractures often pose a challenge for orthopedic surgeons due to the complexity of the required surgery and high rates of complications [1–4,6,7,9–13,22,33,34]. The Ilizarov method has been adopted as one of the techniques used in the treatment of calcaneal fractures [2–14].

The goal of surgical treatment of intra-articular calcaneal fractures is to reduce pain and restore the three-dimensional structure of the calcaneus and the function of the foot [1,2,4–7,22].

Calcaneal fractures may lead to a lowered longitudinal arch, which results in flatfoot [23]. Some authors suggest that the normal shape and restored anatomical structure of the calcaneus determines normal lower-limb biomechanics and gait efficiency [1,2,4,6]. However, other authors reported good clinical and functional outcomes with poor radiological outcomes [1], and others reported poor clinical or functional outcomes with good radiological outcomes [2,7]. Achieving normal musculoskeletal biomechanics—including balance and weight distribution over the lower limbs—following treatment of musculoskeletal pathologies is possible in the case of normal ranges of motion, absence of pain, and restored bone anatomy [15–24]. Typically, weight distribution over the lower limbs is symmetrical [16,17]. In light of the above, it is important not only to conduct clinical and radiological assessments but also to assess balance and weight distribution over the lower limbs, as it is performed in analyzing treatment outcomes in various musculoskeletal pathologies, including injury-induced ones [15–25,31–34,36]. Abnormal biomechanical parameters, including balance and distribution of weight over the lower limbs, may indicate postoperative pain, limited range of motion, and decreased muscle strength, hence the great importance of lower-limb biomechanics assessments following treatment [15–25,31–34,36].

There have been no studies to assess lower-limb biomechanics following the treatment of calcaneal fractures with the Ilizarov method. Authors of earlier studies on gait reported abnormal gait parameters following calcaneal fractures treated with open reduction and internal plate fixation [22–25]. Some authors reported no differences between the treated and the uninjured limbs in terms of the mean contact area in the forefoot and hindfoot in patients after calcaneal fracture treatment with an open reduction and internal plate fixation approach but they assessed neither balance parameters nor percentage weight distribution over the lower limbs [34]. The group of patients who received conservative treatment for calcaneal fractures exhibited abnormal biomechanics between the treated and the uninjured limb in terms of the mean contact area in the forefoot and hindfoot [34]. Other authors reported differences between the treated and the uninjured limbs in terms of maximum pressure and total contact time in patients with calcaneal fractures treated with internal plate fixation [33]. There have been no reports of assessing balance and weight distribution over the lower limbs following calcaneal fracture treatment.

Theoretically, the Ilizarov method is more effective in restoring balance and weight distribution than other available treatments for calcaneal fractures (such as open reduction and fixation with a plate or screws). In comparison with other techniques of calcaneal fracture fixation, the Ilizarov method is less invasive, requires only a small incision, and is associated with a lower risk of infections and other complications [1–4,6,7,9–13]. In comparison with calcaneal fracture fixation with a plate or screws, the Ilizarov method allows patients to bear weight on the operated limb sooner and initiate intensive rehabilitation sooner than with other treatment methods.

Pajchert-Kozłowska et al. used a pedobarographic platform to assess balance in patients following treatment of tibial nonunion with the Ilizarov method [15]. Those authors reported the balance parameters in the experimental group to be comparable with those in healthy volunteers [15]. Another study, which evaluated patients following lower-limb corticotomy procedures with the Ilizarov method, showed poorer balance values in comparison with those in the healthy control group [16]. Analysis of balance following ankle joint arthrodesis with internal fixation or with external fixation with the Ilizarov method showed worse results in the group with internal fixation [17]. Rongies used a pedobarographic platform to assess 21 patients with coxarthrosis and reported balance improvement following rehabilitation [19].

In our group of patients, center-of-gravity displacement was significantly greater than that in the control group of healthy individuals. The area of the center of gravity in the experimental group was greater, though not significantly, than that in the control group. This suggests a lack of balance normalization following calcaneal fracture treatment with the Ilizarov method. Calcaneal fractures may result in swelling, reduced muscle strength, pain, and a limited range of motion [22,24], which may have adversely affected the balance in our experimental group. The balance parameters in our patients were comparable with those reported by authors who assessed patients after corticotomies using the Ilizarov method and after ankle joint arthrodeses using the Ilizarov method [16,17]. The fact that some balance parameters remained abnormal after calcaneal fracture treatment with the Ilizarov method indicates the need for a longer rehabilitation period and exercises for these patients.

In another group of 57 patients treated with lower-limb croticotomy with the Ilizarov method, there were no differences in the percentage weight distribution over the lower limbs between the operated and non-operated limb, and the absolute load values were comparable with those obtained in the healthy control group [16]. Analysis of percentage weight distribution over the lower limbs in patients treated with ankle joint arthrodesis with internal fixation and in those treated with an external Ilizarov fixator revealed no differences between the two groups in terms of weight distribution between the operated and the uninjured limb [17]. Pawik et al. assessed patients with tibial nonunion treated with the Ilizarov method [18]. Those authors observed no differences in the percentage weight distribution between the forefoot and hindfoot of either the operated and uninjured limb in the experimental group or between the experimental and control groups [18]. Güven et al. analyzed 37 patients who underwent surgical treatment of transtrochanteric femoral fractures with partial hemiarthroplasty or proximal femoral nail [31]. Using a pedobarographic platform, those authors assessed the differences in weight distribution between the operated and uninjured limbs in static conditions. The results showed a greater load on the uninjured limb in both analyzed groups [31]. Out of the 26 patients with isolated tarsometatarsal (Lisfranc) joint injuries evaluated by Shepers et al., one-half received surgical treatment and the other half received conservative treatment [32]. Study results showed both groups to have similar percentage weight distribution over the lower limbs. In the case of the injured foot, there was a significantly greater weight distribution on the posterior part of the foot than on the forefoot [32]. Tarczyńska et al. conducted a balance study on 30 patients, assessing the long-term effects of surgical treatment of Achilles tendon injury [36]. They compared two groups of patients: one who sought treatment within 4 weeks of the injury and the other who sought treatment after 4 weeks. Their results showed that delayed treatment of Achilles tendon injury leads to deterioration of balance parameters in long-term follow-up [36].

A fracture reduction that recreates the anatomical structure of the calcaneus helps restore the normal biomechanic parameters and three-dimensional structure of the foot and gain efficiency [1,2,4,6]. Our study showed a symmetrical percentage weight distribution between the operated and the uninjured limb in the experimental group. Similarly, we observed no differences in weight distribution between the operated limb in the experimental group and the non-dominant limb in the control group or between the uninjured limb in the experimental group and the dominant limb in the control group. The only statistically significant difference was in terms of forefoot loading, which was significantly lesser in the operated than in the uninjured limb in the experimental group. This indicates a normalization of percentage weight distribution over the lower limbs following fracture treatment with the Ilizarov method. The patients who underwent calcaneal fracture treatment with the Polish modification of the Ilizarov method achieved comparable percentage values of weight distribution over the lower limbs to those in the control group of healthy volunteers. The results of weight distribution over the lower limbs observed in our study are comparable with those reported in the literature [16–18].

One limitation of our study is its retrospective nature. This is due to the nature of injuries since patients with calcaneal fractures cannot undergo a normal pedobarographic assessment prior to treatment. Other authors also presented retrospective analyses of patients following calcaneal fracture treatment and retrospective pedobarographic analyses [3–6,8–10,12–18,22–25,31,33,34]. Another limitation of our study is the relatively small sample size. This is due to the low incidence of calcaneal fractures and the time constraints for pedobarographic assessments. However, many other authors assessed comparable or even smaller study groups [3–6,8–10,12–15,18–20,23,25,32–34,36]. One of the strengths of our study is the sex-, age-, and BMI-matched control group, a uniform rehabilitation protocol, the follow-up period of over 2 years, and all procedures being conducted by the same surgeon. In the future, we are planning to conduct similar studies in a larger patient population with a longer follow-up period and to assess gait parameters in patients with intra-articular calcaneal fractures treated with the Ilizarov method. We believe it is important to compare the balance parameters and percentage weight distribution over the lower limbs in patients following calcaneal fracture treatment with different fixation techniques (i.e., an external Ilizarov fixator vs. open reduction and internal fixation with a plate and screws). Our study showed that normal balance parameters were not restored following treatment; however, they were similar to those achieved by other patients following treatment with an Ilizarov fixator [16,17]. The fact that some balance parameters did not reach their normal values in our patients may be due to pain, a limited range of motion, swelling, and reduced muscle strength [15–25,31,32]. We are planning to conduct studies to assess the severity of pain, joint range of motion, muscle strength, and quality of life in patients following calcaneal fracture treatment with the Ilizarov method.

Our study showed that some balance parameters did not reach their normal values following calcaneal fracture treatment with the Ilizarov method. We believe that more attention should be paid to patient rehabilitation following calcaneal fracture treatment with the Ilizarov method. These patients should undergo a longer and more intense rehabilitation and have a longer period of follow-up visits. A longer period of post-treatment analgesia and exercises should be considered for patients following calcaneal fracture treatment with the Ilizarov method. Implementing these measures may help reduce pain and swelling and improve range of motion and muscle strength, which would restore normal biomechanical parameters in patients following calcaneal fracture treatment with the Ilizarov method.

5. Conclusions

The use of the Ilizarov method in calcaneal fracture treatment helps achieve normalization of percentage weight distribution in the lower limbs, with the results comparable with those obtained in the healthy control group.

Following treatment, calcaneal fracture patients showed worse mean displacement of the center of gravity than that in the control group, with no differences between these two groups in the mean area of the center of gravity.

Treatment of calcaneal fractures with the Ilizarov method does not help achieve completely normal static parameters of lower-limb biomechanics.

Patients with calcaneal fractures treated with the Ilizarov method require longer and more intense rehabilitation and follow-up periods.

Author Contributions: Conceptualization, M.P. and P.M.; Methodology, M.P., Ł.T. and P.M.; Software, M.P. and Ł.T.; Validation, M.P.; Formal analysis, M.P.; Investigation, M.P., K.K., W.U. and P.L.; Resources, M.P.; Data curation, M.P. and Ł.T.; Writing—original draft, M.P., K.K., W.U., P.L., J.K.-B., G.K. and P.M.; Writing—review and editing, M.P., K.K., W.U., P.L., J.K.-B., G.K. and P.M.; Visualization, M.P., G.K. and J.K.-B.; Supervision, M.P. All authors have read and agreed to the published version of the manuscript.

Funding: Internal project of the Institute of Medical Sciences of the University of Opole P-2022-001 and P-2023-001.

Institutional Review Board Statement: This study was conducted in accordance with the Declaration of Helsinki and approved by the Bioethics Committee of the University of Opole (protocol code UO/0023/KB/2023), date of approval 26 October 2023.

Informed Consent Statement: Informed consent was obtained from all subjects involved in this study.

Data Availability Statement: The data presented in this study are available on request from the corresponding author.

Conflicts of Interest: The authors declare no conflicts of interest.

References

1. Fan, B.; Zhou, X.; Wei, Z.; Ren, Y.; Lin, W.; Hao, Y.; Shi, G.; Feng, S. Cannulated screw fixation and plate fixation for displaced intra-articular calcaneus fracture: A meta-analysis of randomized controlled trials. *Int. J. Surg.* **2016**, *34*, 64–72. [CrossRef]
2. Muir, R.L.; Forrester, R.; Sharma, H. Fine Wire Circular Fixation for Displaced Intra-Articular Calcaneal Fractures: A Systematic Review. *J. Foot Ankle Surg.* **2019**, *58*, 755–761. [CrossRef]
3. McGarvey, W.C.; Burris, M.W.; Clanton, T.O.; Melissinos, E.G. Calcaneal fractures: Indirect reduction and external fixation. *Foot Ankle Int.* **2006**, *27*, 494–499. [CrossRef]
4. Koprowski, P.; Kulej, M.; Romaszkiewicz, P.; Dragan, S.; Krawczyk, A.; Prastowski, A. Assessment of Ilizarov's method in intraarticular calcaneal fractures. *Ortop. Traumatol. Rehabil.* **2004**, *6*, 423–432.
5. Ramanujam, C.L.; Capobianco, C.M.; Zgonis, T. Ilizarov external fixation technique for repair of a calcaneal avulsion fracture and Achilles tendon rupture. *Foot Ankle Spec.* **2009**, *2*, 306–308. [CrossRef]
6. Emara, K.M.; Allam, M.F. Management of calcaneal fracture using the Ilizarov technique. *Clin. Orthop. Relat. Res.* **2005**, *439*, 215–220. [CrossRef]
7. Zgonis, T.; Roukis, T.S.; Polyzois, V.D. The use of Ilizarov technique and other types of external fixation for the treatment of intra-articular calcaneal fractures. *Clin. Podiatr. Med. Surg.* **2006**, *23*, 343–353. [CrossRef] [PubMed]
8. Takahashi, M.; Noda, M.; Saegusa, Y. A new treatment for avulsion fracture of the calcaneus using an Ilizarov external fixator. *Injury* **2013**, *44*, 1640–1643. [CrossRef] [PubMed]
9. Ali, A.M.; Elsaied, M.A.; Elmoghazy, N. Management of calcaneal fractures using the Ilizarov external fixator. *Acta Orthop. Belg.* **2009**, *75*, 51–56. [PubMed]
10. Li, D.; Yin, S.; Wu, P.; Gao, M.; Wen, S.; Xu, Q.; Mao, J. Management of calcaneus fractures by a new "Below-the-ankle" ilizarov frame: A series of 10 cases. *Niger J. Clin. Pract.* **2022**, *25*, 1143–1148. [CrossRef] [PubMed]
11. Paley, D.; Hall, H. Calcaneal fracture controversies Can we put Humpty Dumpty together again? *Orthop. Clin. N. Am.* **1989**, *20*, 665–677.
12. Paley, D.; Fischgrund, J. Open reduction and circular external fixation of intraarticular calcaneal fractures. *Clin. Orthop. Relat. Res.* **1993**, *290*, 125–131. [CrossRef]
13. Mauffrey, C.; Klutts, P.; Seligson, D. The use of circular fine wire frames for the treatment of displaced intra-articular calcaneal fractures. *J. Orthop. Traumatol.* **2009**, *10*, 9–15. [CrossRef] [PubMed]
14. Gupta, V.; Kapoor, S.; Clubb, S.; Davies, M.; Blundell, C. Treatment of bilateral open calcaneal fractures with ilizarov frames. *Injury* **2005**, *36*, 1488–1490. [CrossRef] [PubMed]
15. Pajchert-Kozłowska, A.; Pawik, Ł.; Szelerski, Ł.; Żarek, S.; Górski, R.; Pawik, M.; Fink-Lwow, F.; Morasiewicz, P. Assessment of body balance of patients treated with the Ilizarov method for tibial nonunion. *Acta Bioeng. Biomech.* **2020**, *22*, 131–137. [CrossRef]
16. Morasiewicz, P.; Dragan, S.; Dragan, S.Ł.; Wrzosek, Z.; Pawik, Ł. Pedobarographic analysis of body weight distribution on the lower limbs and balance after Ilizarov corticotomies. *Clin. Biomech.* **2016**, *31*, 2–6. [CrossRef]
17. Morasiewicz, P.; Konieczny, G.; Dejnek, M.; Morasiewicz, L.; Urbański, W.; Kulej, M.; Dragan, S.Ł.; Dragan, S.F.; Pawik, Ł. Pedobarographic analysis of body weight distribution on the lower limbs and balance after ankle arthrodesis with Ilizarov fixation and internal fixation. *Biomed. Eng. Online* **2018**, *17*, 174. [CrossRef] [PubMed]
18. Pawik, Ł.; Pajchert-Kozłowska, A.; Szelerski, Ł.; Żarek, S.; Górski, R.; Pawik, M.; Fink-Lwow, F.; Morasiewicz, P. Assessment of Lower Limb Load. Distribution in Patients Treated with the Ilizarov Method. for Tibial Nonunion. *Med. Sci. Monit.* **2021**, *27*, e930849. [CrossRef]

19. Rongies, W.; Bak, A.; Lazar, A. A trial of the use of pedobarography in the assessment of the effectiveness of rehabilitation in patients with coxarthrosis. *Ortop. Traumatol. Rehabil.* **2009**, *11*, 242–252.
20. Lorkowski, J.; Trybus, M.; Hładki, W.; Brongel, L. Underfoot pressure distribution of a patient with unilateral ankylosis of talonavicular joint during rheumatoid arthritis–case report. *Przegl Lek.* **2008**, *65*, 54–56.
21. Jancova, J. Measuring the balance control system—Review. *Acta Med.* **2008**, *51*, 129–137.
22. Genc, Y.; Gultekin, A.; Duymus, T.M.; Mutlu, S.; Mutlu, H.; Komur, B. Pedobarography in the Assessment of Postoperative Calcaneal Fracture Pressure with Gait. *J. Foot Ankle Surg.* **2016**, *55*, 99–105. [CrossRef]
23. Jandova, S.; Pazour, J.; Janura, M. Comparison of Plantar Pressure Distribution During Walking After Two Different Surgical Treatments for Calcaneal Fracture. *J. Foot Ankle Surg.* **2019**, *58*, 260–265. [CrossRef]
24. Brand, A.; Klöpfer-Krämer, I.; Böttger, M.; Kröger, I.; Gaul, L.; Wackerle, H.; Müßig, J.A.; Dietrich, A.; Gabel, J.; Augat, P. Gait characteristics and functional outcomes during early follow-up are comparable in patients with calcaneal fractures treated by either the sinus tarsi or the extended lateral approach. *Gait Posture* **2019**, *70*, 190–195. [CrossRef]
25. Van Hoeve, S.; Verbruggen, J.; Willems, P.; Meijer, K.; Poeze, M. Vertical ground reaction forces in patients after calcaneal trauma surgery. *Gait Posture* **2017**, *58*, 523–526. [CrossRef] [PubMed]
26. Ataç, A.; Akil Ağdere, S.; Dilek, B. Comparison of the Foot-Ankle Characteristics and Physical and Functional Performance of Racquet Sport Players. *Arch. Health Sci. Res.* **2023**, *10*, 108–114. [CrossRef]
27. Arslan, M.; Görgü, S.Ö. Effect of short-term spinal orthosis and insoles application on cobb angle, plantar pressure and balance in individuals with adolescent idiopathic scoliosis. *Clin. Biomech.* **2023**, *110*, 106121. [CrossRef] [PubMed]
28. Brusa, J.; Maggio, M.C.; Giustino, V.; Thomas, E.; Zangla, D.; Iovane, A.; Palma, A.; Corsello, G.; Messina, G.; Bellafiore, M. Upper and lower limb strength and body posture in children with congenital hypothyroidism: An observational case-control study. *Int. J. Environ. Res. Public. Health* **2020**, *17*, 4830. [CrossRef] [PubMed]
29. Feka, K.; Brusa, J.; Cannata, R.; Giustino, V.; Bianco, A.; Gjaka, M.; Iovane, A.; Palma, A.; Messina, G. Is bodyweight affecting plantar pressure distribution in children? An observational study. *Medicine* **2020**, *99*, e21968. [CrossRef] [PubMed]
30. Scoppa, F.; Messina, G.; Gallamini, M.; Belloni, G. Clinical stabilometry standardization: Feet position in the static stabilometric assessment of postural stability. *Acta Medica Mediterr.* **2017**, *33*, 707–713. [CrossRef]
31. Güven, M.; Kocadal, O.; Akman, B.; Poyanli, O.S.; Kemah, B.; Atay, E.F. Proximal femoral nail shows better concordance of gait analysis between operated and uninjured limbs compared to hemiarthroplasty in intertrochanteric femoral fractures. *Injury* **2016**, *47*, 1325–1331. [CrossRef]
32. Schepers, T.; Kieboom, B.; Van Diggele, P.; Patka, P.; Van Lieshout, E.M.M. Pedobarographic analysis and quality of life after lisfranc fracture dislocation. *Foot Ankle Int.* **2010**, *31*, 857–864. [CrossRef]
33. Schepers, T.; Van der Stoep, A.; Van der Avert, H.; Van Lieshout, E.M.; Patka, P. Plantar pressure analysis after percutaneous repair of displaced intra-articular calcaneal fractures. *Foot Ankle Int.* **2008**, *29*, 128–135. [CrossRef]
34. Kizkapan, T.B.; Yıldız, K.I. The comparison of pedobarographic parameters after calcaneal fractures. *Ulus. Travma Acil. Cerrahi. Derg.* **2022**, *28*, 1521–1526. [CrossRef] [PubMed]
35. Núñez-Trull, A.; Alvarez-Medina, J.; Jaén-Carrillo, D.; Roche-Seruendo, L.E.; Gómez-Trullén, E. Absolute agreement and consistency of the OptoGait system and Freemed platform for measuring walking gait. *Med. Eng. Phys.* **2022**, *110*, 103912. [CrossRef] [PubMed]
36. Tarczyńska, M.; Szubstarski, M.; Gawęda, K.; Przybylski, P.; Czekajska-Chehab, E. Outcomes of Open Repair Treatment for Acute Versus Chronic Achilles Tendon Ruptures: Long-Term Retrospective Follow-Up of a Minimum 10 Years—A Pilot Study. *Med. Sci.* **2023**, *11*, 25. [CrossRef] [PubMed]
37. Machado, G.G.; Barbosa, K.S.S.; Barcelos Oliveira, I.C.; Lobato, D.F.M.; de Oliveira, N.M.L. Protocols of balance assessment using baropodometry in healthy individuals—Systematic review. *Saúde Desenvolv. Hum.* **2021**, *9*. [CrossRef]

Disclaimer/Publisher's Note: The statements, opinions and data contained in all publications are solely those of the individual author(s) and contributor(s) and not of MDPI and/or the editor(s). MDPI and/or the editor(s) disclaim responsibility for any injury to people or property resulting from any ideas, methods, instructions or products referred to in the content.

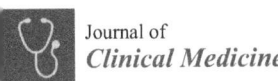

Case Report

Novel Use of a Fibular Strut Allograft with Fibular Head in an Elderly Patient with Proximal Humeral Fracture and Severe Metaphyseal Comminution: An Alternative to Shoulder Arthroplasty

Jun-Hyuk Lim [1], Yeong-Seub Ahn [2], Sungmin Kim [1] and Myung-Sun Kim [1,*]

[1] Department of Orthopedic Surgery, Chonnam National University Medical School and Hospital, Dong-gu, Gwangju 61469, Republic of Korea; ove03@naver.com (J.-H.L.); kimsum83@gmail.com (S.K.)
[2] Department of Orthopedic Surgery, Good Morning General Hospital, Pyeongtaek 17874, Republic of Korea; ysahn84@naver.com
* Correspondence: mskim@jnu.ac.kr; Tel.: +82-62-220-6343

Abstract: Treatment of a comminuted proximal humerus fracture (PHF) in elderly patients with severe osteoporosis is challenging, often leading to arthroplasty (such as hemiarthroplasty or reverse shoulder arthroplasty) as the treatment of choice. However, arthroplasty does not always guarantee favorable outcomes. In contrast, the use of intramedullary fibular strut allografts provides additional reduction stability during locking plate fixation; however, to our knowledge, there is limited literature on the use of fibular strut allografts, including the fibular head. Here we aim to report the advantages of using a fibular strut containing the fibular head in severe osteoporotic PHFs. We present the case of an 88-year-old female patient with severe osteoporosis diagnosed with a left PHF accompanied by severe metaphyseal comminution following a fall from a chair. Rather than shoulder arthroplasty, we performed osteosynthesis using a fibular strut allograft containing the fibular head. At the one-year follow-up after surgery, we observed excellent bony union and a favorable functional outcome without major complications, such as reduction loss. The novel use of a fibular strut allograft containing the fibular head could be promising for PHFs with severe metaphyseal comminution, potentially avoiding the need for arthroplasty.

Keywords: proximal humerus fracture; metaphyseal comminution; intramedullary fibular strut allograft; shoulder arthroplasty

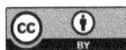

1. Introduction

Proximal humerus fractures (PHFs) frequently occur in elderly women with poor bone quality, typically as a result of low-energy mechanisms. The treatment of PHFs is challenging and controversial [1]. With the aging population, the incidence of PHFs in elderly patients is increasing. Conservative treatment can be considered as an option for PHFs, whether non-displaced or with some degree of displacement, taking into account the patient's age and functional demands [2]. However, complex PHFs often result in poor outcomes with conservative treatment; therefore, surgical treatment is often recommended [3]. The available surgical options, including open reduction internal fixation (ORIF) and shoulder arthroplasty (e.g., hemiarthroplasty or reverse total shoulder arthroplasty), have continuously evolved.

Locking plate fixation for severely comminuted osteoporotic PHFs can lead to various complications. Major complications associated with screw perforation with reduction loss or varus collapse are reported more often in elderly patients because of their poor bone quality [4]. Thus, the importance of medial support is increasingly being recognized [4–6]. Several studies have reported the importance of medial supporting screws for providing medial support [5,6], with recent emphasis being placed on the importance of cement augmentation [7,8] and strut bone grafting to avoid major complications [9,10].

Since its initial report by Gardner et al., who first described how the intramedullary fibular strut allograft could support the medial column and facilitate fracture reduction in unstable PHFs [11], numerous studies have highlighted its advantages. These include providing fixation stability in unstable osteoporotic PHFs during locking plate fixation and reducing various fracture-related complications [12–16].

Meanwhile, with technological advancements and an increase in surgical volumes for shoulder arthroplasty, the use of shoulder arthroplasty in complex PHFs has recently increased. Shoulder arthroplasty may be indicated, particularly in patients aged 70 and above, as well as those with a high risk of avascular necrosis (AVN), such as Neer three-part or four-part fractures, head-splitting fractures, and those with pre-existing rotator cuff tears [17]. Recent studies have reported that, in elderly patients with complex PHFs, the outcomes of reverse total shoulder arthroplasty (RTSA) are superior to those of open reduction and internal fixation (ORIF) [18], with a lower reoperation rate observed in RTSA [19,20]. However, shoulder arthroplasty is considered a joint salvage procedure, and, to date, the long-term outcomes of shoulder arthroplasty in elderly patients with complex PHF remain limited [21]. Moreover, patients with severe osteoporosis face an increased risk of periprosthetic fracture during surgery, leading to potential complications, such as early implant failure [22,23]. This can escalate the likelihood of revision surgery, which, given that the majority of patients are elderly, becomes challenging, complex, and significantly diminishes postoperative shoulder function.

This study aimed to present a novel surgical method through a case report that can serve as an alternative to shoulder arthroplasty in patients with severely comminuted osteoporotic PHFs extending into the metaphyseal area. Instead of shoulder arthroplasty, we opted for joint-preserving surgery using locking plate fixation augmented with an intramedullary fibular strut containing the fibular head, considering the patient's poor bone quality. To the best of our knowledge, there are no reports in the literature regarding the use of fibular strut allografts, including the fibular head, during locking plate fixation of PHFs. We further describe the radiological and functional outcomes of the patient.

2. Case Presentation

The patient was an 88-year-old woman with left arm pain following a fall from a chair. Plain radiography (Figure 1) and computed tomography (CT) (Figure 2) showed a PHF.

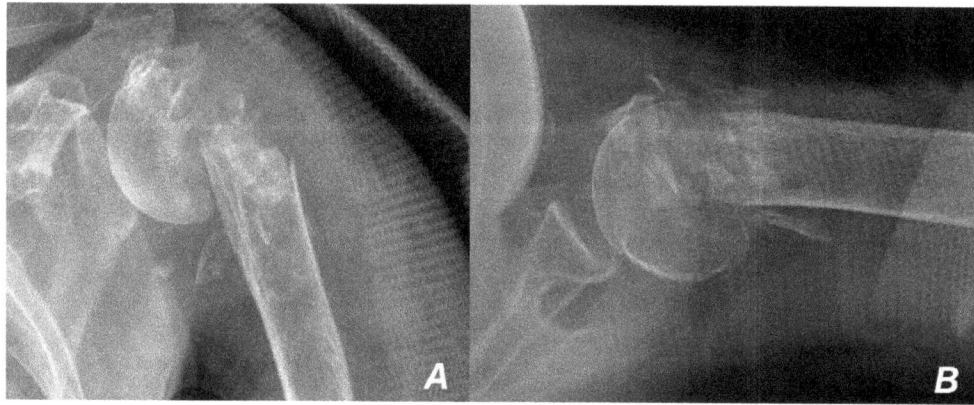

Figure 1. Initial plain radiographs. At the time of the visit, the initial plain radiographs revealed both medial and lateral cortical comminution of the proximal humeral metaphyseal area in the anterior-posterior (**A**) and trans-axillary (**B**) views of the X-ray images.

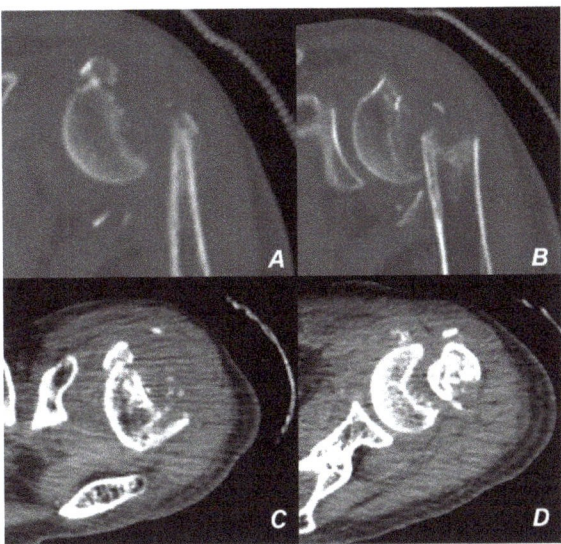

Figure 2. Computed tomographic (CT) slices of the injured arm. The CT slices of the injured arm showed a lesser tuberosity fracture of the proximal humerus, visible in both the coronal (**A**) and axial (**C**) planes. In addition, severe comminutions of the medial and lateral metaphysis areas can be identified in both coronal (**B**) and axial (**D**) planes of the CT slices.

The fracture was diagnosed as a comminuted PHF with varus, flexion, and anteversion of the head of the humerus, with severe medial and lateral metaphyseal comminution and displacement of the lesser and greater tuberosities (Figure 3). Evaluation of bone mineral density revealed severe osteoporosis with a T-score of −4.6 at the femoral neck. Despite being 88 years old, the patient had no significant underlying conditions other than severe osteoporosis and mild hypertension controlled with medication. She maintained a functional demand sufficient for independent household activities and daily living (Table 1).

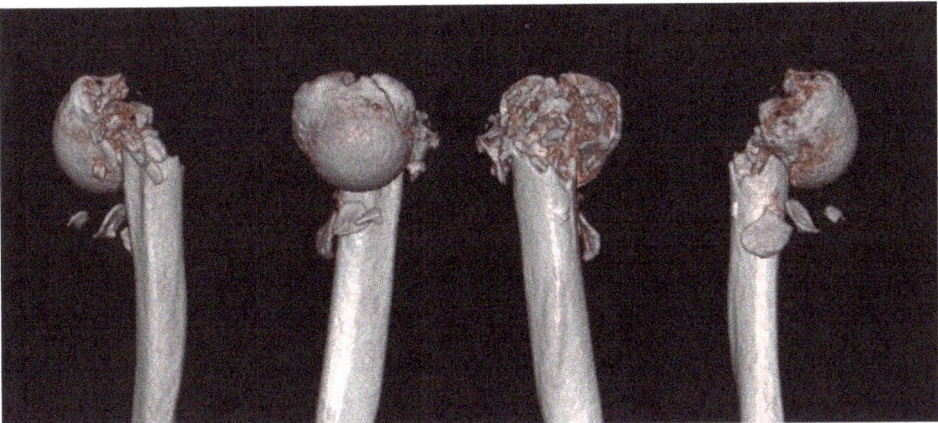

Figure 3. Three-dimensional computed tomography showing the configuration of the patient's injured arm. The three-dimensional computed tomography showed the severe medial and lateral metaphyseal comminution with varus, flexion, and anteversion of the fracture configuration. A displaced fracture of both the lesser and greater tuberosities was also identified.

Table 1. Patient demographic data.

Information	Details
Age at surgery	88
Sex	Female
Diagnoses	Severe osteoporosis (T-score −4.6 at the femoral neck)
	Mild hypertension on medication
	Neer 4-part proximal humerus fracture on the left shoulder
Physical Examination	Decreased painful range of motion in the left shoulder
Functional demand	Independent light household activities
Osteoporosis medication	None
Past medical history	None

The patient had a previous diagnosis of osteoporosis but had not undergone treatments such as medication. We decided to opt for surgical treatment in this patient for several reasons. First, although the fracture line did not directly involve the head, it presented as an unstable fracture pattern with significant displacement and a large gap between the humeral head and shaft. Second, if left to heal conservatively in its current state, it could result in symptomatic malunion, making functional recovery before surgery unlikely. Third, attempting closed reduction to prevent malunion posed a high risk of additional fractures in other parts of the humerus due to severe osteoporosis, and the patient's compliance was inadequate to maintain reduction for several weeks, increasing the risk of reduction loss. Lastly, the patient and their caregiver strongly desired surgery.

Shoulder arthroplasty is a viable option for the management of elderly patients, including this patient with an osteoporotic Neer three- or four-part PHF [17]. However, we determined that arthroplasty would be challenging for several reasons, and we could not assure a favorable outcome post-surgery. First, comminution in both the greater and lesser tuberosities complicated tuberosity healing. Second, considering the very low T-score, the patient was expected to experience severe osteoporotic changes in the glenoid, posing challenges for base-plate fixation. Lastly, the possibility of intraoperative periprosthetic fractures during stem insertion was anticipated, which could significantly impact both short-term and long-term outcomes. Instead, we opted for ORIF with locking plate fixation. To prevent major complications such as reduction loss and varus collapse during locking plate fixation, we ensured adequate insertion of medial supporting screws and utilized additional tension-band suture fixation for augmentation. Additionally, we decided to use an intramedullary fibular strut allograft containing the fibular head, offering robust support for both medial and lateral comminution while adequately filling the void defect within the humeral head using the fibular head.

Surgical Technique

Under general anesthesia, the patient was positioned in the beach chair position. The affected arm was placed on an arm table for easy manipulation and positioning during the procedure. Utilizing a standard deltopectoral approach, a surgical incision of approximately 10–15 cm in length was made just above the coracoid process, tracing along the anterior aspect downward along the beginning of the deltopectoral groove and just above the coracoid process. After identifying the deltopectoral groove and cephalic vein, the pectoralis major and deltoid muscles were located. The deltoid muscle was then retracted laterally, and the pectoralis major muscle was retracted medially. Subsequently, subdeltoid release was performed through finger dissection to create adequate space for plate placement on the lateral side of the proximal humerus.

The humeral head and fragments were retracted, and temporary reduction was attempted to ascertain the anatomical configuration. However, due to severe comminution and bone loss in the medial and lateral metaphyseal area, anatomical reduction and maintenance were deemed impossible without supporting the metaphyseal portion. Due to severe osteoporosis, a void defect was identified within the humeral head. To address these challenges, we supported the medial and lateral metaphyseal defects and the void defect of the humeral head with a fresh-frozen fibular strut allograft including the fibular head (Figure 4A).

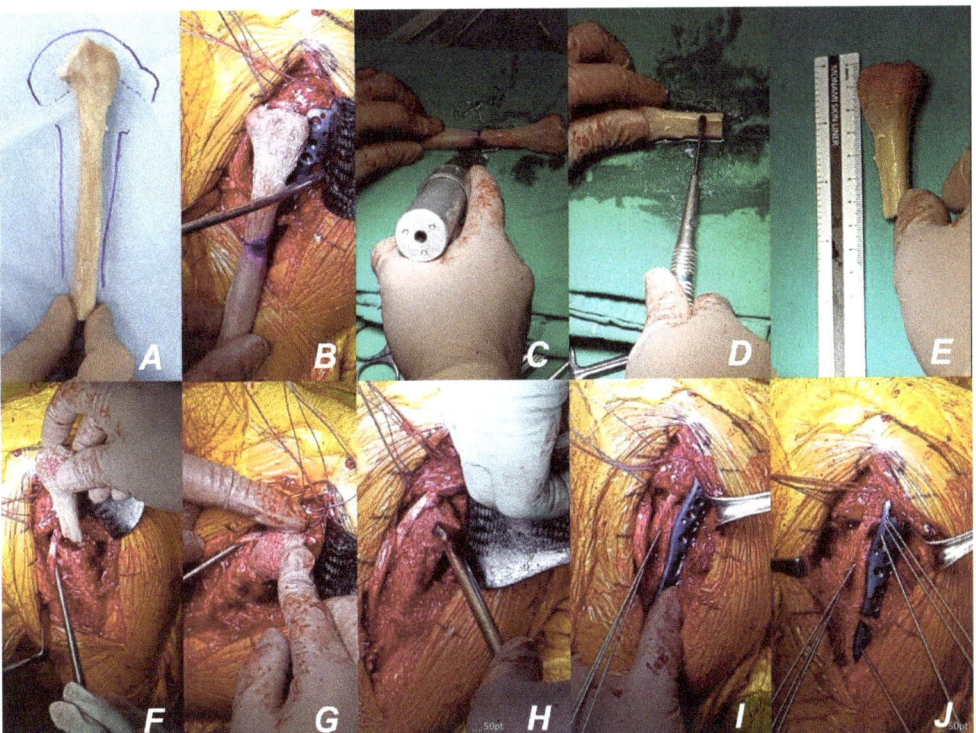

Figure 4. Intraoperative clinical photos of fibular strut allograft preparation. Following the planning of use of the expected configuration with a proximal fibular allograft containing the head (**A,B**), the proximal fibular allograft, including the fibular head, was intraoperatively remodeled and decorticated based on the remaining bone configuration (**C–E**). The refined fibular strut allograft with the head was inserted into the cavity, where severe comminution with bone loss had developed, through the fracture site after canal preparation (**F,G**). The fibular head portion was inserted into the humeral head using a Darrach retractor and an impactor (**H**). After fluoroscopic confirmation of the position of the fibular strut allograft within the proximal humerus, temporary fixation was performed with Kirschner wires (**I,J**).

To ensure optimal fit, we measured the width of the medullary channel of the proximal humeral shaft anteriorly and posteriorly, in addition to the medial and lateral dimensions, before acquiring the fibular strut. The fibular strut, extending from the fibular head to the shaft with sufficient length, was planned to position its metaphyseal area over the main fracture site between the humeral head and shaft (Figure 4A). The distal side of the strut, the shaft portion, was intended to adequately fill the medullary channel of the proximal humerus shaft. Given that the head and metaphyseal area of the fibular strut are relatively thick and the fibular shaft is relatively thin (and fits into the medullary channel of the humerus), we procured a fresh-frozen fibular strut with a shaft corresponding to the smaller size among the measured anterior, posterior, medial and lateral medullary channel widths.

The proximal fibular strut allograft, including the fibular head, was remodeled according to the remaining bony configuration of the patient's proximal humerus. The length of the fibular strut was determined to sufficiently accommodate the distal part of the locking plate, allowing for the insertion of three or more bi-cortical screws. Additionally, to ensure proper insertion of the shaft portion of the strut into the medullary channel without being too loose or too tight, cortical preparation was performed using an oscillating burr. In our patient, the humerus at the proximal shaft level exhibited a large medullary canal close to a circular shape with a thin cortex. Meanwhile, the shaft of the fibular strut was closer to a triangular shape. During passage through the humerus medulla, there were areas where the edges of the strut caught, necessitating smoothing with a burr (Figure 4B–E). The distal portion of the remodeled fibular strut allograft was initially inserted into the intramedullary canal of the meta-diaphysis through the fracture site (Figure 4F,G). The fibular head was then inserted into the humeral head using a Darrach retractor and an impactor. This allowed for the easy and precise insertion of the proximal portion of the fibular strut allograft into the expected portion of the void defect in the humeral head by sliding down while making contact with the Darrach retractor by pushing the impactor (Figure 4H). Upon ensuring proper positioning of the fibular strut allograft inside the proximal humerus, between the meta-diaphysis and humeral head, and confirming via fluoroscopy, temporary fixation using Kirschner wires was performed (Figure 4I,J). The Proximal Humerus Internal Locking System (PHILOS; DePuy Synthes, Raynham, MA, USA) plates were then used to complete the fixation (Figure 5). Additionally, supplementary tension suture fixation using non-absorbable suture materials with two washers (Figure 6) was performed to enhance stability, thus preventing fixation loss and varus collapse [24,25].

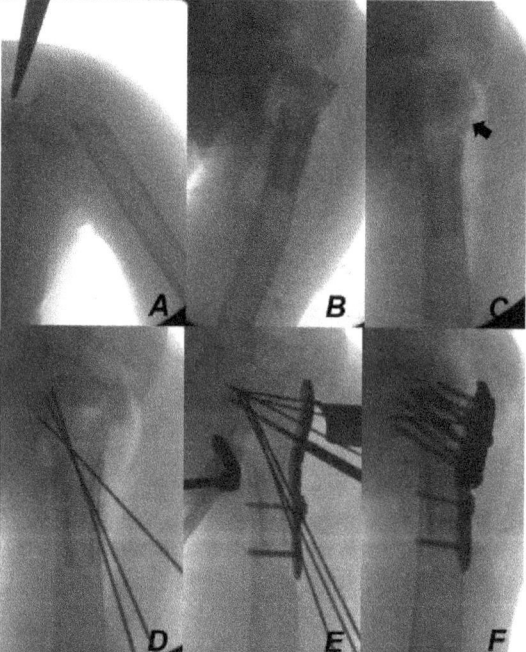

Figure 5. Intraoperative fluoroscopic images of the fixation method using the fibular strut allo-bone-containing head with locking compression plate. After insertion of the proximal fibular strut allograft containing the head (**A**,**B**), humeral head reduction was performed on the allograft (**C**). The defect of the lateral cortex was reconstructed (black arrow) by fibular strut allograft with the head. After confirming via fluoroscopy that the position of the strut bone between the meta-diaphysis and the humeral head was adequate, temporary fixation using Kirschner wires was performed (**D**). While maintaining the reduction state with Kirschner wires, firm fixation was performed using a locking compression plate (**E**,**F**).

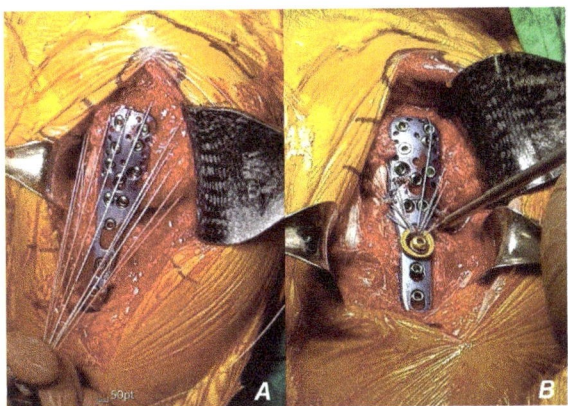

Figure 6. Intraoperative images of locking compression plate application with tension suture fixation. Using non-absorbable suture material, sutures were placed on the subscapularis, supraspinatus, and infraspinatus tendons respectively (**A**). Then, the suture material was passed through two washers. Subsequently, tension was applied to the suture material in the distal direction to its maximum extent, and conventional screw fixation was performed (**B**).

The affected arm was immobilized in a sling for 2 weeks postoperatively, with gradual passive range of motion (ROM) exercises encouraged thereafter. After 4 weeks, active assisted ROM exercises were performed. To mitigate the risk of periprosthetic fracture due to stress concentration at the distal portion of the plate, the patient and their caregiver were informed during hospital visits not to support themselves by touching the ground when standing up using the affected arm. For osteoporosis treatment after surgery, a combination therapy utilizing parathyroid hormone and denosumab was administered for 1 year post-surgery, followed by a decision to continue lifelong denosumab injections every 6 months thereafter. Subsequent follow-ups were conducted at 2 weeks, 6 weeks, 3 months, 6 months, and 12 months. Additionally, serial plain radiographic images were taken during the postoperative follow-up period (Figure 7). At the 3-month postoperative follow-up assessment, CT scans indicated successful bone union (Figure 8). Active ROM in the affected arm was comparable to that of the unaffected arm (Figure 9). By the 1-year follow-up assessment, favorable functional scoring was observed, with a pain Visual Analog Scale score of 1, Constant–Murley score of 64, University of California at Los Angeles shoulder score of 31, American Shoulder and Elbow Surgeons score of 82, and Disabilities of the Arm, Shoulder, and Hand score of 20.

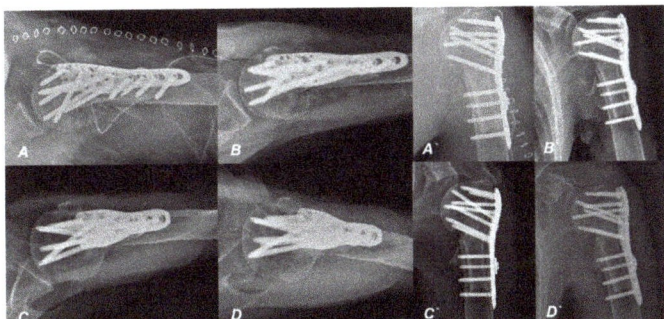

Figure 7. Serial plain radiographic images during the postoperative follow-up period. Continuous radiographic reviews were conducted throughout the outpatient follow-up period following surgery. The images depict radiographs taken at immediate (**A**,**A′**), 3 months (**B**,**B′**), 6 months (**C**,**C′**), and 1 year (**D**,**D′**) postoperatively.

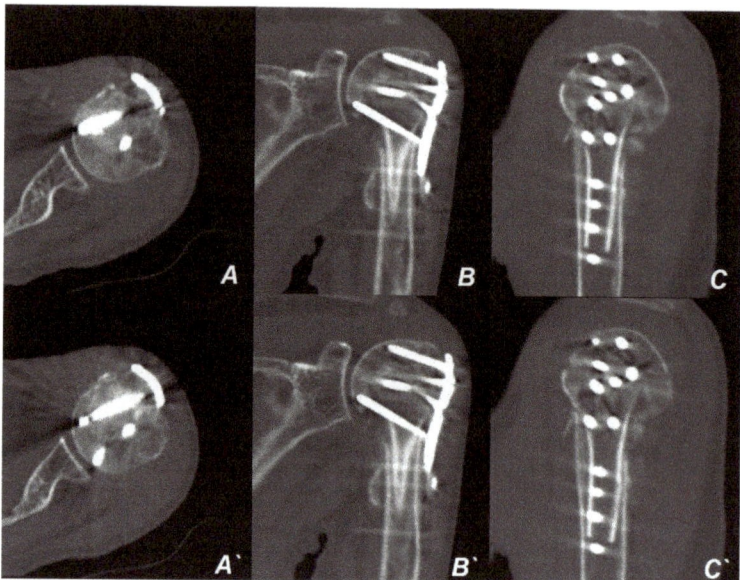

Figure 8. Computed tomography (CT) images performed at the 3-month postoperative follow-up. Progressive bony union was identified in the axial (**A,A′**), coronal (**B,B′**), and sagittal (**C,C′**) slices of the CT images.

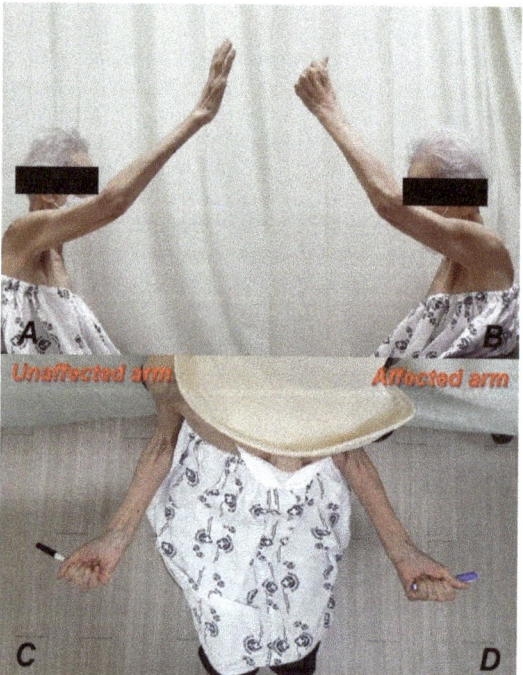

Figure 9. Clinical images of range of motion (ROM) at the last follow-up assessment. The active ROM in the injured arm showed almost the same ROM as that of the unaffected arm, both in forward flexion (**A,B**) and external rotation (**C,D**).

3. Discussion

In our case, we successfully achieved locking plate fixation using an intramedullary fibular strut allograft containing the fibular head as an alternative to shoulder arthroplasty in a patient diagnosed with a severe comminuted PHF extending into the metaphyseal area and complicated by severe osteoporosis.

The patient, being over 70 years old and afflicted with severe osteoporosis, presented with a severely comminuted Neer four-part PHF, potentially indicating shoulder arthroplasty [17]. However, we considered shoulder arthroplasty challenging for several reasons, with concerns regarding achieving favorable functional outcomes in the future. First, the patient's diagnosis of severe osteoporosis, with a femoral neck T-score of −4.6 on bone mineral density, indicated poor glenoid bone quality. Tabarestani et al. have reported a significant decrease in glenoid bone mineral density as the T-score of the femoral neck decreases [22]. Poor bone quality can impact glenoid fixation during reverse shoulder arthroplasty when implanting the glenoid component, thereby increasing the risk of periprosthetic fracture [23,26]. Secondly, the patient exhibited significant comminution and displacement in both the greater and lesser tuberosities, leading us to anticipate challenges in ensuring proper healing. Several studies have reported that tuberosity healing is essential for successful outcomes in procedures such as hemiarthroplasty, and, although not as critical as in hemiarthroplasty, it remains important for future shoulder function in reverse total-shoulder arthroplasty [27–31].

For the reasons mentioned above, we decided to prioritize ORIF with a locking plate for this patient. In our case, we used an intramedullary fibular strut allograft during locking plate fixation to prevent fixation failure. The objective was to achieve optimal anatomical restoration and maintenance of the medial calcar to prevent varus collapse. Several studies have reported that restoring the medial calcar and avoiding varus alignment during locking plate fixation of PHF are the most crucial factors for successful outcomes of locking plate fixation [4,32]. Moreover, elderly patients with osteoporosis or medial column comminution are prone to increased rates of major complications, such as varus collapse and higher re-operation rates [4,33,34]. With advancements in surgical techniques, Gardner et al. [11] first reported using screws to position the fibular strut allograft more medially to improve medial support and maintain fracture fixation stability.

The patient in this case had sever" ost'oporosis and severe comminution around the surgical neck of the humerus, as well as in the medial and lateral cortices. Furthermore, severe osteoporosis resulted in significant hollowing of the humeral head, with minimal subchondral bone remaining; therefore, we used an intramedullary fibular strut allograft containing the fibular head. Each component of the fibular strut served a specific function and has significance. The head of the strut fills the void defect in the humeral head and assists in securely anchoring the locking screw. This approach is consistent with recent studies reporting the advantage of the fibular strut itself in providing vertical support to the humeral head [35]. The metaphyseal area of the strut provides mechanical support to both the medial and lateral columns at the fracture site with comminution. This may allow the thicker metaphyseal area, unlike the shaft of the strut, to contribute more effectively to the stability of the fracture site in both medial and lateral unstable comminuted PHFs, such as in our patient's case. Recent biomechanical studies have demonstrated that fibular strut augmentation during locking plate fixation enhances varus stiffness, torsional stiffness, and maximum load failure [36].

We aimed to ensure a precise fit of the fibular strut within the medullary canal of the humerus. This was achieved by meticulously measuring the dimensions of the canal using preoperative CT axial cuts and procuring a strut that closely aligned with our planned specifications prior to purchase. In general, for upper limb fractures including PHFs, it is recommended to achieve fixation at the distal aspect of the fracture involving at least six cortices. Therefore, we determined the length of the strut to encompass all regions where a minimum of three bi-cortical screws could be fixed for adequate fixation. This approach offers the advantage that the locking screw can be inserted through the sturdy portion of the fibular strut, resulting in a stronger purchase. Although not proven by biomechanical studies, one study reported that the use of a fibular strut reduces the force arm of locking screws, thereby decreasing the possibility of screw breakage [35].

We encountered no technical difficulties during surgery as we obtained a fibular strut of the expected size through preoperative planning. In case of size-related errors during the procedure, the advantage lies in the ability to easily resolve the situation through burring, allowing for a straightforward surgical procedure. Salzman et al. recommended the use of additional structural graft when the void defect of the humeral head is sufficiently large enough to make impaction of the strut shaft difficult. Additionally, they suggested contouring the distal portion of the fibular strut using an oscillating saw to ensure stable placement of the strut at the fracture site [37]. Another study reported a technique in which the fibular strut shaft can be placed in the desired position using a K-wire guidewire, which is then used to temporarily hold the fibular strut in place during plate fixation [12]. However, this method may pose technical challenges, as there is a risk of the strut being damaged during K-wire guidewire fixation or slipping into the medullary canal. On the contrary, our fibular strut has a sufficiently large fibular head size, minimizing the need for additional grafting. It provides stable support to the head and is large enough to cover the entire medulla. Once successful grafting is achieved, the surgeon can focus solely on locking plate fixation, offering a technical advantage.

However, several considerations should be taken into account when using fibular strut allografts. First, it does not prevent the risk of AVN in the humeral head, the most significant fracture-related complication that can occur during locking plate fixation. Nonetheless, given our priority of joint-preserving surgery, revision surgery via shoulder arthroplasty can be performed at any time if AVN occurs. This approach preserves bone stock compared to revision arthroplasty due to shoulder arthroplasty failure and makes revision surgery easier. One study reported a mean time of approximately 8.5 months for the detection of global AVN in the humeral head [8]. Fortunately, in up to 1 year post-surgery, AVN of the humeral head has not been detected in our patient. Second, we cannot completely rule out fresh-frozen allograft-related complications such as the transmission of infection or rejection through strut allografting. Lastly, legal restrictions in some countries may result in the unavailability of fibular struts. One study reported that the use of fibular strut allografts was associated with longer surgical times and higher costs compared to groups that did not use fibular struts. There was no significant difference reported in clinical outcomes between the group that used fibular struts and the group that did not [38]. However, this study was limited to two-part and three-part PHFs, and it did not compare the strut allograft group with the shoulder arthroplasty group, indicating its limitations. Most studies commonly describe the advantages of fibular strut augmentation during locking plate fixation in unstable PHFs [9,11–16]. Additionally, fibular strut augmentation is cost-saving compared to shoulder arthroplasty.

We recommend that surgeons facing challenging cases of severe comminuted PHFs with severe osteoporosis, where shoulder arthroplasty may be difficult or may not yield favorable outcomes, consider the use of an intramedullary fibular strut allograft containing the fibular head. Our novel surgical method is valuable, as it not only provides structural and volumetric support during locking plate fixation, but also enhances fixation stability, potentially reducing the need for shoulder arthroplasty, facilitating faster bony union and enabling early rehabilitation. However, our study has several limitations. It is a short-term follow-up case report, and the patient had an intact rotator cuff, which may have contributed to achieving a favorable functional outcome separate from bony union issues. Additionally, we used additional techniques, such as tension band suture augmentation, to prevent varus collapse and reduction loss, which could potentially influence the results.

4. Conclusions

In conclusion, our novel intramedullary fibular strut allograft, incorporating the fibular head, presents an attractive option for facilitating early bony union and favorable functional outcomes in patients with severe comminuted osteoporotic PHFs undergoing locking plate fixation. It serves as both volumetric support and a strong structural support, providing an alternative to shoulder arthroplasty in challenging scenarios where such an alternative may not be feasible. This approach promotes early bony union and improves functional outcomes for patients.

Author Contributions: Conceptualization, J.-H.L. and M.-S.K.; Methodology, Y.-S.A.; Software, S.K.; Validation, J.-H.L., S.K. and M.-S.K.; Formal Analysis, S.K. and Y.-S.A.; Resources, S.K.; Data Curation, J.-H.L. and S.K.; Writing—Original Draft Preparation, J.-H.L.; Writing—Review and Editing, J.-H.L. and M.-S.K.; Visualization, S.K.; Supervision, M.-S.K. All authors have read and agreed to the published version of the manuscript.

Funding: This research received no external funding.

Institutional Review Board Statement: The study was conducted in accordance with the Declaration of Helsinki and approved by the Institutional Review Board of the Chonnam National University Hospital (IRB No. CNUH-EXP-2020-373, approval date 11 December 2020). The Chonnam National University Hospital Institutional Review Board does not require formal consent for this type of study.

Informed Consent Statement: The Chonnam National University Hospital Institutional Review Board does not require formal consent for this type of study.

Data Availability Statement: The data presented in this study are available on request from the corresponding author. The data are not publicly available due to privacy.

Acknowledgments: This study was supported by grants (BCRI-23063, BCRI-24086) from Chonnam National University Hospital Research Institute of Clinical Medicine.

Conflicts of Interest: The authors declare no conflicts of interest.

References

1. Iglesias-Rodríguez, S.; Domínguez-Prado, D.M.; García-Reza, A.; Fernández-Fernández, D.; Pérez-Alfonso, E.; García-Piñeiro, J.; Castro-Menéndez, M. Epidemiology of proximal humerus fractures. *J. Orthop. Surg. Res.* **2021**, *16*, 402. [CrossRef] [PubMed]
2. Martinez-Catalan, N. Conservative treatment of proximal Humerus fractures: When, how, and what to expect. *Curr. Rev. Musculoskelet. Med.* **2023**, *16*, 75–84. [CrossRef]
3. Lopiz, Y.; Alcobía-Díaz, B.; Galán-Olleros, M.; García-Fernández, C.; Picado, A.L.; Marco, F. Reverse shoulder arthroplasty versus nonoperative treatment for 3-or 4-part proximal humeral fractures in elderly patients: A prospective randomized controlled trial. *J. Shoulder Elb. Surg.* **2019**, *28*, 2259–2271. [CrossRef] [PubMed]
4. Gardner, M.J.; Weil, Y.; Barker, J.U.; Kelly, B.T.; Helfet, D.L.; Lorich, D.G. The importance of medial support in locked plating of proximal humerus fractures. *J. Orthop. Trauma* **2007**, *21*, 185–191. [CrossRef]
5. Wang, Q.; Sheng, N.; Rui, B.; Chen, Y. The neck-shaft angle is the key factor for the positioning of calcar screw when treating proximal humeral fractures with a locking plate. *Bone Jt. J.* **2020**, *102*, 1629–1635. [CrossRef] [PubMed]
6. Jung, W.-B.; Moon, E.-S.; Kim, S.-K.; Kovacevic, D.; Kim, M.-S. Does medial support decrease major complications of unstable proximal humerus fractures treated with locking plate? *BMC Musculoskelet. Disord.* **2013**, *14*, 102. [CrossRef]
7. Kim, D.-Y.; Kim, T.-Y.; Hwang, J.-T. PHILOS plate fixation with polymethyl methacrylate cement augmentation of an osteoporotic proximal humeral fracture. *Clin. Shoulder Elb.* **2020**, *23*, 156. [CrossRef]
8. Foruria, A.M.; Martinez-Catalan, N.; Valencia, M.; Morcillo, D.; Calvo, E. Proximal humeral fracture locking plate fixation with anatomic reduction, and a short-and-cemented-screws configuration, dramatically reduces the implant related failure rate in elderly patients. *JSES Int.* **2021**, *5*, 992–1000. [CrossRef] [PubMed]
9. Kim, D.-S.; Lee, D.-H.; Chun, Y.-M.; Shin, S.-J. Which additional augmented fixation procedure decreases surgical failure after proximal humeral fracture with medial comminution: Fibular allograft or inferomedial screws? *J. Shoulder Elb. Surg.* **2018**, *27*, 1852–1858. [CrossRef] [PubMed]
10. Lee, S.-J.; Hyun, Y.-S.; Baek, S.-H. Strut support with tricortical iliac allografts in unstable proximal humerus fractures: Surgical indication and new definition of poor medial column support. *Clin. Shoulder Elb.* **2019**, *22*, 29. [CrossRef]
11. Gardner, M.J.; Boraiah, S.; Helfet, D.L.; Lorich, D.G. Indirect medial reduction and strut support of proximal humerus fractures using an endosteal implant. *J. Orthop. Trauma* **2008**, *22*, 195–200. [CrossRef] [PubMed]
12. Cui, X.; Chen, H.; Ma, B.; Fan, W.; Li, H. Fibular strut allograft influences reduction and outcomes after locking plate fixation of comminuted proximal humeral fractures in elderly patients: A retrospective study. *BMC Musculoskelet. Disord.* **2019**, *20*, 511. [CrossRef] [PubMed]
13. Kim, J.Y.; Lee, J.; Kim, S.-H. Comparison between MIPO and the deltopectoral approach with allogenous fibular bone graft in proximal humeral fractures. *Clin. Shoulder Elb.* **2020**, *23*, 136. [CrossRef] [PubMed]

14. Zhao, L.; Qi, Y.m.; Yang, L.; Wang, G.r.; Zheng, S.n.; Wang, Q.; Liang, B.; Jiang, C.z. Comparison of the effects of proximal humeral internal locking system (PHILOS) alone and PHILOS combined with fibular allograft in the treatment of Neer three-or four-part proximal Humerus fractures in the elderly. *Orthop. Surg.* **2019**, *11*, 1003–1012. [CrossRef] [PubMed]
15. Myers, D.M.; Triplet, J.J.; Warmoth, P.J.; Passias, B.J.; McGowan, S.P.; Taylor, B.C. Improved outcomes using a fibular strut in proximal humerus fracture fixation. *Orthopedics* **2020**, *43*, 262–268. [CrossRef] [PubMed]
16. Tuerxun, M.; Tuxun, A.; Zeng, L.; Wang, Q.; Chen, Y. Locking plate combined with endosteal fibular allograft augmentation for medial column comminuted proximal humeral fracture. *Orthopedics* **2020**, *43*, 367–372. [CrossRef] [PubMed]
17. Kelly, B.J.; Myeroff, C.M. Reverse shoulder arthroplasty for proximal humerus fracture. *Curr. Rev. Musculoskelet. Med.* **2020**, *13*, 186–199. [CrossRef] [PubMed]
18. Fraser, A.N.; Bjørdal, J.; Wagle, T.M.; Karlberg, A.C.; Lien, O.A.; Eilertsen, L.; Mader, K.; Apold, H.; Larsen, L.B.; Madsen, J.E. Reverse shoulder arthroplasty is superior to plate fixation at 2 years for displaced proximal humeral fractures in the elderly: A multicenter randomized controlled trial. *JBJS* **2020**, *102*, 477–485. [CrossRef]
19. Luciani, P.; Procaccini, R.; Rotini, M.; Pettinari, F.; Gigante, A. Angular stable plate versus reverse shoulder arthroplasty for proximal humeral fractures in elderly patient. *Musculoskelet. Surg.* **2020**, *106*, 43–48. [CrossRef] [PubMed]
20. Greiwe, R.M.; Kohrs, B.J.; Callegari, J.; Harm, R.G.; Hill, M.A.; Boyle, M.S. Open reduction internal fixation vs. reverse shoulder arthroplasty for the treatment of acute displaced proximal humerus fractures. *JSES* **2020**, *30*, 250–257. [CrossRef]
21. Antonios, T.; Bakti, N.; Phadkhe, A.; Gulihar, A.; Singh, B. Outcomes following arthroplasty for proximal humeral fractures. *J. Clin. Orthop. Trauma* **2020**, *11*, S31–S36. [CrossRef] [PubMed]
22. Tabarestani, T.Q.; Levin, J.M.; Warren, E.; Boadi, P.; Twomey-Kozak, J.; Wixted, C.; Goltz, D.E.; Wickman, J.; Hurley, E.T.; Anakwenze, O. Preoperative glenoid bone density is associated with systemic osteoporosis in primary shoulder arthroplasty. *JSES* **2023**, *33*, 727–734. [CrossRef]
23. Casp, A.J.; Montgomery Jr, S.R.; Cancienne, J.M.; Brockmeier, S.F.; Werner, B.C. Osteoporosis and implant-related complications after anatomic and reverse total shoulder arthroplasty. *JAAOS-J. Am. Acad. Orthop. Surg.* **2020**, *28*, 121–127. [CrossRef] [PubMed]
24. Kim, K.-C.; Rhee, K.-J.; Shin, H.-D. Tension band sutures using a washer for a proximal humerus fracture. *J. Trauma Acute Care Surg.* **2008**, *64*, 1136–1138. [CrossRef] [PubMed]
25. Cho, C.-H.; Jung, G.-H.; Song, K.-S. Tension suture fixation using 2 washers for proximal humerus fractures. *Orthopedics* **2012**, *35*, 202–205. [CrossRef]
26. Terrier, A.; Obrist, R.; Becce, F.; Farron, A. Cement stress predictions after anatomic total shoulder arthroplasty are correlated with preoperative glenoid bone quality. *J. Shoulder Elb. Surg.* **2017**, *26*, 1644–1652. [CrossRef] [PubMed]
27. Marin, R.; Feltri, P.; Ferraro, S.; Ippolito, G.; Campopiano, G.; Previtali, D.; Filardo, G.; Marbach, F.; De Marinis, G.; Candrian, C. Impact of tuberosity treatment in reverse shoulder arthroplasty after proximal humeral fractures: A multicentre study. *J. Orthop. Sci.* **2023**, *28*, 765–771. [CrossRef] [PubMed]
28. Schmalzl, J.; Jessen, M.; Sadler, N.; Lehmann, L.-J.; Gerhardt, C. High tuberosity healing rate associated with better functional outcome following primary reverse shoulder arthroplasty for proximal humeral fractures with a 135° prosthesis. *BMC Musculoskelet. Disord.* **2020**, *21*, 35. [CrossRef] [PubMed]
29. Takayama, K.; Yamada, S.; Kobori, Y.; Shiode, H. The clinical outcomes and tuberosity healing after reverse total shoulder arthroplasty for acute proximal humeral fracture using the turned stem tension band technique. *J. Orthop. Sci.* **2022**, *27*, 372–379. [CrossRef]
30. Rivera, A.R.; Cardona, V. Reverse total shoulder arthroplasty for complex proximal humerus fracture in the elderly: Clinical and radiological results. *JSES Rev. Rep. Technol.* **2023**, *3*, 131–136. [CrossRef]
31. Hackett Jr, D.J.; Hsu, J.E.; Matsen III, F.A. Primary shoulder hemiarthroplasty: What can be learned from 359 cases that were surgically revised? *Clin. Orthop. Relat. Res.* **2018**, *476*, 1031. [CrossRef] [PubMed]
32. Solberg, B.D.; Moon, C.N.; Franco, D.P.; Paiement, G.D. Locked plating of 3-and 4-part proximal humerus fractures in older patients: The effect of initial fracture pattern on outcome. *J. Orthop. Trauma* **2009**, *23*, 113–119. [CrossRef] [PubMed]
33. Gupta, A.K.; Harris, J.D.; Erickson, B.J.; Abrams, G.D.; Bruce, B.; McCormick, F.; Nicholson, G.P.; Romeo, A.A. Surgical management of complex proximal humerus fractures—A systematic review of 92 studies including 4500 patients. *J. Orthop. Trauma* **2015**, *29*, 54–59. [CrossRef] [PubMed]
34. Sproul, R.C.; Iyengar, J.J.; Devcic, Z.; Feeley, B.T. A systematic review of locking plate fixation of proximal humerus fractures. *Injury* **2011**, *42*, 408–413. [CrossRef] [PubMed]
35. Nie, W.; Wang, Z.; Gu, F.; Xu, S.; Yue, Y.; Shao, A.; Sun, K. Effects of fibular strut augmentation for the open reduction and internal fixation of proximal humeral fractures: A systematic review and meta-analysis. *J. Orthop. Surg. Res.* **2022**, *17*, 322. [CrossRef] [PubMed]
36. Chang, H.-H.; Lim, J.-R.; Lee, K.-H.; An, H.; Yoon, T.-H.; Chun, Y.-M. The biomechanical effect of fibular strut grafts on humeral surgical neck fractures with lateral wall comminution. *Sci. Rep.* **2023**, *13*, 3744. [CrossRef] [PubMed]

37. Saltzman, B.M.; Erickson, B.J.; Harris, J.D.; Gupta, A.K.; Mighell, M.; Romeo, A.A. Fibular strut graft augmentation for open reduction and internal fixation of proximal humerus fractures: A systematic review and the authors' preferred surgical technique. *Orthop. J. Sports Med.* **2016**, *4*, 2325967116656829. [CrossRef] [PubMed]
38. Davids, S.; Allen, D.; Desarno, M.; Endres, N.K.; Bartlett, C.; Shafritz, A. Comparison of locked plating of varus displaced proximal humeral fractures with and without fibula allograft augmentation. *J. Orthop. Trauma* **2020**, *34*, 186–192. [CrossRef] [PubMed]

Disclaimer/Publisher's Note: The statements, opinions and data contained in all publications are solely those of the individual author(s) and contributor(s) and not of MDPI and/or the editor(s). MDPI and/or the editor(s) disclaim responsibility for any injury to people or property resulting from any ideas, methods, instructions or products referred to in the content.

MDPI AG
Grosspeteranlage 5
4052 Basel
Switzerland
Tel.: +41 61 683 77 34

Journal of Clinical Medicine Editorial Office
E-mail: jcm@mdpi.com
www.mdpi.com/journal/jcm

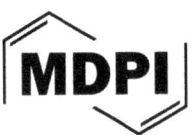

Disclaimer/Publisher's Note: The statements, opinions and data contained in all publications are solely those of the individual author(s) and contributor(s) and not of MDPI and/or the editor(s). MDPI and/or the editor(s) disclaim responsibility for any injury to people or property resulting from any ideas, methods, instructions or products referred to in the content.